THE AROMA OF RIGHTEOUSNESS

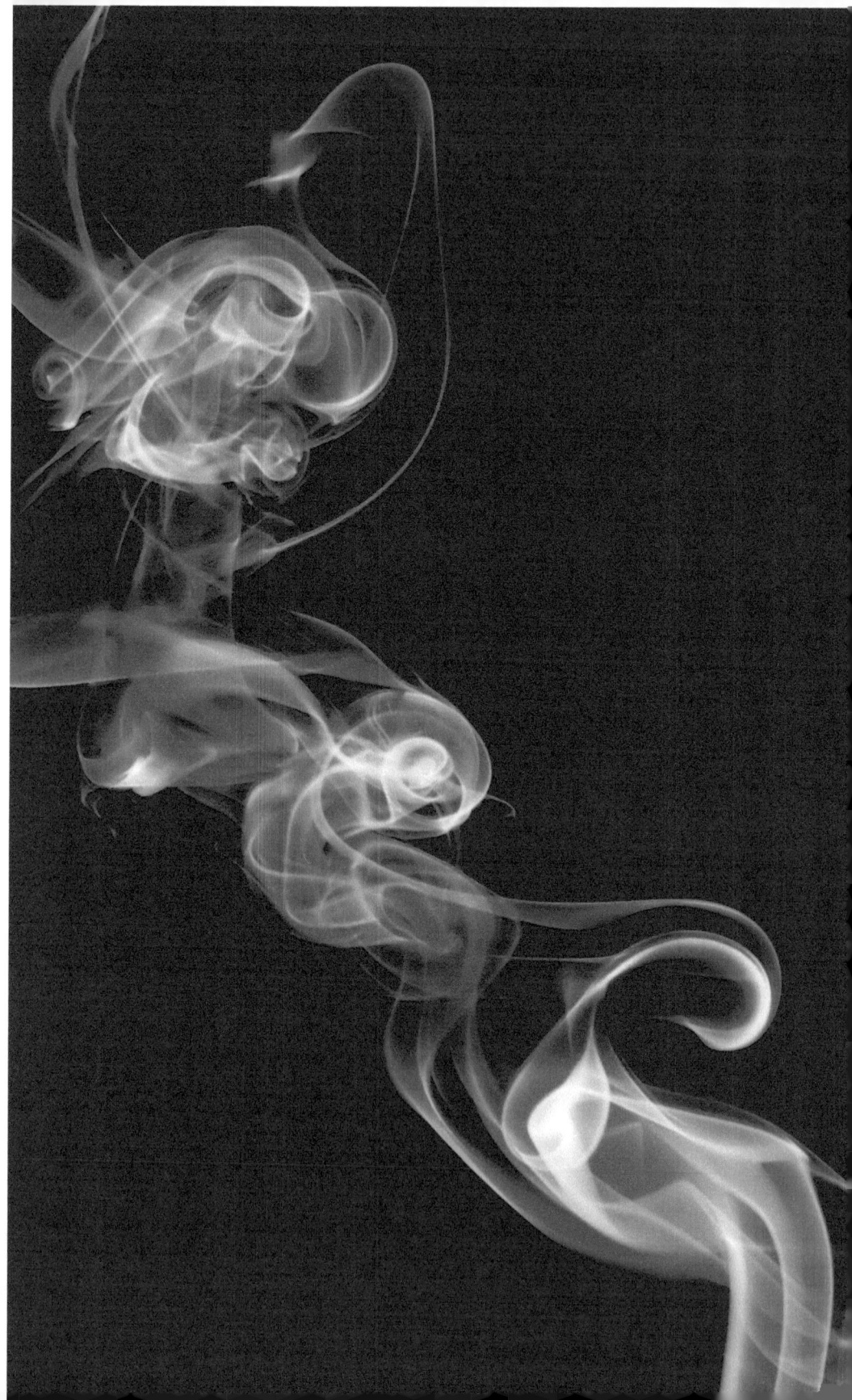

DEBORAH A. GREEN

THE
AROMA
OF
Righteousness

Scent and Seduction in Rabbinic Life and Literature

The Pennsylvania State University Press
University Park, Pennsylvania

Library of Congress Cataloging-in-Publication Data
Green, Deborah A.
The aroma of righteousness : scent and seduction in
rabbinic life and literature / Deborah A. Green.
      p.   cm.
Includes bibliographical references and index.
Summary: "Studies aroma in Jewish life and literature in
Palestine in the late Roman and early Byzantine periods.
Uses the history and material culture of perfume and
incense as a lens to view daily activities"
—Provided by publisher.
ISBN 978-0-271-03767-7 (cloth : alk. paper)
ISBN 978-0-271-05066-9 (pbk : alk. paper)
1. Odors in the Bible.
2. Perfumes—Religious aspects—Judaism.
3. Rabbinical literature—History and criticism.
4. Bible. O.T.—Criticism, interpretation, etc.
5. Jews—Palestine—Social life and customs.
6. Judaism—History—Post-exilic period,
586 B.C.–210 A.D.
I. Title.

BS1199.O34G74 2011
296.1'208152166—dc22
2010039072

Copyright © 2011 The Pennsylvania State University
All rights reserved
Printed in the United States of America
Published by The Pennsylvania State University Press,
University Park, PA 16802-1003

It is the policy of The Pennsylvania State University Press
to use acid-free paper. Publications on uncoated stock
satisfy the minimum requirements of American National
Standard for Information Sciences—Permanence of
Paper for Printed Library Material, ANSI Z39.48–1992.

FOR *Reuben and Joshua*

CONTENTS

LIST OF ILLUSTRATIONS   ix

ACKNOWLEDGMENTS   xi

NOTE ON STYLE   xv

1

Tracking the Trail of Scent:
An Introduction   1

2

The Aroma of Daily Life:
Aromatics in Roman and Rabbinic Culture   19

3

Election and the Erotic:
Biblical Portrayals of Perfume and Incense   64

4

Spicy Ideologies:
Fragrance and Rabbinic Beliefs   116

5

Soothing Odors:
Death, Suffering, and Sacrifice   169

6

Ephemerality and Fragrance:
Desire for Divine Immanence   197

NOTES   209

BIBLIOGRAPHY   257

SOURCE INDEX   271

GENERAL INDEX   275

ILLUSTRATIONS

Figure 1   Unguentarium, 50–75 C.E. Collection of The Corning Museum of Glass, Corning, New York. 64.1.27.   23
Figure 2   Unguentarium, first century C.E. Collection of The Corning Museum of Glass, Corning, New York. 50.1.14.   25
Figure 3   Candlestick unguentarium, late first to third century C.E. Collection of The Corning Museum of Glass, Corning, New York. 69.1.19. Gift of Honolulu Academy of Arts, Hawaii.   26
Figure 4   Pyxis, first century C.E. Collection of The Corning Museum of Glass, Corning, New York. 55.1.69a, b.   27
Figure 5   Collection of glass bottles on display at The Corning Museum of Glass, Corning, New York. Courtesy of Steven Fine, Yeshiva University.   29
Figure 6   Dropper flask, third to fourth century C.E. Collection of The Corning Museum of Glass, Corning, New York. 52.1.63.   35
Figure 7   Unguentarium, first century to early second century C.E. Collection of The Corning Museum of Glass, Corning, New York. 54.1.53. Gift of I. C. Elston Jr.   44
Figure 8   Jar, third to fourth century C.E. Collection of The Corning Museum of Glass, Corning, New York. 53.1.6.   45
Figure 9   Rectangular ceramic incense shovel from Sepphoris, Middle Roman period. With permission from the Joint Sepphoris Project, Eric and Carol Meyers.   50
Figure 10   Oval-shaped ceramic incense shovel from Sepphoris, Middle Roman period. With permission from the Joint Sepphoris Project, Eric and Carol Meyers.   51
Figure 11   Cosmetic flask, fourth to fifth century C.E. Collection of The Corning Museum of Glass, Corning, New York. 54.1.47. Gift of I. C. Elston Jr.   54

ACKNOWLEDGMENTS

There are those who say that writing a book is like giving birth to a child. It is true that writing sometimes feels like labor pains and the process does change us in unexpected and permanent ways, but now that I have given birth during the writing of a book I can state with confidence that the two events are nothing alike. Most assuredly a book requires more quiet time, more patience, and the involvement of many more people. And it is to those people who have been most intimately involved with this project that I wish to express my gratitude here.

The beginning of this project coincided with my arrival at the University of Oregon, where I have found a warm and productive professional home among colleagues and friends. In the Department of Religious Studies, Daniel Falk, Stephen Shoemaker, Mark Unno, Rick Colby, Veena Howard, Tariq Jaffer, Erin Cline, David Reis, Michael Slater, and Jonathan Seidel have graciously engaged me in dialogue and supported me throughout this project. I am deeply grateful to Judith Baskin, who, in her role as the founding director of the Harold Schnitzer Family Program in Judaic Studies, has been instrumental in much of the success I have enjoyed thus far in my career. More important, Judith is a good friend and a wise and nurturing mentor.

Institutional support has been critical for this project. In the early stages, while in graduate school, I received research and dissertation grants from the Divinity School and the Martin Marty Center of the University of Chicago, the Dorot Fellowship, and the Memorial Foundation for Jewish Culture. The seeds for this more recent project were planted during the year I spent in Israel as a graduate student (2000–2001). While there, I worked in the National Library, studied at the Hartman Institute, and was afforded the opportunity to attend weekly sessions at the Institute of Advanced Studies at Hebrew University. As a result, I received not only help and encouragement but the sustenance of wonderful conversations and connections with a host of scholars from Israel and the United States. Although I do not have room to list them all, at the moment of this writing I have learned of the recent passing of Hanan Eshel (ז"ל) and must take at least a few lines to remember him. Hanan and Esther ("Esti") Eshel warmly extended themselves to me from the moment I met them at the bus stop in Jerusalem. Hanan strongly encouraged me to pursue the archaeological evidence for perfume and incense—even to the point of dropping the occasional article or journal on my desk at the National Library and copying an out-of-print source for me from his own library. Those references appear in this volume thanks to him. Conversations with others throughout that year, including Yairah Amit, Menachem Lorberbaum, Moshe Halbertal, Israel Knohl, Jan Willem van Henten, Adele Reinhartz, Greg Sterling, Tessa Rajak, Cana Werman, Michael Swartz, Esther Chazon, Betsy Halpern-Amaru, Dena Ordan, Daniel Stökl Ben Ezra, Søren Holst, and Raquel Ukeles, were also invaluable.

More recently, grants from the Oregon Humanities Center and the University of Oregon Office of Research, as well as time off from teaching responsibilities, have ensured that I was able to focus on my work and travel as necessary. To the Catacomb Society, to Laurie Brink in particular, and to the entire "Grateful Dead" team, I am extremely appreciative. Meeting and traveling with them was invaluable to my research; getting to know them, a delight (thank you, Laurie, David Balch, John Bodel, Patout Burns, Amy Hirshfeld, Robin Jensen, Tanya Luhrmann, Margaret Mitchell, Carolyn Osiek, Richard Saller, Susan Stevens, and Andrew Wallace-Hadrill). I also want to express my gratitude to Annal Franz and Karen Stern for their perceptive and helpful responses to my paper at the Shohet Conference.

My experience with the "Grateful Dead" team encouraged me to continue my pursuit of material culture, and to that end I am indebted to Gideon Avni (and the Israel Antiquities Authority), Steven Fine, Esther Jacobson-Tepfer, Jodi Magness, Sarah McClure, Carol Meyers, Eric Meyers, and Zeev Weis for their insights, comments, and advice. Closer to my intellectual home, in the area of the study of the senses and religion, I have received a warm reception from those who have trodden this ground ahead of me. Among those of special note are Georgia Frank, who invited me to comment on Susan Ashbrook Harvey's book at the Byzantine Studies Conference. There I was able to meet Susan, whom I am pleased to thank for her book and for her support. I also wish to thank Phyllis Granoff, who invited me to participate in the Senses of Religion conference at Yale University. This conference helped me to keep my focus on the broad contours of the role of the senses in religion as I trained my lens on the particulars of my topic. Scent is a broad topic, and so I have found myself on several occasions outside the study of religion altogether. I have found answers to my questions in the fields of biology, physiology, and psychology as well as in history, classics, philosophy, and literature. In these pursuits, my father, Harry Green, has amiably answered my questions and pushed me to frame others, as have Jack Maddox, David Luebke, Malcolm Wilson, Steve Shankman, Mark Johnson, and Louise Westling.

In my own field, conversations and correspondence with, among others, Charlotte Fonrobert, Christine Hayes, Yair Hoffman, Diana Lipton, Jon Schofer, and Steve Weiss have had significant influence and been of critical help. That said, I cannot thank enough those who read part or all of the manuscript: Judith Baskin, Steven Fine, Michael Fishbane, Mary Jaeger, Derek Kruger, Laura Lieber, Jodi Magness, Jenifer Presto, Michael Satlow, and the anonymous readers at the Press. All of their comments were a helpful guide as I made revisions, and I apologize for those infelicities that I know still remain. With the indulgence of the reader, I linger for a moment on the name of my teacher, Michael Fishbane. In the early stages of working with him, Professor Fishbane unlocked for me the doors to Judaism's most exquisitely elusive texts and guided my study so that I might one day walk through those doors myself. But more than that, as mentor and friend, Buzzy has remained a constant guide to me both professionally and personally, and I know that I may always count on him and Mona to lend an understanding ear and to give wise counsel. I would be remiss if I did not also acknowledge two other teachers, John Collins and Tikva Frymer-Kensky (ז״ל). Sadly, Tikva's voice is now silent, but I feel fortunate to be able to continue to seek safe harbor from the somewhat intimidating waters of academia in John's candor and advice.

To make a book from a manuscript takes an awful lot of work, and to that end I am very appreciative of the team at Penn State Press—Patrick Alexander, Kathryn Yahner, Laura Reed-Morrisson, Jennifer Norton, and Suzanne Wolk—for shepherding my manuscript through the publication process. I recall that I first spoke to Patrick about this project in 2005. I didn't know then how really pleased I would be now that we have been able to work together on its publication. To the administrative staff at the University of Oregon, Heidi Gese and Carol Kleinheksel, and to my student Elizabeth Shulman, thank you for your help in getting the manuscript out the door. A special thank-you as well to Steven Fine, the Corning Museum of Glass, and Eric and Carol Meyers for the use of their photographs.

In one very important respect, giving birth and the writing of this book have been the same; I have been buoyed—well, really sustained—by my friendships and the love and patience of my family. My friends have listened, listened some more, and then listened yet again: Laura Lieber, Denise Mandel-Becker, Colleen Murphy, Pete Nixen, Jon Schofer, Jenifer Presto, Gina Hermann, Priscilla Yamin, Dawn Marlan, Jill Dupont, Esther Jacobson-Tepfer, and Gary Tepfer. To the "Dads' Club," this book wouldn't have gotten done without you and your little ones. Admittedly, "thank you" is a wholly inadequate expression of the sentiment I feel toward my sister, Cindy Anderson, my brother-in-law, Paul Anderson, and my parents, Harry and Carol Green. Without the love, generosity, work ethic, and sheer tenacity that they have demonstrated in the example of their own lives, I would not have had the opportunity to pursue this second career, much less found the resolve to continue this line of research. I dedicate this book to Reuben and Josh Zahler. I believe the greatest gift I have been given is my life with Reuben, my husband and my true partner in the world. To be able to be Josh's mom on top of that—well, it just doesn't get any better. You two teach me every day how to smile, how to laugh, and how to live. Your patience is abounding, and I am lit up and alive in your arms.

NOTE ON STYLE

Transliterations follow the "general purpose style" of the *SBL Handbook of Style* (28) for words and names, except in cases in which a more familiar spelling prevails (e.g., R. Akiba, *mitzvot*). Abbreviations of biblical books and of tractates and other rabbinical works follow the "style of abbreviation" of the *SBL Handbook of Style* (73–74, 79–80).

All translations of biblical and rabbinic texts are the author's, unless otherwise noted.

In order to distinguish between biblical quotations and midrashic text in chapters 4, 5, and 6, biblical quotations that appear within indented block quotations are in italics.

Tracking the Trail of Scent: An Introduction

Rabbi Eliezer's brothers were once plowing on the plain, while R. Eliezer plowed on the mountain. R. Eliezer's cow fell and was maimed. It proved fortunate for him that his cow was maimed, because he fled from his brothers and came to the famed R. Yoḥanan ben Zakkai to study. But now R. Eliezer was poor and had nothing to eat, so he ate clods of dirt until his mouth had a bad odor. The other students went to their teacher and complained about their fellow student's bad breath. The rabbi turned to his odiferous student and said, "Just as the odor of your mouth caused you to smell bad for the sake of Torah, so will the fragrance of your learning go from one end of the world to the other."[1]

This brief narrative describes the sacrifice of a young rabbinical student and the prediction by his teacher of that rabbi's future greatness. To accomplish its goal, the narrative relies on our personal experience—not with how difficult it may be to plow a mountain, or the distress with which a family might receive news of its cow being lame; these are explained within the context of the narrative.[2] Rather, the climax and resolution of the vignette depend upon our firsthand knowledge of bad breath. And this remains unexplained. That is, the narrator relies on our personal experience so that we will empathize with the students, for we all know how repulsive bad breath in others can be. At the same time, because we know how difficult it is to perceive bad breath in oneself, we might also have sympathy for R. Eliezer (as if his being destitute and eating clods of dirt weren't enough to render us compassionate). More intriguing, however, is R. Yoḥanan ben Zakkai's response, which turns bad odor into a positive—even worthy—attribute. R. Eliezer may emit an offensive odor in pursuit of Torah, but once he has acquired knowledge and begins the teaching of Torah he will emit a perfumed fragrance to which people will be drawn. Bad or offensive odor is rendered not only positively but as perfume. The rabbi's odor wafts abroad, attracts students to him, and draws them in. They, in turn, teach the rabbi's teachings and spread the perfume from one end of the world to the other. Bad breath becomes fragrance, and fragrance is Torah. What appears to be a simple legend is, on closer perusal, a deeply encoded metaphor and lesson. Sacrifice and suffering for Torah operate in the world as perfume, seducing others to believe.

This book examines rabbinic imagery of fragrance and explores how the ancient rabbis employed aromatic images to propagate their social, theological, and religious claims. It focuses on the many midrashim[3] that mention specific spices, such as frankincense, myrrh, and balsam, and those that reference the more general language of perfume, incense, anointment, and fumigation. At its most poetic, this study uses the lens of aroma to examine rabbinic reflections on such topics as love, righteousness, death, the Divine, and the "other." At its most mundane, it explores and describes the utterly quotidian. That is to say, it seeks out the impulse for these comparisons and finds them in everyday experience: the fumigation of clothing and rooms, the use of incense in the rituals of various religions, the application of medicinal unguents and ointments, and the bathing and anointing of the body with oil. In the late Roman and early Byzantine periods, these daily activities meant that one inhaled the scents of exotic places in the marketplace, the bathhouse, and the home. These experiences, along with rabbinic reflections upon them, which ranged from the apprehensive, to the soothing, to the sublime, form the backdrop for the astounding layers of metaphor and meaning found in the many "aromatic" midrashim.

When I first began my work on fragrance, I believed that the Hebrew Bible served as the primary impetus for rabbinic images of fragrance. After all, the ancient rabbis interpreted every element of Scripture. I therefore spent much time and energy locating almost every reference to olfaction, aroma, and particular spices in the Hebrew Scriptures. I evaluated the terms, studied clusters of terms, and noted that these groupings quite naturally gravitated to spheres of priestly, royal, or erotic *topoi*. I explained that these groups sometimes overlapped and that the terms themselves often served as the bridge from one metaphor to another. I then turned my attention to the rabbinic interpretive literature, and there it appeared that the rabbis picked up these biblical terms, along with their associated meanings and valences,[4] and transformed them solely on the basis of "rabbinic" understandings of the biblical literature. I analyzed these midrashim and unpacked their thickly layered metaphors.

As other studies have done, my work demonstrated that these rabbinic interpretations and perceptions were multivocalic and often at odds with one another within and across the tradition and historical periods of redaction. Further, it appeared that early midrashim incorporated "shorthand" descriptions of the same images that were amplified in later interpretive collections.[5] Most important, this work served as an initial demonstration of the serious consideration the ancient rabbinic voices gave to olfaction and fragrance. These voices employed the biblical terms as well as the characteristics and other features that had adhered to those terms and deployed them with finesse and subtlety in the interpretations.

In the midst of that project, however, I began to notice that the rabbis embedded several scent images within a single midrash. In some cases it seemed to me that this level of creativity would have required an intimate acquaintance with the initial image in order to build and layer these metaphors one on top of the other. As I moved from one midrash to the next, I began to intuit that the rabbis had a tradition of how aroma operated and a deep cultural understanding of what particular scents meant. I began to wonder whether some of the rabbis might have had firsthand experience with these particular smells and whether the force of the imagery, whether it concerned erotic arousal or beatific death, came from their own intimate knowledge. While I attempted to address and incorporate some of the cultural questions that arose during the course of the initial project, it became increasingly clear that this avenue of investigation was better suited to another study, which has become this book.

In this book I investigate the relevant history, archaeology, and cultural data that serve to enlarge and deepen our understanding of these remarkable rabbinic interpretations. Although I am not formally trained in history, archaeology, or anthropology, I believe that work in these areas is of critical importance to students of texts if we want to comprehend the full scope and profundity of any given rabbinic interpretation. This work uncovers and organizes the social science data, reviews the biblical texts, and then turns its attention to the midrashic literature in order to demonstrate that the words and associations of the biblical text, the mores of the larger society, and the experience of the rabbis themselves shape the interpretations, their images, and their didactic force.

Some readers will find ample rationale for this study in the synthesis of information and methods from a variety of disciplines. Such an interdisciplinary pursuit has the potential to inform not only the literary analysis, thereby presenting a more complete picture of the texts, but also may change how we understand the history and daily life of the rabbis of the late Roman and early Byzantine periods (roughly the second through the fifth century C.E.). But there are those who will no doubt question the value of such a study, and still others who may applaud interdisciplinary pursuits of one kind or another but see little value in studying the concept of aroma in rabbinic literature. It is true that the rabbis did not use scent as an organizing principle in either of the Talmuds, and they have no overarching opinion, theory, or consensus about fragrance. So why study scent at all, and why pleasant aroma in particular?

First, odor, whether pleasing or foul, enters almost every aspect of our lives—its subtle pervasiveness affects our attitudes and judgments toward both the mundane and the sacred. In the rabbinic worldview, where almost every daily activity became a locus of theological discussion, interpretation, or legislation, aroma was quite naturally part of the discourse. Second, olfaction is one of the primary modes of interaction and communication with God in the Hebrew Bible. Each properly performed sacrifice is described as a "soothing odor before the Lord," and God's chosen leaders are identified through anointing with perfumed oil. Both king and savior are referred to as messiah, "anointed one." Even the Bible's most secular book, the Song of Songs, is replete with sensual images of wafting perfume and seductive spices. The rabbis of the late Roman and early Byzantine periods, who inherited and transformed many of these biblical images in order to express their own theology and values, lived in a milieu in which spices and perfumes were in common use and carried a variety of cultural meanings. To ignore scent—where it appears in the interpretive texts or in the social world of the rabbis—is to exclude one of the most pervasive and influential themes of rabbinic discourse. I would also argue that the study of the foul is just as important as that of the fragrant, but limits on time, space, and the reader's endurance require that this subject be addressed elsewhere.

Problems in the Study of Odor

As important as this undertaking is to the field of the history of Judaism specifically and of religion more generally, it is also rife with difficulties. Our understanding of ancient cultures is most commonly derived from an interpretation of their material remains and history. Spices and perfumed oils do not endure over long periods of time, however, and the destruction of incense, through burning, is integral to its employment. Only the containers (bottles, jars, burners) or implements of formulation (oil presses, mortars and pestles, molds) of these substances survive, and these in very small quantities. Add to this the nature of archaeological science, in which only a few select sites can be thoroughly excavated, and the evidence from the material record becomes quite sparse. Further, our construction of social history for the ancient world is derived in large measure from the interpretation of textual sources. Issues surrounding source selection and interpretation are only the beginning of the difficulties the social scientist faces. For the literary researcher who wishes to study olfaction and fragrance, even language becomes a problem.

Intuitively, one may understand scent images as categorically different from auditory or visual descriptions. Scents are most often described by simile, metaphor, or metonym. While this may be true for visual and auditory images as well, further description of those images is also possible. The visual simile "her cheeks are like pink roses" can be described further by elucidating the details of "her cheeks" or of "pink roses." The additional descriptions may include the aspects of softness, size, or precise hue. Such supplemental descriptions are not only difficult with scent; they are almost impossible to grasp if one has not previously experienced the scent. A bar of soap may smell like a rose, but it is difficult to describe precisely what "rose" smells like to anyone who has not already experienced this fragrance, and further descriptions of the object will seek to include visual, tactile, or other perceptual clues of the "bar" or "soap" rather than of the "rose."

Without an aesthetic lexicon for aromas, a textual analysis may be reduced to simple repetition of the text. In addition, concentration on the memory of a visual image enables the subject to see the image in his or her mind. Scent does not lend itself to this kind of memory. Most of us cannot smell the fragrance of an orange by mentally concentrating on the idea of an orange.[6] In literature spanning several centuries, continents, and cultures, however, the emotional and recollective reaction to specific scents, such as Marcel Proust's reaction to the madeleine in *The Remembrance of Things Past,* is so striking as to inspire consideration of scent's pervasive hold on our emotions and memory. Further study on these initial problems reveals their origin in the physiological mechanics of olfaction. The nature of human olfaction, in turn, triggers several important cultural developments—a short review of which is necessary if we are to be able to suspend the judgment of our own culture and historical moment in order to understand those of the late Roman and Byzantine periods.

The Physiology of Smell

In her popular book *A Natural History of the Senses,* Diane Ackerman gives one of the most lucid descriptions of olfaction:

> Odor molecules float back into the nasal cavity behind the bridge of the nose, where they are absorbed by the mucosa containing receptor cells bearing microscopic hairs called cilia. Five million of these cells fire impulses to the brain's olfactory bulb or smell center. Such cells are unique to the nose. . . . If you damage neurons in your eyes or ears, both organs will be irreparably damaged. But the neurons in the nose are replaced about every thirty days and, unlike any other neurons in the body, they stick right out and wave in the air current like anemones on a coral reef.[7]

As one can detect from Ackerman's description, the physical act of olfaction is unique in comparison with the other senses.[8] The neurons in the nose are constantly replenished, making the sense of smell less susceptible to physical damage or the frailties of old age. In addition, since the molecules actually enter the body cavity and are deciphered directly by the brain, olfaction can be considered an unmediated activity.

Most scholars agree, though, that our senses are "mediated experience"; that is, when we experience an event through our senses, our brain interprets that experience. This interpretation may involve our personal history (our experience of that sensation before), our generation, our culture, our religion, or any number of factors.[9] With olfaction, this second order of experience (the interpretation of what we have smelled) occurs so quickly that we experience the two steps as one reaction, and our reflection on the interpretation seems to disappear.

In part, this phenomenon may be due to the physical location in which our experience of scent resides. Once the brain encounters an odor, it sends a message directly to the limbic system, that "mysterious, ancient, and intensely emotional section of our brain in which we feel, lust, and invent."[10] This repository of our olfactory experiences is also the warehouse in which we store emotions and many of our deepest memories. As a result, each time we smell something familiar, emotions and memories associated with that odor return practically instantaneously. In fact, because scent is stored in the limbic system, it may have the strongest link to memory of any of the senses. Memories of our other sense experiences can almost be considered short term, because they are easily replaced or forgotten.[11] A scent, by contrast, because it is stored in the limbic system, is better retained in the memory.

Because the olfactory bulb is located so "far down" (medial and inferior) in the brain, while sight and hearing take place in the outer (cortical) layer of the brain, many researchers theorize that olfaction is the "oldest" of our senses.[12] As Ackerman observes, it is the olfactory bulb sticking right out of our ancestors' heads when still swimming in the sea that became the mammal's brain. These two factors, that the sense of smell is the oldest of our senses and that the experience of sight and hearing occurs in a different place in the brain, may account for the perception that olfaction is more "animal-like" than vision or hearing—or at least that it was more useful to humans in their earlier developmental period. Taste can be included with smell in this respect, as it requires that the subject be close to the object (as smell often does) and does not exist in all its nuances and varieties without smell. On its own, taste includes only the basic sensations of salty, sweet, bitter, and sour; it requires interaction with smell to derive all other flavors.[13] It is easy to see how these two senses may have worked in tandem in early human development, given the importance of avoiding poison. Smell and taste are the two primary indicators of what should and should not be ingested.[14]

The wellspring of emotions found in the limbic system may account for the disconnection between scent and language. Many researchers agree that we seem to have emotional reactions to scent far more quickly than we can articulate them. But it also appears that our inability to describe odor goes beyond this emotional reaction, for even long after we experience them, we most often describe scents by metaphor, simile, or simply naming the scent. William Miller, in his work on disgust, elaborates:

> The lexicon of smell is very limited and usually must work by making an adjective of the thing that smells. Excrement smells like excrement, roses like a rose, rotting flesh like rotting flesh. Sometimes we attempt description by saying that rotting flesh smells like feces, or that a perfume smells like a rose. What is missing is a specially dedicated qualitative diction of odor that matches the richness of distinction we make with the tactile as with squishy, oozy, gooey. . . . Odor qualifiers, if not

the names of the things emitting the odor, are usually simple adjectives and nouns expressing either the pleasantness or unpleasantness of the smell, most of which merely mean bad or good smell. . . . Olfactory and gustatory reduce us to saying little more than yum or yuck.[15]

In response to Miller, one might ask whether this lexical insufficiency pertains only in English (or Hebrew or Aramaic, as I discovered). Dan Sperber clarifies that "even though the human sense of smell can distinguish hundreds of thousands of smells and in this regard is comparable to sight or hearing, in none of the world's languages does there seem to be a classification of smells comparable, for example, to colour classification."[16] Sperber argues that unlike vision or hearing, there is no "semantic field of smells." We know and recognize thousands of scents but have virtually no ability to describe them or place them in semantic categories. Further, Ackerman points out that with 23,040 breaths a day, we use our sense of smell almost as much as our sense of touch.[17] We smell while we sleep, eat, exercise—while we do everything and anything. We can't turn smell off, and we can't seem to describe it either.

The physiological phenomena regarding olfaction do not end where the "trail of scent" stops. Work in recent years on pheromones has shown that we are smelling even when we are not consciously aware of it. Pheromones may explain many mysteries once thought to be purely social, such as common menstrual cycles in collectives of women who either live or work together, mate selection, group leadership dynamics, and common fear responses, to name a few.[18] Considering the physiological phenomena, researchers' interest in olfaction, scents themselves, and the operation of pheromones is not surprising. Recent years have seen an avalanche of information on scent, how it operates in the human body, and which scents (or pheromones) elicit and affect which behaviors.[19] In the humanities, though, far fewer studies have been undertaken. This is surprising, especially in the study of ancient religion and culture, where odors must have dominated rites of sacrifice. This oversight may have more to do with our own cultural attitudes toward scent than with its physiological aspects.

Philosophy and Psychology and the Sense of Smell

The study of olfaction in the humanities has been hindered largely by the inculcation of Western philosophy and early psychology into the various fields of the humanities. Nowhere is this more evident than in the study of religion, where research should include investigation of all aspects of human existence and expression: intellectual, emotional, and physical or sensorial. In fact, most definitions of religion mention "ritual" as an attribute. And what is ritual if not the physical and sensorial expression of religious belief? If it is nothing else, "practice" is sensual.

In the past several years this lacuna has been greatly rectified by scholars studying the "embodiment of religion," mostly in religions other than Christianity and Judaism. Until very recently studies of the senses, and specifically of olfaction, were often considered frivolous, even laughable, by many scholars of these two Western religious traditions.[20] These negative attitudes can be traced back to a history of devaluation of the senses in Western philosophy and psychology. With respect to philosophy, Hans Rindisbacher points out that

> the epistemology of the senses has its origins in Plato and Aristotle. It is with Plato in particular and his forms that the emphasis in the dyad of perception and cognition is placed in favor of the latter and thus shifted from the concrete to the abstract; and it is in the opening lines of Aristotle's *Metaphysics* that the sense of sight is extolled in both its usefulness and its pleasure-giving function. It is Aristotle also who, by acknowledging the senses' potential for both knowledge and pleasure, places them at the beginning of a road that will soon bifurcate into the cognitive-scientific and the hedonistic-aesthetic realms. With the emergence of Christianity and its ambivalent attitude, to say the least, toward the world of the senses, this division is reinforced and undergoes a shift in emphasis: Augustine . . . redraws the line between the disembodied, spiritual, and transcendental realm on the one hand and the corporeal, sensual, and immanent on the other.[21]

This bifurcation becomes so entrenched in the predominant denominations of Christianity that it naturally enters the humanities and the study of religion by way of those who perform the research. This division, which becomes a binary oppositional organization that values the incorporeal over the corporeal, the spiritual over the sensual, and aligns rational thought with the transcendent and emotion with the immanent, seems to act subliminally upon investigators. As a result, scholars who are otherwise reasonable, open, and objective fail to see how their own values and assumptions prevent them from evaluating religious practice and belief by any other structure or in any other way. Thus, it is not surprising that the issues of "embodiment" and "the senses" are infants in the study of Western religions—particularly the history of Judaism, which seems to lag somewhat behind the history of Christianity in this respect.

When the senses are studied at all, sight is the most commonly emphasized.[22] Occasionally, one may encounter a study on "hearing," in part because the Hebrew Bible itself tries to propagate, at least in certain sections, the idea that God is heard and not seen (Deut 4) and in part because scholars of the Bible have come to understand textual traditions as having their basis in oral traditions. Until recently, however, studies on the other senses (touch, taste, and smell) have been rare. Rindisbacher would likely attribute this omission to the further demotion of these senses brought about by Kant and Hegel. These two philosophers include only vision and hearing in their constructions of an aesthetic realm.[23] Hegel asserts that the "sensual in art is limited to the two theoretical senses of vision and the ear whereas olfaction, taste, and touch are barred from aesthetic enjoyment." These three senses are linked too closely with "the material and the unmediated sensual qualities of matter."[24]

It is not surprising, when one considers the interconnectedness among the various areas of the humanities, that, excluded from the developing category of aesthetics in philosophy, the three "lower" senses would receive less attention than vision and hearing in the field of religion. Olfaction becomes linked with matter, rather than intellectual complexity, and is therefore less interesting to religious scholars. Philosophy alone, however, is not responsible for the neglect of the study of scent. The discipline of psychology and the Western cultural construct of "good taste" that evolved in the eighteenth and nineteenth centuries have also played significant roles.

The eighteenth century witnessed the emergence of writing and research on scent, as a rising bourgeois class became obsessed with elements of "good taste" and sanitary conditions. An increasing perception of smell (good and bad) in the family circle was extended to the public arena.[25] Western society was transformed as odors—particularly bad, offensive, and "unhealthy" odors—were scrutinized, researched, and catalogued. Attempts were made to control odors in every realm of society. But what seemed so important in everyday life, and what the "scientific" community responsible for public health focused on, was considered an unacceptable topic of conversation, intellectual pursuit, and possibly even literature. This trend continues today, as evidenced by the overwhelming number of deodorants and cleansers stocked in our grocery stores to rid our bodies and homes of any conceivable "bad" smell. The abundance of perfume counters and the glut of new perfumes on the market also testify to our desire to cover up unwanted body odor. Ultimately, our obsession with "bad" odors has led to the desire to create an environment that has no scent at all. While I hope to the contrary, it would seem to follow that a society that values "odorlessness" would produce scholars in the humanities who find it unnecessary, possibly unintellectual, and even undesirable to study scent.

Whether or not our culture's values hold sway over academic study, the study of scent in the humanities was dealt another blow when Freud and other sexual researchers first defined the psychology of scent and the human sense of smell. Freud supposed that as man became more civilized, he sought to repress his erotic desires, which were constantly triggered by the scents of women. Freud pointed to man's evolution into a being who walked upright (without "his nose to the ground") as the development that freed him from the scent of female genitalia.[26] The implications of Freud's assertions are staggering. Scent, having already been connected to the "sensual," devalued as an aesthetic category, and relegated to the corporeal, now became entwined with the erotic and animalistic. By virtue of this association, aroma was relegated to the dark recesses of the human mind and body and consigned to the uncivilized, bestial world—the world that was repressed in the civilizing process and that required vigilant suppression. By standards of "good taste" and polite society, discussion of the erotic, much less erotic behavior, became taboo among the cultural and intellectual elite.

The study of scent came to be an area of research on the subhuman, or on the human in its most rudimentary forms. Repression of the erotic thus took place at both the individual and the social level. Scent took on an added stigma given its liminal nature and our inability to control leaking odors, particularly bodily odors. Freud's view of smell caused studies of scent in connection to psychology to focus on pathology: sexual dysfunction, disease, and mental illness. An understanding of human development that transformed the nose into an anachronistic sexual organ that had to be repressed was easily translated into a theory that humans do not need their sense of smell, or need it less than they did in earlier stages of development.[27] As a result, people with a keen sense of smell could be considered less human and more akin to the animals who are unable to repress their sexual desires.

It is noteworthy that some academics have feminized the study of olfaction. It makes sense to them that a woman would study scent because, as a few of them have remarked, "women have a keener sense of smell." My research has yet to uncover any evidence for this assertion.[28] I can only surmise that this view is the result of those links forged early on by philosophy and psychology that connected aroma, the erotic, and the feminine. Other scholars sidestep the issues surrounding the eroticism of smell and maintain that our olfaction does not work as well as it did in ancient times. Proponents of this theory seem to have absorbed a "lay" understanding of Darwinism, coupled with an obvious misconception of history.[29] Nevertheless, the number of academics who claim that humans are not able to smell as well as they used to is astounding—especially since there is no scientific evidence for this view. Smell is an adaptive sense, which means that our ability to detect odor may be infinite![30]

But the philosophers and psychologists were not all wrong. Some of their rational and intuitive assessments of olfaction have been verified by scientific discoveries on the neurological aspects of smell. The philosophers were correct in describing olfaction as categorically different from vision and hearing. These two senses first appear at a later stage in human development, they take place at a distance from the object of discernment, and their language pathways seem to be more developed. On this last point, the philosophers correctly ascertained that we have few methods for organizing ideas about scent; we lack a "lexicon" for categorizing scents.[31] And just as smell is the oldest of the senses, it is also a direct experience in terms of the molecules entering deeply into the body. That the memory of a scent is stored in the limbic system, "the seat of emotion,"[32] means that both the philosophers and Freud were fair in their assessment of scent as difficult to intellectualize, or as in some way related to the "unmediated sensual qualities of matter."[33] Our responses to scent are tied directly to emotions that are not easily articulated, and memories associated with scent are also very strong and often associated with early childhood experiences, whether positive or negative. Freud was not wrong in positing a connection between scent and the repression of feelings and desires, a normal part of the human maturation process. He was also correct in defining a connection between scent and the erotic; this has been verified by the scientific discovery of pheromones. As a result of scent's special liminality in the psyche and body, its unwieldy ephemerality, and the development of our own cultural prejudices, the lack of research until recently is not so surprising. But now that physical, biological, and social scientific research on scent and olfaction is "blossoming," the time has come to look at this important sense perception in terms of its cultural, historical, and religious significance.

Studies of Scent

Many influences have contributed to recent studies on olfaction and aroma. The postmodern period has witnessed a new trend toward individualism and a blurring of the lines between pop and high culture. The line between the biological and social sciences has also eroded, as a resurgence of scientific study on scent and pheromones continues to uncover the physiological, emotional, and psychological importance of scent in our lives. In addition, more positive lay attitudes in the West toward scent are evolving through experiences with holistic health practices, homeopathy, and Eastern medicine. These developments have opened new avenues of research in each of the humanities and have promoted interdisciplinary studies. A significant rise in the number of women in the academy, along with major achievements in feminist studies and theory, has also had widespread positive effects on research in virtually every area, smell and scent included. Some of the longest-standing and most misogynistic claims about women are simply read and dismissed without hesitation, thereby inviting us to investigate the same material with new methods and from different viewpoints.

Several excellent studies have been published on aroma. Each has a unique focus and methodology, and almost all have supplied valuable insight and data for this project. Works on social history by Alain Corbin and William Ian Miller have encouraged me to reflect on the daily lives of the ancient rabbis. In addition, Miller has explored the changes we may experience psychologically when some action, object, or type of behavior moves from the public to the private sphere. What prompts disgust at the public level provokes a different reaction at the level of intimacy, particularly sexual intimacy. By analogy, this line of thinking is helpful in considering many different unpleasant and agreeable odors. I have also found helpful Hans Rindisbacher's literary analysis of the operation of smell in nineteenth- and twentieth-century German literature. Remarkably, the triangulation of scent, *eros,* and *thanatos* that he perceives in German literature appears in some rabbinic midrashim. In addition, *Aroma: The Cultural History of Smell,* by Constance Classen, David Howes, and Anthony Synnott, demonstrates the deep connections of history, culture, and religion with fragrance. The authors also address the question of how culture-specific our evaluation of scent can be; one culture may identify a scent as abhorrent while another finds it pleasurable. Such reversals and inversions appear in rabbinic literature as well. Finally, an important article by David Howes, "Olfaction and Transition," helped me to clarify my thinking about olfaction, ritual and life transitions, and perfume and liminality.

A handful of sense-specific studies on the Bible, Judaism, and Christianity have also been immensely informative.[34] The most important of these is Susan Ashbrook Harvey's *Scenting Salvation: Ancient Christianity and the Olfactory Imagination.* I assumed that as I moved toward the later rabbinic literature, I would find that the later rabbis had less direct experience with incense and perfume than their earlier Roman-period counterparts. The Roman Empire, with its vast employment of spices for adorning the body, fumigation, and sacrifices to the gods, changed fundamentally under Christian leadership. But Harvey maintains that although the early church fathers may have had ambivalent attitudes toward perfuming the body, incense and perfume were used liberally in the Christian communities of the East, particularly from the fourth century onward. This discovery demanded that I reconsider the late Palestinian material, which until then I thought had been a period of aromatic unadornment. It also encouraged me to reevaluate the Babylonian material, as I realized that Babylonia would have had continual access to these spices long before, during, and after the Sassanid dynasty and the corresponding height of the Roman and Byzantine periods in Palestine. Harvey's work also led me to the important research of Béatrice Caseau, and the strong tie between perfume and medicine in the ancient world—also evident in the rabbinic literature.

I hope that this volume will add to an ever-expanding discussion of the senses, and the role of olfaction more specifically, in the history of religion. Although the rabbis' use of aromatics is primarily nonritualistic, rabbinic interpretations reveal deeply encoded cultural constructions of what perfume, incense, and spice represent. In some cases, as in the midrash on R. Eliezer with which this introductory chapter begins, understanding the midrash depends entirely on these structures. This study thus seeks to unpack the layers of these midrashim by demonstrating how scent operates in them. To that end I have relied on a methodology that combines literary contextual analysis with an examination of the role of aromatics in the society in which these texts were produced.

Method and Organization

The sheer number of passages concerning scent and the difficulty in deciphering the meanings behind these literary and cultural representations require a system of categorization and evaluation. Drawing on the groundbreaking work of the classicist Marcel Detienne, my analysis of rabbinic texts reveals a profoundly complex social encoding of scent images and layering of the ideas, or valences, that adhere to those images.[35] Perfume, for example, which is often associated with romance, sexuality, and tranquility, can be viewed quite positively when referring to God (with attendant images of mercy and memory) but may have strong negative associations (witchcraft and idolatry) when applied to women.

Rabbinic images of fragrance (most often articulated by means of perfume, incense, and spice) and their attendant characteristics (good, bad, dangerous, erotic) are not purely literary productions, however. The perfumed substances and their environments (people, bathhouses, altars) are part of the *realia* of daily life. As such, they possess and attract distinct characteristics and valences of their own, and these too find their way into the literature. As a result, a thorough understanding of everyday practices involving fragrance is critical to unraveling the full meaning of the texts.

To identify these practices, one must turn to the archaeological record and the textual sources. Fortunately, a solid pathway has been trudged by several experts in late antique Jewish written and material evidence, and this allows us to form a synthesized understanding of the culture. By reading literature alongside historical, archaeological, and social evidence, these scholars have transformed our understanding of the cultural landscape of rabbinic Judaism.[36]

Several literary and historical studies have noted that rabbinic literature, both *halakhic* (legal) and *aggadic* (nonlegal), often reveals the worldview of the rabbis themselves, or at least their desire that the world be seen in a particular way. And these rabbinic attitudes and viewpoints often stand in sharp contrast to how the world actually operated. For example, historians have raised the issue of self-referential rabbinic ascendancy for times during which the political situation must have been otherwise. Other investigations have demonstrated rabbinic accommodation to widespread practice, the preponderance of legislation that was probably ignored by the Jewish community, and the unreliability of the rabbinic interpretation of history.[37]

In order to paint an objective picture of the community in which the rabbis lived, then, we need to examine the broad external evidence and compare it to the archaeological, historical, and social record of the immediate culture.[38] First and foremost, however, we must choose which rabbis to study and find out where and when they lived. The large group of midrashim taken up later in this volume is found primarily in the books of *Genesis Rabbah* and *Song of Songs Rabbah*. *Genesis Rabbah* is a collection of interpretations that follow the biblical book of Genesis line by line. It was redacted in Palestine during the fifth century C.E. but incorporates much earlier material. *Song of Songs Rabbah*, by contrast, which interprets its biblical namesake, was probably not redacted before the middle of the sixth century C.E. Although *Songs Rabbah* is considered a somewhat late compilation, its sources also include much older material (from the Mishnah, several *baraitot*,[39] the Palestinian Talmud, and, most important, *Genesis Rabbah*). The interpretations cross numerous generations of rabbis, primarily from the third through the fifth century C.E., and present a wide range of interests and opinions.[40] In light of the strong presence of Palestinian tradents[41] in this literature, combined with the redaction of the Mishnah, Tosefta, and Talmud Yerushalmi in Palestine, those cities, towns, and villages that had significant Jewish populations and most likely a rabbinic presence during these centuries seem to be the best places to study. This study thus focuses on the cities of Caesarea, Tiberias, and Sepphoris, as well as smaller Jewish towns such as Meiron, Gush-Halav, and Beit She'arim from approximately the second through the fifth century C.E.[42]

As has often been noted, the term "rabbis" is problematic because it implies a group in universal agreement on many, if not all, issues. As almost every aspect of rabbinic literature so far studied has revealed, however, particular rabbis and groups of rabbis had particular views, often in sharp disagreement with one another. Thus, it is not unreasonable to assume that the rabbis disagreed about issues surrounding fragrance or that their views changed in this respect over the course of the several centuries represented in the literature, as well as across geographic regions. When and in what manner aromatic spices should be used, or whether the employment of incense and perfume by gentiles could have a negative influence on Jews are two questions about which there was undoubtedly disagreement. In her work on scent in early Christianity, Harvey discusses the variety of opinions about, and reactions to, perfume among the early church fathers.[43] Although attitudes as strident as those of some of the church fathers appear only occasionally in rabbinic literature, negative opinions are expressed and occasionally forcefully argued. More common, however, is the absence of opinion on fragrances and their employment, and in these cases the literary material should be read neither prescriptively nor proscriptively.

Nevertheless, the general outlook that may be derived from the literary and material evidence indicates widespread familiarity with, acceptance of, and employment of pleasurable aromas on the part of the rabbis and their communities. To that end, chapter 2 reviews the cultural, archaeological, and literary evidence of perfume and incense use in the eras before and during the Tannaitic and Amoraic periods (the rabbinic periods most closely aligned with the late Roman and early Byzantine periods) in Palestine. This evidence is organized around the contexts of daily life in which fumigants could be found: the marketplace, the bath, the home, and burial. In this chapter I seek to draw as complete a picture as possible of the everyday uses of spices. Not only do rabbinic customs, rituals, and attitudes surrounding aromatics conform in large measure to those of the wider society, but these everyday uses, experiences, and attitudes often underlie and serve as the impetus for the metaphors and images incorporating scent that are deployed in rabbinic interpretive texts.

Examination of the material and cultural underpinnings of daily life and the sensory experience of scent in this period lays the groundwork for the subsequent chapters. The literary analysis in succeeding chapters is informed by discussion of everyday practices such as bathing, eating, fumigating garments, and burial, as well as by broader issues, such as the spice trade, economic realities, and the dynamics of urban life. In addition, chapter 3 departs slightly from rabbinic issues to review the scent images found in the Hebrew Bible and to explore how inner-biblical reinterpretation combines erotic metaphors about perfume with those of sacred incense, primarily in the books of the Prophets. Although this chapter appears to take several steps backward, historically speaking, its method of literary analysis conforms closely to that employed in the subsequent chapters on midrash, and it focuses on the key passages and images that form the basis for rabbinic interpretations involving fragrance, primarily from Song of Songs. For this reason I have placed chapter 3 just before my analyses of rabbinic interpretation.

Chapter 4 presents the variety of scent interpretations that the sages of the rabbinic period employed in their elucidations of key values about people, places, and history. For example, the rabbis interpret Song of Songs, in which the young woman describes her beloved as flowing myrrh, while he describes her as a garden of spicy delights, allegorically as referring to the relationship between Israel and God. Drawing on this meta-metaphor, rabbinic interpretation assigns the role of the beloved variously to biblical characters (Abraham and Jacob), the righteous of the world, and even the rabbis themselves. These interpretations are heavily laden with fragrance imagery and reveal deep-seated feelings among the rabbis. The section in chapter 4 on perfume and "the other," for example, illuminates rabbinic attitudes toward women (both as virtuous and as licentious) by means of perfume. Likewise, the rabbis subtly compare the aroma of perfume and the substance of perfumed oil so as to raise questions of who is righteous and how rabbis should behave.

Because rabbinic literature transforms so many biblical images of perfume, spices, and love into images of erotic death or sacrifice and eventual redemption, chapter 5 assesses rabbinic material concerned specifically with sacrifice, death, and martyrdom. Here the "bundle of myrrh" worn by the beloved in Song of Songs is transformed into the suffering servant, whose death by fire serves as both atoning sacrifice and redemption for Israel.

Chapter 6 discusses the implications of what has gone before, looking primarily at how we might reconsider rabbinic theology in light of both the material-cultural evidence and rabbinic literary constructions of the erotic, death, and suffering. During the fourth century C.E., we see not only a rise in the use of aromatic imagery but also a new thread of this imagery that views Israel's persecution as inherent in her intimate relationship with God.

2

The Aroma of Daily Life:
Aromatics in Roman and Rabbinic Culture

In the Talmud Bavli, R. Isaac interprets a prophecy in Isaiah about the women of Jerusalem, who are haughty not only in their demeanor but in their dress as well. These women were said to make a tinkling sound with their feet when they walked. Of that sound,

> R. Isaac of the house of R. Ammi said: "This teaches that they (i.e., the women of Israel) put myrrh and balsam in their shoes and would walk in the marketplaces of Jerusalem. And when they approached the young men of Israel, they kicked the ground and splashed [it] on them. They instilled in them an evil urge like the poison of a serpent."[1]

As a method of applying perfume, the practice of putting perfume in one's shoes is virtually unattested in the ancient sources. Nevertheless, R. Isaac's teaching is instructive. He imagines that the already ancient city of Jerusalem had marketplaces similar to those of his own city, and that these markets might be dangerous to one's morality and even to one's life because of the perfumed women one might encounter there. But what if R. Isaac, who is purported to have lived in Tiberias, Caesarea, and Babylonia during the late third and early fourth centuries C.E.,[2] is not the author of this midrash? What if, centuries later, an anonymous redactor heard several different versions of this narrative,[3] embellished it on his own, and included it in the Bavli in a lengthy discussion about which articles might be carried on the Sabbath? Would it then be any less instructive or useful? On the contrary, for all of its apparent fantasy and negative stereotyping of women, this midrash depicts, in passing, many of the cultural, historical, and even physiological characteristics of perfume that the rabbis and other Romans express in their writings. The midrash describes particular spices (myrrh and balsam); its setting is a locale in which one might smell perfume (the marketplace); and it draws a picture of how perfume operates (it is smelled by those in close proximity and seems to turn off their rational minds and excite within them lustful desires).

This chapter explores the historical, archaeological, and textual evidence of perfume and incense and explores the cultural institutions and attitudes surrounding aromatics. It begins with a brief account of aromatics in the land of Israel and beyond, with particular attention to the use of spices in the Roman Empire. The second half of the chapter focuses on Palestine (primarily the Galilee) during the late Roman and early Byzantine periods, drawing together the material remains and the rabbinic legal literature that refers to aromatics. My purpose is not to evaluate the arguments or explicate the legal minutiae set forth, but rather to glean from the passages the aromatic cultural information referred to in passing. The goal is to examine the contexts in which the Palestinian rabbis experienced these pleasing fragrances and to demonstrate how thoroughly steeped in perfume and incense they must have been. In the succeeding chapters, we will begin to see how these experiences came to influence and shape rabbinic interpretive endeavors.

From Israel to Rome: Cultures of Spice

The employment of spices by those who lived in and around Israel's vicinity long predates the period of the Hebrew Bible.[4] While the use of spices is described in texts that date to much later periods, archaeological evidence of incense burners and perfume vials is incontrovertible. Archaeologists have found incense burners at pre-Israelite and Israelite sites most often associated with cultic contexts.[5] Among a variety of forms and decorations, incense altars with horns that project from the corners (similar in style to sacrificial altars) dating to the tenth century B.C.E. have been found at Megiddo, Tel Qedesh, and Lachish, among other places.[6] One particular incense burner has sparked the interest of archaeologists and biblical scholars alike. Found in Taʿanach and also dated to the tenth century B.C.E., this incense burner may depict Canaanite Asherah, a female consort of the male Israelite god.[7]

In addition to cultic employment, much material evidence of perfume use has been discovered in burial sites. Small ceramic bottles, juglets, and *amphoriskoi* are commonly found in burial sites from the middle Bronze Age onward among all the groups present in this area—namely, the Canaanites, Egyptians, Philistines, and later Phoenicians and Israelites, among others.[8] Less common, but of great beauty, are containers made of *alabastra* or bone. The small size of these bottles and their narrow openings indicate that they contained precious liquids. This observation, read in conjunction with later Hellenistic art in which these bottles are clearly depicted as being used for fragrant oil (i.e., perfume), has led most archaeologists to concur that they are unguentaria. Because these unguentaria are found alongside other pottery, such as cooking pots and storage jars, anthropologists and archaeologists have variously suggested that the substances inside were intended to travel with the deceased or were used for meals by visitors to the graves. No definitive judgment has been made with respect to the perfume bottles, which, like the other grave goods, appear among the small finds of excavated settlements.[9]

Modern readers may think it obvious that people of the ancient world used perfume and incense because they were aware that they and their homes "smelled bad," but in fact this does not seem to be the case. Rather, perfumery had more to do with dry skin and the social convention of "smelling attractive" than with masking some displeasing body odor. The water used in ablution was rich in minerals and alkalis that would dry the skin, so creams and oils were needed to alleviate the drying effects of washing.[10] These unguents were scented with spices from exotic places. Similarly, although clothing and rooms might take on foul odors easily alleviated by means of fumigation (i.e., lighting incense), it appears that people also fumigated their clothing and dining areas as an aphrodisiac or simply to make an occasion more festive.

In Greece in the fourth century B.C.E., emphasis on the body meant a close connection between bathing and athletics, and many *palaestras* and *gymnasia* had bathing facilities attached. Michal Dayagi-Mendels explains that "before the competition, the athletes would oil their skin and sprinkle it with a powder appropriate for the kind of sport they were doing. This oily layer was removed after the game with a strigil, a scraper made specifically for this purpose."[11] Material remains related to bathing, such as strigils and pottery or stone *aryballoi* (short oil bottles), date to the sixth century B.C.E., and in some cases earlier. Much of the information on perfume practices comes from "literary sources and depictions on vase paintings."[12] For example, some paintings portray banquet scenes in which footbaths can be seen under the table. Bathing the feet regularly entailed not only the washing of the feet but the application of scented oil afterward. Dayagi-Mendels notes that in Greece, "anointing the body with oil was a routine matter, often replacing washing or bathing."

As Alexander the Great crossed the Mediterranean, conquering the coastal cities, moving south and west to Egypt and then east through Babylonia, Parthia, and regions beyond, Greek culture, as well as the cultures of these conquered areas, spread. With this exchange came access to plentiful, new, and exotic aromatic spices. Long in use in Egypt, Arabia, and throughout the Near East, the bounty of aromatic spices that Alexander's armies discovered in these lands must have been a delight to them and the societies that followed.

In the Near East, the spice trade was controlled by the Nabataeans, whose trade routes wove from the southern tip of Arabia, north (through the territory of Israel) to Syria, east along the Euphrates, and west across the Red Sea to Egypt and other parts of Africa. Nabataean control of the spice trade was likely in place long before Alexander and his empire emerged. It probably began in the Persian period and was certainly firmly entrenched by 312 B.C.E., when Petra became the Nabataean capital.[13] With Pompey's entrance into the land and politics of Judea in 63 B.C.E., it was only a matter of time until Rome would take over the spice trade. In 106 C.E. Rome annexed Nabataea and named the region Arabia Petraea. The absorption of Nabataea allowed the Roman emperors to charge a uniform duty on the entire commerce in spices.[14] And so trade in spices, primarily for aromatics but later as condiments for food as well, became one of the most important elements in the Roman economy.[15]

This rise in the manufacture and trade of spices probably received a significant boost from technological changes in glassmaking, and consequently in the fabrication of perfume bottles, which occurred at roughly the same time. During the first century C.E., glassblowing superseded the older methods of core or rod forming and chip casting as the preferred method of glass production, and this change made glass much more widely available.[16] Glass quickly became the preferred container for storing precious liquids such as perfumes because, unlike ceramic ware, it is nonporous (see fig. 1).[17] But glass is also much more fragile than pottery, and so it is not surprising that, in comparison to pottery finds, far fewer bottles have been found intact among the remains of populated areas. For this reason, much of the best evidence for perfume bottles has been found in graves.

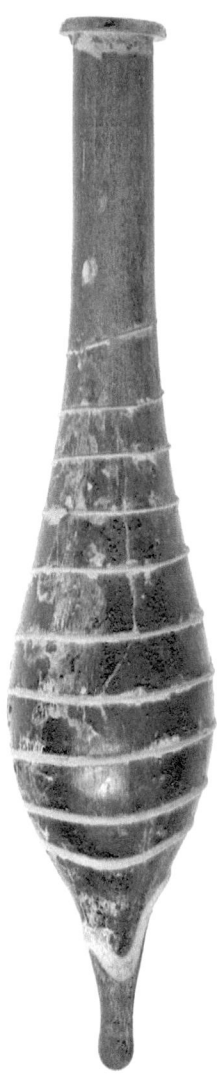

Figure 1 Unguentarium, 50–75 C.E. Collection of The Corning Museum of Glass, Corning, New York. 64.1.27.

Containers for scented oil include small bottles, miniature bottles, and even small jugs, or "juglets." In the Hellenistic period, pottery unguentaria are usually described as fusiform in shape (i.e., spindle shaped), but in the first century C.E., piriform (pear-shaped) bottles become more common.[18] Similarly, glass bottles of the first century C.E. were often piriform (fig. 2), while the candlestick shape (i.e., a flat base with a long, thin neck; fig. 3) is more common for unguentaria from the first through the third century C.E.[19] In addition, small glass jars or "boxes" (*pyxides*) were probably used to store unguents of a more solid nature, such as lotions or creams (fig. 4).

Rome could not seem to satiate its ever growing appetite for perfumery, whether in the form of oil, cream, or resin. Seeing itself as the cultural beneficiary of ancient Greece, Rome adopted and then transformed many of the Hellenistic practices surrounding perfume and incense.[20] Roman architects refined the public bathhouse and designed a *hypocaust* system that allowed water to be heated to various temperatures via underground vents. The design of the public bath often included a special room for the application of perfumed oils and unguents, variously called an *aleipterion, destrictarium,* or *unctorium*.[21] Women and men frequented the baths regularly, usually in the afternoon. They might partake in light exercise before the bath, and this would involve oiling and scraping the body.[22] The regular application of perfumed oil and scented unguents took place after bathing in hot water.

The wealthy of both sexes anointed the head and hair before being seen in public. For women, having one's hair coiffed and anointed was a regular part of getting dressed for the day. At banquets, hosts and hostesses might present their guests with special aromas with which to adorn themselves or scented wreaths to wear upon their heads; they would light incense and have flowers strewn on the tables and floors. The wealthy took advantage of every conceivable opportunity to imbue the dining room with fragrance. And while Rome grew some of its own aromatic plants (e.g., the rose), the exotic scents of the far reaches of the empire and beyond were much more enticing. Myrrh and frankincense from Arabia, spikenard from India, galbanum from Syria, and cinnamon, thought to be from "some distant coast on the Indian Ocean,"[23] were exciting and arousing not only because they smelled earthy, floral, musty, or spicy but also because they were foreign and strange, from unfamiliar places, and so sparked the imagination and awakened physical desire. The aromas of faraway places were not confined to the domestic sphere; on the contrary, Romans recognized that the erotic spices of bath and banquet were fit more for the gods than for humans.

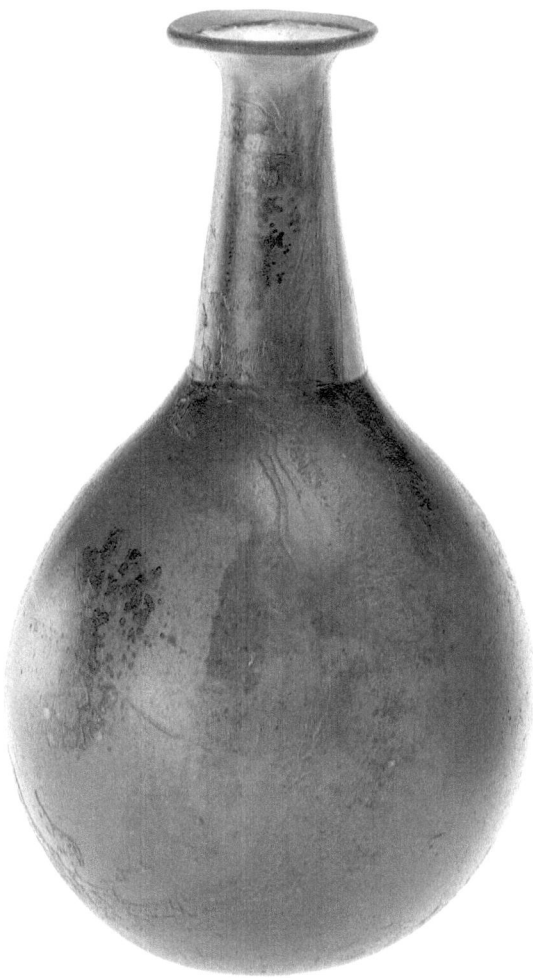

Figure 2 Unguentarium, first century C.E. Collection of The Corning Museum of Glass, Corning, New York. 50.1.14.

Accordingly, they adorned the statues of the gods with scented wreaths and anointed the likenesses of the gods with oils.

In the Roman period, the use of perfume became so common that the wealthy bought custom-made potions, while the poor and slaves wore ready-made perfumes. There were those, however, who took issue with Rome's lifestyle of excess. Stoics, Platonists, and satirists alike denounced what they saw as the overuse of, and exorbitant expenditures on, perfume.

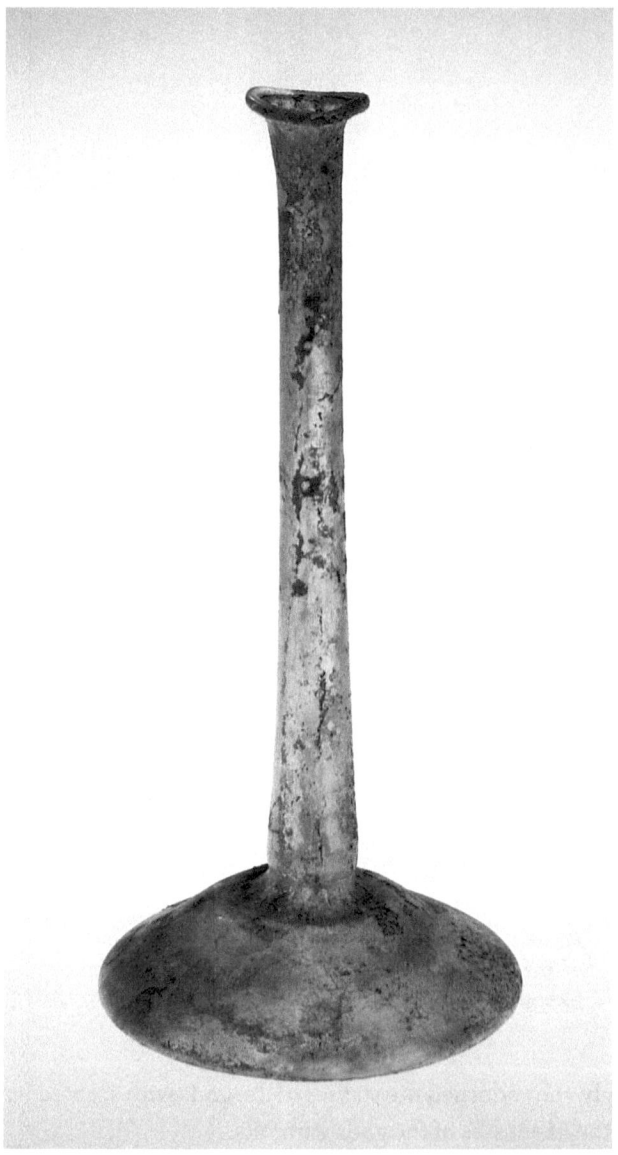

Figure 3 Candlestick unguentarium, late first to third century C.E. Collection of The Corning Museum of Glass, Corning, New York. 69.1.19. Gift of Honolulu Academy of Arts, Hawaii.

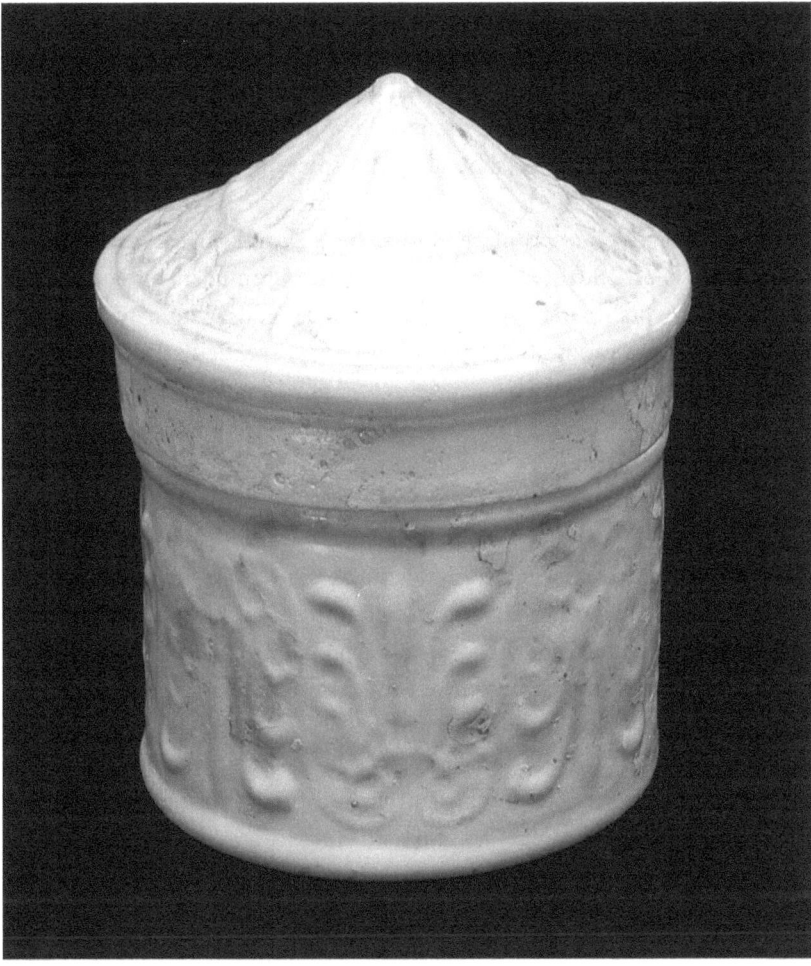

Figure 4 Pyxis, first century C.E. Collection of The Corning Museum of Glass, Corning, New York. 55.1.69a, b.

For some, spice used to excess—either in adornment or in food—revealed an obvious incongruity, a "stench" of moral depravity.[24] This dissoluteness could be spied not only at the banquet but at the bath as well. Often situated near areas of ill repute and prostitution, the baths, and therefore overindulgence in fragrance, were closely associated with licentiousness and promiscuity. Likewise, men who wore too much oil in their hair might be seen as effeminate. But these attitudes were the minority opinion and inconsistent even in those who voiced them.[25]

Not surprisingly, aromatics were used in the bedroom, both to rid the area of disagreeable odors and as aphrodisiacs. In addition, specific scents and oils were identified and prescribed by physicians as treatments for particular ailments.[26] Perfumed oils could be purchased at the spice shop in the local market. The spice shop also sold spices in liquid, resinous, hard, and powdered forms for use as incense. The ingredients would be laid atop burning charcoal that was placed either on a shovel or in a covered container with holes. The three primary contexts for burning incense were daily sacrifice and worship of the gods; aristocratic funerals, where it was laid on the pyre; and as a room fumigant and freshener—particularly at the dining table—in order to create a more celebratory atmosphere.

Aromatics in Roman and Byzantine Palestine

From the testimony of her authors, it would seem that Rome was constantly bathed, fumigated, anointed, and rubbed in pleasant aromas. But most of this evidence comes from those writers who lived at the hub of society in Rome or very nearby. Is there proof for perfumery in the provinces—in Palestinian Jewish communities in particular? Unfortunately, remnants of perfume, incense, or spices are only occasionally recoverable from material remains. For example, Joseph Patrich and Benny Arubas thought they had found a juglet containing balsam extract in the area of Qumran, but the chemical tests proved inconclusive.[27] The findings of Yizhar Hirschfeld are also uncertain. Hirschfeld has argued that the Qumran site (where most archaeologists believe the Essenes worked, lived, and wrote the Dead Sea Scrolls) was a fortified manor house in the style of other early Roman manor houses in Judea, and that one of its main products was balsam.[28] However, this claim appears to be unsubstantiated.[29]

In the absence of organic materials, we must search instead for the instruments, containers, and other furnishings related to aromatics (see fig. 5) and for any literary evidence that might describe how, when, and where they were used.[30] Fortunately, in the case of Palestine in the Roman and Byzantine periods, this evidence is bountiful—principally in cities and towns, at graves, and in the rabbinic texts themselves. The cities of Caesarea, Tiberias, and Sepphoris are of special interest because they had large Jewish populations and were most probably areas of rabbinic concentration.[31] But many other Jewish towns and cemeteries in the Galilee provide evidence in

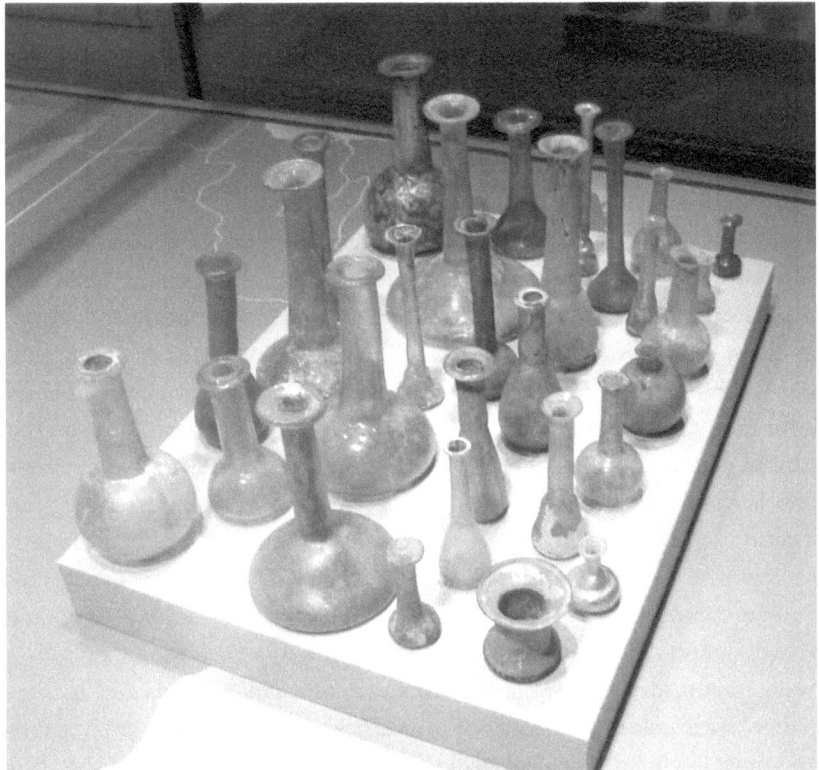

Figure 5 Collection of glass bottles on display at The Corning Museum of Glass, Corning, New York. Courtesy of Steven Fine, Yeshiva University.

both their small finds and their larger structures and spaces that perfumes and incense were used in the same places that rabbis frequented.[32]

Briefly, Caesarea Maritima was founded by King Herod in the first century B.C.E. to honor his friend Augustus and to provide revenues through the establishment of a large commercial harbor (Sebastos).[33] The design of the city was purely Roman in its layout and furnishings. Herod had built a beautiful palace on the sea, a hippodrome, an amphitheatre, and other typical Roman urban structures. It is likely that the rich lived upwind (that is, west) of the rest of the city, while the poor lived inland. The ruins of several mansions with warehouses have been found along the coast. Finished near the time of the king's demise, Caesarea and its man-made port grew. The emperor Vespasian named the city a Roman colony,[34] and in the second century C.E. Caesarea became the provincial capital, a status it held for six hundred years.[35] There, between the third and fourth centuries C.E., a large

Jewish minority could be found that participated along with Greeks, Romans, Christians, and Samaritans in the array of activities the city had to offer.[36]

Just up the coast and inland (northeast) of Caesarea is the region of the Galilee, home to two important Jewish centers in late antiquity, Tiberias and Sepphoris. Situated on the western edge of the Sea of Galilee, Tiberias was founded in the first century C.E. by Herod Antipas, King Herod's son, to serve as his capital. Thirty kilometers west of Tiberias and already probably a powerful city in the first century B.C.E., we find Sepphoris.[37] After the destruction of the Second Temple in 70 C.E., the Galilee witnessed a large immigration of Jews, and migration to the Galilee increased again after the Bar Kokhba revolt (ca. 132–35 C.E.).[38] As a result, Tiberias and Sepphoris both grew, and around 200 C.E. Judah ha-Nasi (the patriarch) moved the patriarchate from Beit She'arim to Sepphoris. The patriarch lived in Sepphoris from ca. 200 to ca. 217 C.E.,[39] and that city is also thought to be the location where he redacted the Mishnah. Between the third and the fifth century C.E., Tiberias and Sepphoris became not only Jewish but rabbinic urban centers.[40] Each city had distinguished *batei midrash* (rabbinic schools), and each could boast of being home to several famous rabbis.[41] Scholars consider it likely that the Talmud Yerushalmi was redacted in Tiberias.[42] Nevertheless, each city was also distinctively Roman in architecture and most likely in culture as well, with very few exceptions. Each city had a typical Roman layout for its streets, one or more marketplaces, and various public buildings. And, unlike the smaller Jewish towns or villages in the Galilee, the temples of these cities indicate that Jews would have been exposed to one or more different religions, and most of these probably employed incense or perfume or both in their rituals.[43]

That said, a perusal of even a modicum of rabbinic literature reveals that the rabbis held quite negative opinions of many Roman social and religious practices and of those whom they considered "pagan." For example, the texts depict non-Israelite characters from the Hebrew Bible as hedonists who had licentious lifestyles. *Genesis Rabbah* 86:3 variously portrays Potiphar as a priest in Egypt who "uncovers himself" as part of his cultic practice or who purchases Joseph in order to have sexual intercourse with him. In *b. Meg.* 13a, we are told that Esther and her counterparts in the harem soaked in myrrh for six months in order to depilate their bodies, one of the implications being that foreign kings liked their women to look like young girls. Opinions like these are easily transposed onto Rome. In addition, comments about religious practices portray the prevailing cultic activities as uncomplicated idol worship—an almost "pan-Roman" religion.⁴⁴ The rabbis also appear to hold in contempt specific Romans, such as Hadrian, who reigned as emperor during the Bar Kokhba revolt. Sometimes their animosity is directed at Roman culture more broadly. For example, the rabbinic voices are often loud and uncharacteristically united in their condemnation of Rome by identifying it with Esau and Edom.⁴⁵ Esau, considered the ancestor of Edom, sought to kill his brother, Jacob, the namesake and progenitor of Israel. Thus the rabbis came to see Roman civilization as pagan, ruthless, homicidal, and in every way loathsome.

It appears that the rabbis were nonetheless quite Roman in many aspects of their lifestyle and daily habits, and their literature is full of references to customs, practices, and cultural behaviors that they carried out in much the same way as other Romans throughout the empire.⁴⁶ One example is the use of the public bathhouse, which, with its innovative *hypocaust* system for heating water and its other accoutrements, was distinctively Roman in character. In other cases, it seems that the forebears of the rabbis, like other Jews, exhibited these behaviors independently, long before Rome entered Judea and maybe even before Alexander conquered the Near East. The fumigation of clothing and anointment with perfumed oil are two activities that appear in the biblical text and were well known as part of daily life in the Near East and the Mediterranean. Likewise, burial of the dead with perfumed oil is well attested throughout these regions.

This part of the study, therefore, reviews the contexts for the use of aromatics in Palestine: the marketplace (and the city at large), the bath, the home, and burial. It begins with a review of the terms used for aromatics in the rabbinic texts and cites those passages that refer either to aroma directly or to related practices or behaviors. The goal is to tease out from the texts rabbinic attitudes toward fragrance. While the rabbis regularly came in contact with spices and were for the most part favorably disposed toward them, the texts often contain hints of ambivalence. This is particularly true of the Talmud Bavli, which in several cases reorganizes the passages from the Yerushalmi and dramatically changes their emphasis.

Most of the passages presented here are from the Mishnah, Tosefta, and Talmud Yerushalmi. All three documents originate in the Galilee during the second through the early fifth century C.E. and were redacted in Palestine. A few of the passages come from the Talmud Bavli, as these exhibit familiarity with Palestinian customs and mores or appear to originate with Palestinian tradents. Two other factors call for the inclusion of these more remote texts. Harvey has demonstrated conclusively that the employment of aromatics increased in Christendom as the power of the church increased in the Byzantine period. It is thus possible, even likely, that the later texts actually exhibit more rather than less direct experience with perfume and incense in Palestine. In addition, although the great schools of Babylonia probably lacked direct interaction with a widespread Christian culture, they may still have had intimate knowledge of perfume and incense. Babylonia had a spice culture that predated even the earliest Israelite sources, and it appears that a significant number of rabbis traveled between Babylonia and Palestine. The references both to the material remains and to the texts included here are meant to be illustrative rather than exhaustive. They demonstrate rabbinic knowledge of, and experience with, aromatics, and from them we may also begin to observe and identify other images or cultural valences that adhere to perfume and incense.

The Terms

The rabbinic literature uses a variety of terms to indicate specific spices, perfume, incense, and fragrance. Many of these terms appear in the Bible, but their precise definitions in either corpus are difficult to pin down. One such term, *bosem* (בשם), can mean spice, balsam, or perfume. Sometimes the plural is used, as in the phrase "the chief of spices" (*ra'shei besamim*, ראשי בשמים).[47] This expression no doubt refers to balsam specifically, for that spice, also known as opalbalsam (*Commiphora opobalsamum*), was one of the most coveted in the empire. Until the Great Revolt (67 or 68 to 73 C.E.) and perhaps even afterward, Judea seems to be the sole producer of balsam within the empire, making the spice both rare and costly. While Theophrastus (371–287 B.C.E.) mentions that balsam "grows in the valley of Syria,"[48] Pliny (23–79 C.E.) is more forthcoming:

> Every other scent ranks below balsam. The only country to which this plant has been vouchsafed is Judaea, where formerly it grew in only two gardens, both belonging to the king; one of them was of not more than twenty iugera in extent and the other less. This variety of shrub was exhibited to the capital by the emperors Vespasian and Titus; and it is a remarkable fact that ever since the time of Pompey the Great even trees have figured among the captives in our triumphal processions. The balsam-tree is now subject of Rome.[49]

Pliny goes on to describe how the Jews attempted to destroy the balsam gardens, presumably during the Great Revolt, but were stopped by Roman authorities.

Josephus too refers to balsam production in Palestine. He imparts the tradition that the queen of Sheba brought balsam to King Solomon as a gift[50] and mentions two orchards, one in or near Jericho and the other near the Dead Sea at Ein Gedi.[51] While Josephus does not describe the attempted destruction of the balsam trees, he does tell of a raid by the Zealots on Ein Gedi during which they supposedly killed upward of seven hundred women and children.[52] It is possible that either Pliny or Josephus assumed the wrong motivation for this sequence of events, or that each author recounted certain facts according to his own interests. Ze'ev Safrai notes that while it appears that balsam production in Jericho was greatly limited at some point (perhaps soon after the Great Revolt), literary sources regarding production in the area of Ein Gedi prove otherwise.[53] It is clear, however, that production of balsam ceased completely at some time during or after the Byzantine period.

The importance of this spice in the land of Israel can be seen in the range of its syntactical usage, for *bosem* (בשם) is also used to mean "spice" or any general reference to spices. For example, the phrase *'atsei besamim* (עצי בשמים), which literally means "woods of balsam," "woods of spices," or "trees of spices," is usually understood to mean "fragrant wood" or "spiced wood" and so can refer to any spice.[54] In other cases the term for "spices" is combined with the word for oil (*shemen*, שמן) to mean any perfume or scented oil (*shemen besamim*, שמן בשמים). Other names for perfume include sweet, pleasing, or mixed oil (*shemen 'arev*, שמן ערב) and good oil (*shemen tov*, שמן טוב).[55] One can also be "perfumed" or "scented" (*mevusam*, מבושם).[56] And although a spice used for food is almost always referred to as *tevel* or *tavla'* (תבל/תבלא), the expression for spiced wine uses the expression "perfumed" (*yayin mevusam*, יין מבושם), hence "fragrant wine."[57]

In addition to *bosem*, other terms for balsam are also popular in the literature, and the various texts demonstrate preferences for some expressions over others.[58] For example, the word *afarsemon* (אפרסמון), which also means balsam, appears twelve times in the Talmud Bavli, but only twice in the Yerushalmi and not at all in the Mishnah or Tosefta. Two additional terms that may or may not be related to balsam are *qetaf* (קטף) and *tsori* (צרי). Both spices are commonly associated with resin that is used as an aromatic.⁵⁹ Most of the other spices mentioned in the rabbinic literature are connected in some way to the Bible; of these, the most prevalent are frankincense (*levonah*, לבונה) and myrrh (*mor*, מור).

The substance we would generally associate with incense is most frequently cited as *mugmar* (מוגמר), while the holy incense used in the Temple retains its biblical name, *qetoreth* (קטורת). In addition, words related to aroma are also useful for study. These include the verb "to anoint" (*sukh*, סוך) and its passive form "to be anointed" or "to be perfumed" (*nisakh*, ניסך). The passive form appears only once in the Mishnah and twice in the Tosefta, but nine times in the Talmud Bavli and twelve times in the Yerushalmi. Other related terms include the verbs "to scrape" (*gared*, גרד); "to crush" or "to pound" (*pittem*, פיטם), as in spices pulverized by the apothecary or perfumer (the *pattam*, פטם, or *bosem*, בשם); to "bathe" (*rahats*, רחץ); and the term for "bathhouse" (*beit rahtsah*, בית רחצה, or *dimusin*, דימוסין).⁶⁰

The Spice Dealer and the Marketplace

As in Greek and Roman literature, the perfumer, the apothecary, and the spice dealer appear to be either the same person or at the very least persons well acquainted with one another who may have also worked closely together.⁶¹ As a result, references to these professions, to the spice shop, and to the implements of the trade (e.g., mortar and pestle, perfume bottle, etc.; fig. 6) are scattered throughout the literature.⁶²

As for the professionals involved in the production of aromatics, one of the best examples comes from a discussion on laws that apply to the sabbatical year: "R. Yehudah ben Isaiah, the Perfumer (*habasam*, הבשם), testified before R. Akiba, in the name of R. Tarfon, that the law of sabbatical applies to *qetaf*."⁶³ Here we not only see the perfumer as consultant to one of the most famous rabbis, but the advisor is none other than a rabbi himself! Another reference to the profession appears in a comment on the compounding of Temple incense: "Bar Qappara taught: The perfumers of Jerusalem would say, 'If one were to put a small amount of honey into it (i.e., the incense), the whole world would not be able to endure its scent.'"⁶⁴ Bar Qappara's recollection of the perfumers of Jerusalem presents them as an organized body whose job included preparing the incense for daily offering in the Temple. A more metaphorical reference appears in *Avot d'Rabbi Natan* 18.5, in which R. Judah compares five sages to various things; among these are nuts or stones, a storehouse, and a spice peddler's basket:

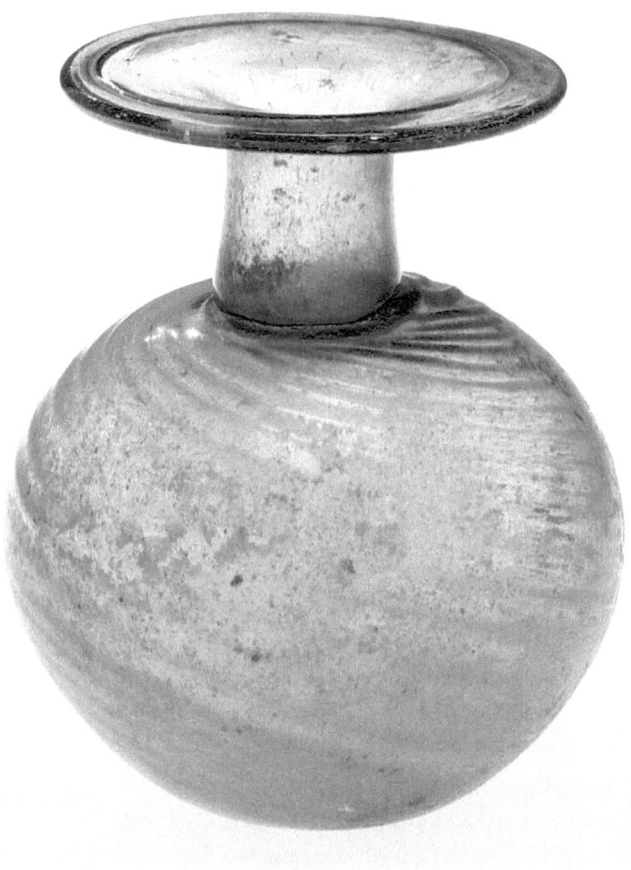

Figure 6 Dropper flask, third to fourth century C.E. Collection of The Corning Museum of Glass, Corning, New York. 52.1.63.

He called R. Eleazar ben Azariah a [spice] peddler's[65] basket (קופה של רוכלים). And why was R. Eleazar like a spice peddler who carries his basket and enters the province? Because the men of the province come to him and say to him, "Do you have good oil (שמן טוב) with you? Do you have ointment (פולייטין)? Do you have balsam (אפרסמון)?" And they would find he had all [these things]. Just so was R. Eleazar ben Azariah when students would come to him. If [the student] asked about Scripture, he told him; about Mishnah, he told him; about Midrash, he told him; about Law, he told him; about

Aggadoth, he told him. When [the student] went out, he was filled with good and blessing.[66]

In this passage, several different terms, all related to fragrance, are employed to describe the various subjects of the rabbi's expertise. The rabbi is analogized as a spice peddler who has come to town to sell his aromatics. When the student leaves the rabbi, the student is perfumed in the sense of exuding the pleasing odor of the teachings. Of note, unlike the first two examples of perfumers, the spice peddler is not a regular resident of the town. It would seem that he passes through as a traveling salesman might. As for what he proffers, the midrash presents three different types of products: perfume, ointment, and a specific spice.

Each of the passages so far examined implies rabbinic familiarity with a profession or trade connected with spices and perfume. In addition, each example radiates positive valences; that is, it either portrays a positive attitude toward aromatics or the perfumer's expertise, or it is employed in ways that affirm the use of perfume. R. Judah would not have compared R. Eleazar to something he felt negatively about in order to praise the rabbi's knowledge. Several undercurrents may also be detected in the texts. The first is that the profession seems to be respected, at least in the area of its own expertise. There is no evidence of mistrust or disapproval of this line of work. If there are negative attitudes toward the burning or application of fragrant spices, they do not appear to apply to the people who sell or compound products. The second undercurrent is related to this first point; the spice peddler in the last example is an itinerant. This in itself could make him a somewhat suspicious character, but he is not depicted in this light at all. On the contrary, his association with R. Eleazar carries only positive connotations. As a result, rather than see the peddler as strange or untrustworthy and so deserving of suspicion, he is depicted as interesting and exotic.

The marketplace itself is more ambiguous. There, the spice dealer might not be Jewish. A comment on the spices of gentiles can be found in the Mishnah. The discussion follows a series of disputes between the houses of Hillel and Shammai about the order in which blessings are said at evening meals on the Sabbath and festivals. The reference is elliptical both because it has nothing to do with meals and because its language and structure are unusual: "One may not bless over the lamp or over the spices of gentiles,[67] or over the lamp or over the spices of the dead, or over the lamp or over the spices [placed] before idolatry. One may not bless over the lamp until one can use it for light."[68]

The law contains a four-part structure. The first three injunctions focus on lamps and spices: those belonging to non-Jews (or idolaters), those for the dead, and those for idolatry. The last section seems to be an addition to the foregoing—namely, that as for lights and occasions on which one does say a blessing over a lamp, one does not do so until the light is lit. As for the law regarding lamps and spices for the dead, which is wedged between the laws on lamps and spices of the gentiles (or idolaters) and idolatry, we will return to this injunction below. For purposes of this discussion, the rabbinic voices seem to stipulate a difference between those lamps and spices *owned* by gentiles or idolaters and those actually *used* in idolatrous practices. One does not say a blessing for either, but nevertheless a distinction is made.

While the passage clearly delineates a difference between idolaters and idolatry, it does not explain that difference. Therefore, the Yerushalmi attempts to clarify the laws through amplification: "R. Jacob stated before R. Jeremiah: One may bless over spices of gentiles. [On] what does he differ? It is confirmed that he burns [spices] in front of his store."[69] R. Jacob points out that, contrary to the Mishnah, one does say a blessing over the spices of gentiles. He gives the case of a gentile who owns a spice shop and burns spices in front of the store to alert customers to the presence of the store and so draw them inside. A Jewish passerby who smells the scent wafting in the air should say a blessing in appreciation of the pleasant experience regardless of who owns the spices.[70] These spices are categorically different from those of idolatry, which may smell the same but are being put to heretical use.[71]

On the whole, the references to spices and smelling incense in the market appear to be neutral. Even the passing reference to gentiles and their spices is not negative, although the Yerushalmi's discussion highlights a disagreement within the rabbinic tradition. Admittedly, though, smelling perfume at the spice shop is not the same experience as smelling someone who has intentionally perfumed him- or herself; nor is it akin to perfuming oneself. Indeed, being smelled in the marketplace—or more generally in public—may be fraught with danger.

The Tosefta and Yerushalmi both discuss the situation in which the dinner attendant who brings the incense after the meal has his head rubbed with the oil by the host.[72] If the attendant is a student (תלמיד חכם), however, oil is not smeared on his head, because "there is no profit (שבח) in a student who goes out perfumed (מבוסם)."[73] The implication is that it is not seemly for students to be perfumed in public. The Talmud Bavli uses much stronger language to express this view: "it would be *shameful* (or disgraceful, גנאי) for a student to go to the marketplace (שוק) when he is perfumed (מבושם)."[74] This passage is the second in a series of three *baraitot*. The next *baraita* continues in this vein by establishing six things that are shameful for a student to do, all of which occur in public. The first is a repetition of the injunction on being perfumed, and here the Talmud comments:

> R. Abba the son of R. Ḥiyya bar Abba said in the name of R. Yoḥanan, "[This is with regard] to a place where there is a suspicion of lying with a male." R. Sheshet said, "That is said only about one's clothing, but as for one's body—it passes sweat." R. Papa said, "And one's hair is like one's clothing." But others say, "It is like one's body."[75]

On the surface it would seem that, according to R. Yoḥanan and his followers, a scholar may go to the market perfumed, with the caveat that he not go to places where men who engage in homosexual activity may be found, as his perfumed body is likely to attract those of untoward desires. R. Sheshet responds that the problem arises with the scholar who fumigates his garments; fumigation of clothing seems to cross the boundary of acceptable behavior—at least in public.[76] Anointing the body, however, is not an issue, for perfumed oil aids in getting rid of sweat. The passage concludes with a discussion of whether the hair is considered more like clothing (R. Papa's position) and so off limits for perfuming, or whether it is part of the body (the anonymous voices) and therefore allowed.

Here we see the same apprehensive view of the marketplace that we saw in the passage on the perfumed women of Jerusalem that opened this chapter. As a public place with a mixed population, the market is dangerous and can be morally hazardous. The rabbinic voices are well aware that the power and authority they enjoy in less crowded or private spaces (e.g., a home, a field, or the *beit midrash*) is mitigated or nonexistent in the marketplace. In addition, there is a strand in the texts that exhibits anxiety over the sexual vulnerability of students, and this too is related to space in two ways. The first concerns anointment and fumigation. While it would seem logical that the anointed body presents a greater problem in public than the fumigated garment does, the reverse is actually the case. The aroma of the anointed body can be detected only when one is in close proximity to it, and if a strigil was used to scrape the body, only a little of the scent would remain. The fumigated garment, by contrast, can be smelled from a distance, and as one walks by dressed in such garments, the scent is likely to linger.[77] Second is the relationship between aroma and areas of the city associated with people of ill repute or licentiousness. This correlation among aroma, public space, and moral corruption appears in the Roman literature as well, and therefore seems to indicate a certain reality of city life for all Romans.

One distinctive aspect of the description of city life in rabbinic literature concerns "idolatrous incense." Other Roman authors had no objection to incense used for ritual purposes, and it is unlikely that rabbis in small towns or villages populated entirely by Jews had direct experience with the rituals of other religions. Therefore, the passages suggest either an urban rabbinic setting in which rabbis regularly came into contact with temples, or that "idolatry," as articulated by the rabbis, means practices performed by Jews of which the rabbis disapprove. Regardless of their origins, these passages clearly demonstrate that anointing with oil was regularly practiced by rabbis, that rabbis visited spice shops, and that they knew of and might have been in regular contact with perfumers. To be sure, they may have objected to the fumigation of clothing and to other public encounters with aromatics, but they anointed their bodies and hair much as other Romans did.

The Bath

The public space most likely to conjure negative reflection in some Roman literature was the bathhouse. A public place in which men and women appeared naked and relaxed, where one could not help but smell the pleasing aroma of scented unguents and oils made from exotic spices, the bathhouse was seen as closely associated with lasciviousness and certain types of lewd behavior. The location of brothels nearby probably didn't help matters. But the bathhouse was also often a public place of great beauty, and that people went there to relax, bathe, meet and greet each other, partake in exercise, and in some cases even hear a lecture or read a book in the library, meant it had many positive associations as well.

If the rabbis were truly like everyone else in the empire, they had personal knowledge of the bathhouse from daily or weekly visits. They would have moved through the structure from the *apodyterium* (the room for changing from street clothes into bathing attire), to the *frigidarium* (the room for the cold bath), to the *caldarium* (the room for the hot bath). If the bathhouse was somewhat small, the rabbis might have returned to the *apodyterium* for the application of oils and creams. If it was very large, they would probably have proceeded to the *unctorium* for the application of oils and a massage. In a larger bathhouse, a rabbi could go for a swim in one of the large pools or into a hall for some light exercise. Even the briefest investigation of the rabbinic texts reveals that the rabbis not only knew of the quintessentially Greco-Roman practice of bathing but participated in it as well. The archaeological evidence also confirms Jewish, if not rabbinic, contact with the bathhouse.

The public Roman bathhouse was usually a large complex centrally located in the city. In the private sphere, the bath existed as an amenity for the wealthy. The remains of public bathhouses are often easy to recognize, particularly if their *hypocaust* systems are identified. These underground heating systems were made by erecting small pillars under the floor in order to create a space through which heat could travel. Even in cases where the flooring has long since been destroyed, the pillars, or parts of the pillars, often remain. However, the domestic baths of Roman and Byzantine Palestine are somewhat more difficult to categorize. When found in predominantly Jewish areas, the domestic bath may appear to be a *miqveh* (Jewish ritual immersion bath). In places like Sepphoris, where many Jews are known to have lived, archaeologists continue to debate whether the baths found there are regular private baths or examples of *miqva'ot*. In the case of Sepphoris, this debate has carried over from the private bath to the public bathing complex as well, as archaeologists indicate that one of the two public baths found in Sepphoris seems to have had a *miqveh* associated with it.[78] Some archaeologists interpret the stepped baths (i.e., *miqva'ot*) found in the domestic quarters as evidence not only of Jewish presence but of the presence of priestly families.[79] Others argue that Jews other than priests (i.e., rabbis) may have also used the baths for ritual immersion. Still others argue that, whether priestly, rabbinic, or neither, it is likely that these baths were used for more "profane" bathing as well as for ritual immersion.[80]

The bathhouse at Tiberias, which was found in early excavations, looms large in rabbinic literature. So too do the bathing facilities of Ḥammat Tiberias, a small town just south of Tiberias whose hot springs were famous in antiquity.[81] While early literature, such as the Mishnah, refers occasionally to the baths and bathing, the later literature of the Talmud Yerushalmi is much more explicit and verbose.[82] There, several long expositions may be found on the adventures of rabbis at the baths. On the topic of condolences and eulogies, for example, the Yerushalmi includes a discussion of rabbis coming and going from the Galilee. In one case, R. Yassa (Assi) visits the barber and then decides to take a bath at the public bathhouse in Tiberias.[83] Another example recounts that R. Joshua b. Levi would regularly listen to his grandson recite the weekly portion (his lesson) every Friday afternoon. On one occasion, however, the rabbi forgot and went to "bathe in the bath at Tiberias." [84] When he remembered his grandson's lesson, he left the bath. The Yerushalmi provides many other references to the baths at Tiberias as well as those at Ḥammat Tiberias.[85] Magical or disturbing events at the baths are often recorded in the rabbinic texts, and, as in the Roman literature, traces of mistrust about the baths—the danger they represented both physically and morally—is also present. The *hypocaust* system could be treacherous to one's life, and instances of floors collapsing were well known. As a result, the rabbis discuss which prayers should be said upon entering and leaving the baths.[86] Other frequenters of the baths could also pose problems. Thieves might steal one's possessions from the *apodyterium*. As for the moral dangers, these were essentially the same as those of the marketplace: one might encounter people with whom it was considered ill advised to consort.

But the bath might present another problem, one to which perfumed oil is directly connected:

> Rabbi was praising R. Ḥiyya the Elder before R. Ishmael ben Yossi. . . . One time R. Ishmael saw him (Ḥiyya the Elder) at the bathhouse, but he (Ḥiyya) did not rise to pay his respects. . . . Rabbi said, "Why did you do thus?" He (Ḥiyya) said to him, " . . . I didn't know. At the time I was going over matters of the *aggadah* from the whole book of Psalms." From that time on, he (Rabbi) assigned two students to accompany [Ḥiyya] into the unctorium.[87]

In this narrative, R. Ishmael feels insulted by R. Ḥiyya's behavior at the bathhouse, for he thinks R. Ḥiyya has snubbed him by not standing up to pay his respects. When Rabbi inquires as to the reason for this rudeness, R. Ḥiyya explains that his mind was on *aggadah* and that he was unaware of Rabbi Ishmael's presence. From that time on, Rabbi assigns two students to assist the rabbi when he is in the *unctorium*.

For purposes of studying rabbinic encounters with perfume, the mention of the *unctorium* is significant. Of all the rooms in the bathhouse, it is in the *unctorium* that a person was most likely to reflect deeply and randomly, as the pervasive aroma of the oils imbued the room with such pleasant and soothing qualities as to focus the mind. Or it may be that the perfume, combined with the massage that regularly took place in this room, created such a feeling of well-being that the rabbi forgot entirely the requisite decorum due his colleague. Either way, Rabbi seems to think that engagement with the students would help keep R. Ḥiyya's mind on track and ensure that he remain within the bounds of appropriate conduct for a rabbi in the bathhouse.

The passage also raises some interesting questions and concerns, not least whether R. Ḥiyya was dressed when R. Ishmael saw him. This is important in light of *t. Ber.* 2:20, where we learn that if a person is in an area of the bathhouse in which people are dressed, then one is allowed to greet his colleagues and to pray. If one is in a room in the bathhouse in which people are naked, however, then one should neither greet colleagues nor pray. Finally, if this person is in an area of the bathhouse in which some people are dressed and others undressed, then he may greet his colleagues, but he may not pray. In our passage, R. Ishmael expects the rabbi to afford him the usual respect due him; therefore, we must assume that R. Ḥiyya is in an area of the bathhouse either where people are dressed or where some are dressed and some are not. If R. Ḥiyya is in an area of the bathhouse in which all the people are dressed, then why the need to ruminate on *aggadah*? If, however, R. Ḥiyya is in an area of the bathhouse in which some people are dressed and others are not, then it is more likely that he is "dressed" (i.e., wearing some kind of covering) but is so engrossed in his meditation that he fails to greet R. Ishmael. The text is ambiguous, but it seems to suggest that in the *unctorium*, rabbis wore some kind of covering.[88]

References to perfumed oil, spices, and the bathhouse appear in a few other places in the rabbinic literature with reference to other rabbinic laws and customs. For example, in the Tosefta's version of the disagreement between the houses of Hillel and Shammai, the comment is made that one does not say a blessing over the wood and spices of the bathhouse.[89] With reference to the Sabbath, we find that one may not anoint his head and then go to the bath, but he may anoint his entire body and then wipe his body limb by limb.[90] The Tosefta also includes several references to oil being placed on a marble table that a person then rolls around on in order to anoint himself. While the passages are somewhat abstruse (e.g., concerning a priest and oil of heave offering or gentiles preceding Jews on such a table), they all seem to refer either to scented oil in general or to the perfumed oil found at the bathhouse.[91]

The next example does not mention the bathhouse directly, but it does portray another convention considered to be purely Greco-Roman and intrinsically connected to the baths: the sport of wrestling. In reference to the Sabbath, the Mishnah says that certain exercises associated with wrestlers were not permitted: "They may oil and massage their stomach but not exercise and not scrape. They may not go down to the *kordimah* (a certain kind of exercise area of mud and clay) and may not use artificial emetics."[92] Both oil and scraping are mentioned here. And, while the rabbis permit oiling of the body, they do not allow scraping on the Sabbath. Likewise, one may not engage in other specific exercises.

The final example comes from a *baraita* found in the Talmud Bavli. The subject is ownership and the passage seeks to determine what the term "takes possession" (*ḥazakah*, חזקה) means. Although the text that precedes this passage concerns real estate, the discussion then turns to slavery:

> What was it that was taught? How [does ownership occur] by "taking possession"? [If] he put on his shoes for him, or loosened his shoes for him; or [if] he carries his vessels after him to the bath, and undresses him, and washes him, anoints him, scrapes him, and dresses him, puts on his shoes.[93]

In this passage, the slave's work is described in terms of the activities of bathing. All the steps of the bath are described, first in order of undress and then in order of dress. The passage contains details rarely seen in rabbinic literature; that is, it seems to be usual practice that if one has a slave, this person brings the unguents and oils necessary at the bath. (These "vessels" would include bottles and jars. See figs. 7 and 8.) We would expect, therefore, that those who do not have slaves bring their own accoutrements. The passage also depicts anointing and scraping as customary and regular activities that occur after washing. Although we find observations in both rabbinic and other Roman literature that indicate the reverse (i.e., anointing and then washing), it is likely that at least some people anointed both before and after washing, depending on their physical activity at the bath.[94]

These passages demonstrate that the rabbis were quite familiar not only with the bathhouse and bathing but also with activities of exercise (e.g., wrestling), anointing, and scraping. Their experience with perfumed oil is personal, and they seek to regulate anointment with oil as they would other activities of daily life.[95]

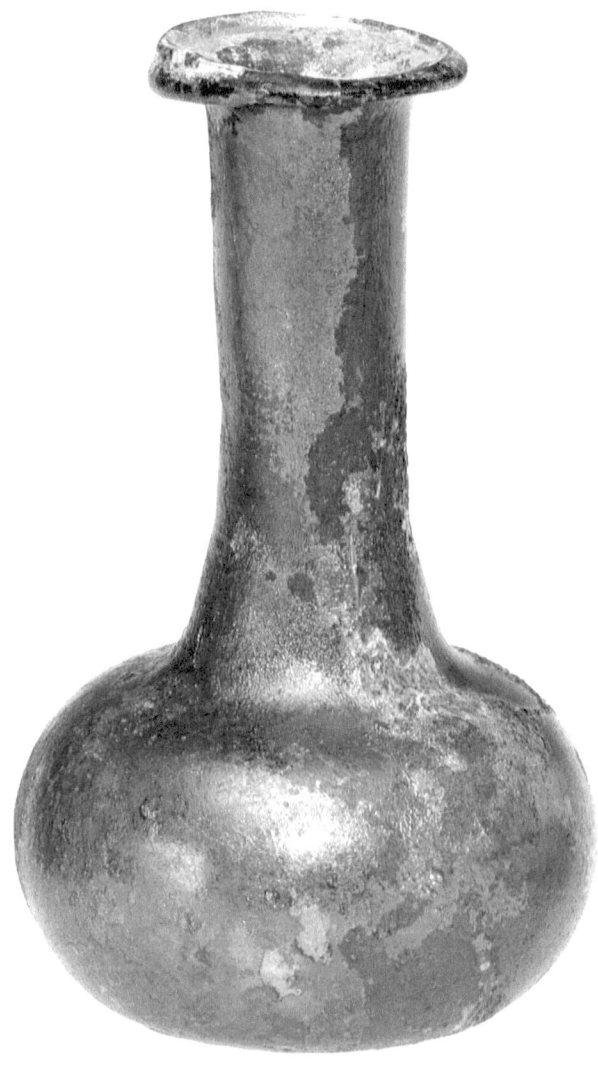

Figure 7 Unguentarium, first century to early second century C.E. Collection of The Corning Museum of Glass, Corning, New York. 54.1.53. Gift of I. C. Elston Jr.

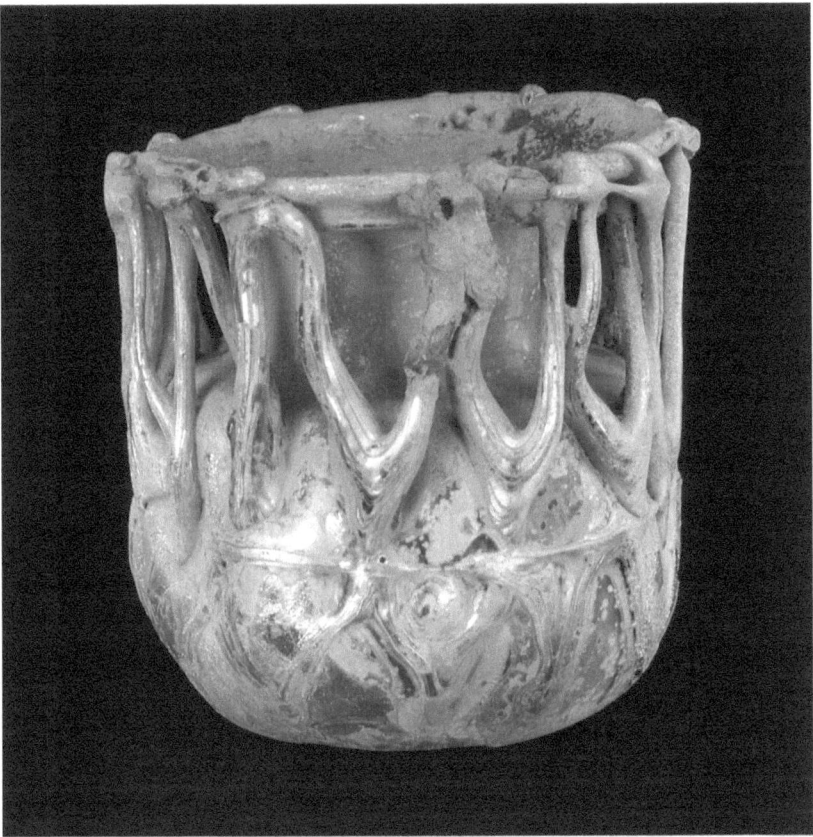

Figure 8 Jar, third to fourth century C.E. Collection of The Corning Museum of Glass, Corning, New York. 53.1.6.

In the Home

The home was the hub of daily life for almost all the inhabitants of the city, and most people, especially women and children, spent more time at home than anywhere else. One ate, slept, and often worked at home. For a complete assessment of rabbinic contact with aroma, we must therefore ascertain to what extent pleasant scents were found in the home. Given the evidence from the marketplace and the bathhouse, it seems logical to assume that the rabbinic home was also its own fragrance center, and indeed the vast majority of references to perfume, incense, and fumigation concern the home or its inhabitants.

First and foremost, the house itself was regularly fumigated. This was most common after meals, when one might want to clear the air of the smell of food, but, more important, fumigation was an act of festivity that added to the enjoyment of the evening.⁹⁶ The incense employed was probably either a soft resin or an oily substance placed on top of lit coals. The example mentioned above from *b. Ber.* 43b, in which the attendant brought incense into the dining room after the meal and then had some wiped on his forehead, refers to a discussion in the Mishnah on which blessings are said for which items and includes the following dictum:

> [If] they are sitting to eat, each one [by himself], each blesses for himself; if they recline (i.e., eat together), then one blesses for everyone. If wine is brought to them during the meal, each one blesses for himself. [If wine is brought to them after the meal], one blesses for everyone. And he says the blessing over the incense (מוגמר), even though they are brought in only after the meal.⁹⁷

This passage suggests that when incense is brought, the person who said the blessing over the wine also blesses the incense. These occasions seem to be ones of formal dining at which the Roman custom of reclining in the *triclinium* is being practiced.

On the issue of blessing the spices, the Yerushalmi (*y. Ber.* 6.6, 10d) asks, "What is the difference between incense (*mugmar*, מוגמר) and wine?" The answer is, "Everyone smells incense. Each one tastes wine." The Talmud understands both the collective and individual aspects of the sense of smell; that is, each person smells the incense even though it is a single portion. The experience of smelling incense is somewhat different from tasting wine, as with wine each person ingests from his own portion.

The Yerushalmi continues with a debate on which blessing is said when the smoke rises. R. Ze'ira says, " . . . who gives good scent to pleasant oil" (ריח טוב לשמן ערב), while Rav Jeremiah corrects him: " . . . who gives good scent to spiced wood" (עצי בשמים).⁹⁸ Others weigh in on the issue, until Geniva says, "oil that is for filth (זיהומה), one does not bless."⁹⁹ Heinrich Guggenheimer notes that this oil is used primarily for cleaning (e.g., rubbing one's hands with oil after a meal) and so no blessing is said.¹⁰⁰ The Talmud Bavli makes this point a bit differently, asserting that if the fragrant substance is used primarily for something other than "smelling" (i.e., enjoyment of scent), then no blessing is said.¹⁰¹ This rule would seem to hold for other substances as well, including an unguent or resin that was sprinkled onto the floor for cleaning or sweeping.¹⁰² The discussion ends with Rav

Ḥisda's remark that one says the blessing for "spiced wood" over all fragrances except musk. Over musk, one blesses God for the "good smell of all kinds of spices" (במיני בשמים). Notably, the same discussion in the Talmud Bavli is quite long and detailed and contains many suggestions about which blessings should be said over which pleasant spices. There, reference is made both to the balsam groves of R. Judah and to those of Caesar.[103]

For some, like Rabban Gamaliel, lighting incense was so important that a ruling was necessary to ensure that incense could be used on festival days (when no lighting can occur): "Now he (Rabban Gamaliel) also pronounced leniently on three things: they [may] sweep between the couches and put on the spices on a festival day, and they may make a helmeted[104] kid on the nights of Passover. But the sages forbid [them]."[105] The Mishnah presents both Rabban Gamaliel's lenient rulings and the rescission of these decisions by a group of anonymous sages. The Tosefta also visits this issue but goes to great lengths to mitigate the sages' pronouncement:

> Concerning the house of Rabban Gamaliel, they would place the incense in a *megufah* (מגופה).[106] R. Eleazar ben Rabbi Ṣadoq said, "Many times I ate at the house of Rabban Gamaliel and I didn't see them put incense in the *megufah*. Rather, [the incense] would be burning in a *partasqa'oth* (פרטסקאות)[107] from the evening of the festival day. When the guests entered, they would bring [it] in and open it up." [The rabbis] said to him, "If this is so, it is permitted to do this on the Sabbath."[108]

R. Eleazar ben Ṣadoq is able to defend Rabban Gamaliel by clarifying how incense was enjoyed on festival days. The problem is that even if the coals are already lit, placing the incense on them is considered "kindling." Instead, the rabbi explains, the incense was placed in a special type of container and lit the evening before. On the festival day, as the guests arrived, the container would be unstoppered so the smoke could come out.

The description found in the Talmud Bavli[109] is similar to that in the Tosefta (above) but describes the container as being made out of iron and having its air holes stopped up the night before the festival. On the festival day the air holes would be unplugged and the room would be filled with fragrance. In addition, the Talmud frames this passage with an explanation from R. Assi, who asserts that the original dispute between Rabban Gamaliel and the rabbis concerned fumigation of a room as a consequence of fumigating garments, and such work is not allowed on a festival day (or Sabbath).[110] Presumably the spices used for clothing are like those used in cleaning the hands; they are not burned for pleasure but are utilitarian in nature. Still, they must have emitted a scent similar to that of incense, for both the Yerushalmi and the Bavli stipulate that no blessing is said for fragrances wafting in Sepphoris or Tiberias before or after the Sabbath because these derive from fumigating garments.[111] If the odors were not similar, one would not be likely to say a blessing by mistake. This mistake could also be made during the Sabbath because the perfuming of garments may begin before the Sabbath begins at sundown and continue throughout the night and next day.[112] It would seem, then, that according to R. Assi, Rabban Gamaliel allowed the burning of incense for room fumigation to continue from the night before the festival day, but he did not allow the perfuming of clothing, even though this was allowed on the Sabbath if begun the night before.

From the rabbinic discussion on these types of fumigatory spices and from passing references to the oils and spices used for cleaning the hands and floor, it is clear that the rabbis had direct contact with perfume and incense in the home. These practices—lighting incense, fumigating clothing, wiping the hands—were part of the routines of daily life in the Roman Empire. What makes the rabbis different from at least some other Romans is their desire to articulate thanksgiving for these small pleasures (ברכות נהנים). Their practice of saying a blessing each time they smell incense that is lit for purely pleasurable purposes seems to be unique within the empire.

Spices of another sort are worth mentioning here, because they too are most frequently experienced in the home. The Mishnah records, "The House of Shammai say[s], 'Light, food, spices (*besamim,* בשמים), and *havdalah.*' And the House of Hillel say[s], 'Light, spices, food, and *havdalah.*' The House of Shammai say[s], '. . . who created the light of the fire' and the House of Hillel say[s], '. . . who creates the lights of the fire.'"[113] *Havdalah* (meaning "distinction" or "division") is the blessing that identifies the transition from the Sabbath to a regular workday. In this passage the houses of Hillel and Shammai agree that the *havdalah* blessings may be said in conjunction with the blessings over food that follow the last meal of the Sabbath. They disagree, though, about the order of these blessings. The Shammaites would say the blessing over the spices after the blessings for food, while those from the house of Hillel would bless over the spices before the blessings for food.

Praxis follows Hillel, whose rulings are often more lenient than Shammai's. Both rulings, however, as presented in the Mishnah, would allow the ignition of the spices, because both agree that the blessing over the lights (and therefore their ignition) has already taken place when the spices are blessed. The Sabbath is technically over, and one is therefore allowed to light other materials. Despite this permission, however, from the medieval period on, we have evidence (in the form of spice boxes) that some groups of Jews did not light the spices employed during the *havdalah* ceremony; they simply inhaled the fragrance of the raw spices.[114]

A clue to this discrepancy between cultural norms and ritual praxis may be found as early as the Tosefta, wherein R. Judah asserts that the houses of Hillel and Shammai agreed that the blessings for the meal came first and that those for the *havdalah* came last. What they disagreed about was the order of the blessings for the lights and spices. Shammai argued for lights first and then spices (which would have allowed the fumigation of the spices), while Hillel opted for blessing the spices first (the fumigation of which would have violated the Sabbath law).[115] If practice follows the ruling of Hillel, then the spices must remain unlit. The Yerushalmi depicts yet another permutation. There, Shammai is said to bless the spices first and then the light, while Hillel is said to do the reverse. These statements are followed by a pronouncement not seen in the earlier passages: "R. Ba and R. Judah [said] in the name of Rav, 'The law is according to the one who says, "spices and after that light."'"[116] This declaration uncharacteristically affirms Shammai and explains why the spices are not lit.[117]

The smelling of these spices at *havdalah* is one of the few ritual uses of spices or performative acts of olfaction found in the rabbinic corpus.[118] Because of the proximity of these rulings to others surrounding meals, and because of the inclusion of this blessing with a particular meal, it is likely that this ritual grew out of the regular custom of lighting incense at the end of a meal.[119] It is even possible that some groups ensured that they recognized the official end of the Sabbath in order to light the spices. Over time, it appears that the spices became more strongly associated with the end of the Sabbath rather than with the meal.[120]

With all the fumigation and perfuming that the sources describe as taking place in the home, it may seem odd that few implements have survived. As mentioned above, the fact that unguentaria were made of glass during this period means that relatively few examples survive intact in areas

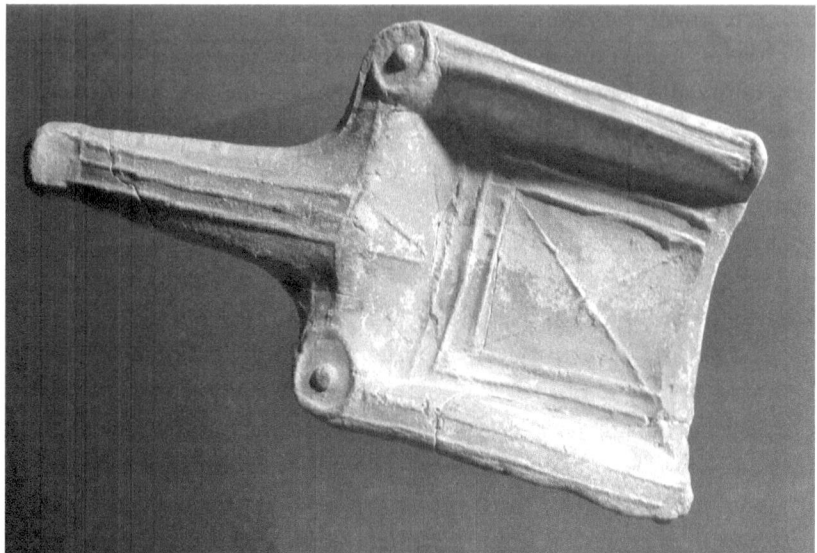

Figure 9 Rectangular ceramic incense shovel from Sepphoris, Middle Roman period. With permission from the Joint Sepphoris Project, Eric and Carol Meyers.

that were heavily trafficked (e.g., the market, the bath, the home).[121] Nevertheless, archaeologists regularly attest to significant numbers of small unguentaria-like bottles and glass sherds from similar bottles.[122] But what of those accoutrements related to incense—the standing burners, censers, and shovels? As for these, only a few incense burners have been found in all the land of Israel, and these are of bronze.[123] Of the iron burner that the Bavli describes, we have no evidence.

One of the most intriguing finds at Sepphoris, however, is a cache of incense shovels found in the domestic quarters of the city, in a neighborhood that archaeologists consider quite upscale and Jewish. The house in question had a large courtyard, storage facilities, and a bath (or *miqveh*). The approximately fifteen shovels (some rectangular and some oval) and fifty shovel fragments date from the second through the third century C.E. Some of the shovels have lids with holes that would facilitate the burning of incense. Because this is the largest collection of shovels found in Palestine to date, because they are ceramic, because they are the only shovels to have been found in a controlled excavation, and because they resemble—to a remarkable degree—many late Roman and early Byzantine depictions of incense shovels from the Temple, they have been the center of much speculation (see figs. 9 and 10).

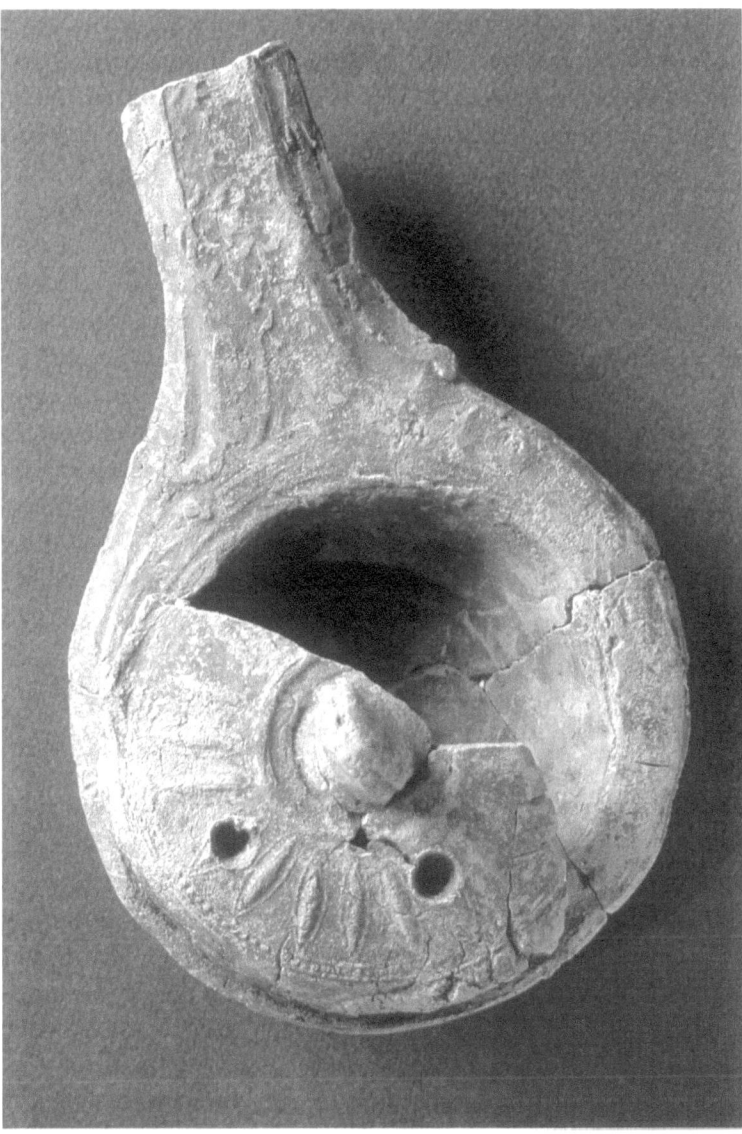

Figure 10 Oval-shaped ceramic incense shovel from Sepphoris, Middle Roman period. With permission from the Joint Sepphoris Project, Eric and Carol Meyers.

To heighten the mystery and conjecture surrounding the finds, the team's geologist and provenience specialist, Eric Lapp, and the team's ceramist, Marva Balouka, disagree on the condition of the shovels. Balouka, the first person to study the shovels in detail, considered that all the lids on the shovels had burn marks on their interior sides.[124] Some years later, however, when Lapp and Eric Meyers looked at the shovels again, Lapp described all the fragments as appearing to be "brand-spanking new" and made of a type of clay different from that used for other objects found at Sepphoris.[125] Of the black slip that appears on one fragment, Leonard Rutgers posits that the shovel was blackened during the original firing or was later thrown into a fire on purpose.[126]

These shovels and sherds, in addition to the shovel fragments that James Strange has reported finding, have led Rutgers to suggest that the shovels represent an interim stage between the actual incense shovels (*mahtoth*) used in the Temple and the depiction of Temple shovels seen on the floors of synagogues in Palestine of the late Roman and early Byzantine periods.[127] Rutgers concludes that the shovels were owned by a well-to-do priestly family but were not actually used because the Temple no longer existed.[128] In response, Eric Meyers has postulated that while the shovels, baths, and rabbinic sources suggest the presence of priestly families in Sepphoris, the shovels were probably used in the home to fumigate clothing and freshen rooms. He suggests that rather than burning spices (i.e., incense), the owner of the shovels filled the containers with herbs, spices, and other dry fumigants, and then carried or placed this potpourri (Meyers's term) throughout the home.[129]

Both Rutgers and Meyers depend upon Lapp's assessment that the shovels were never used, and both archaeologists associate the shovels with the priesthood—evidently by means of the late Roman and early Byzantine synagogue depictions of the Temple and its cultic furniture, and the findings of stepped baths in the domestic quarters of Sepphoris. Rutgers interprets the evidence and associations to mean that the shovels could not have been used in the domestic context in which they were found. Meyers, by contrast, while also employing the evidence and its associations with the priesthood, argues that something found in a domestic context was likely to have been used in that context. This argument seems eminently plausible.

Meyers's conclusion could be pushed a bit further, though. The appearance of these incense shovels and those that Strange has found in domestic areas should not surprise us; as we have seen, incense was used extensively for fumigating rooms and clothing throughout the Roman period. Apparently, some shovels were made of pottery and others of bronze. The fumigation of clothing required a receptacle with a handle because one needed to wave the fumigant in the air. For those who regularly used ceramic implements, this waving of the shovel and the fact of pottery's fragility meant that replacements would be needed owing to breakage. As for the connection to the priesthood, the presence of a stepped bath and the fact that some shovels look like those depicted on synagogue floors do not necessitate a priestly connection. Many people bathed, and it is likely that Jews other than priests practiced ritual bathing as well. But even if the *miqva'ot* at Sepphoris are an indication of a priestly presence, this does not mean that the shovels were necessarily for cultic use; any wealthy priestly family would have used incense in the home. As for the similarity of the shovels to depictions of Temple shovels on synagogue floors, this should not be surprising. It seems logical that artists would depict the incense shovels used in the Temple as similar to those with which they were most familiar.[130]

In addition to the shovels, archaeologists at Sepphoris and other towns throughout the Galilee have discovered many small finds related to cosmetics and adornment (see, e.g., fig. 11). At first glance, these do not appear to be related directly to aromatic practices, but rabbinic discussions about the home, women, and adornment would naturally overlap with those about cosmetics, personal hygiene, and aroma. This connection is most clearly discerned in discussions surrounding the Sabbath. For many Jews of this period, the cessation of regular work activities on the Sabbath must have meant more time at home. As a result, the home became a natural reference point for several Sabbath restrictions. Most of these limitations involve items that might or might not be taken outside the house, or worn, or moved from place to place during the Sabbath, and several of these prohibitions mention cosmetic receptacles, jewelry, and spice or perfume. For example, those who take out oil for anointing even the tiniest part of the body are culpable of breaking the Sabbath.[131] Likewise, someone who carries something larger than the foot of a small mortar used for grinding spices is also culpable.[132]

More directly, the Mishnah presents the case of women carrying spices outside the home in small perfume vials or in brooches or other jewelry that might have contained perfume.[133] Using terminology from the period of the Second Temple, Rabbi Meir finds these women liable for a "sin-offering," but the other anonymous rabbis allow some of these items. In the Talmud Bavli, Rabbi Eliezer indicates some cases in which these women are allowed to go abroad scented, although the argument he puts forth is less than flattering. He maintains that women who have a foul odor and so regularly use jewelry or other perfume containers to mask their odor are not culpable for

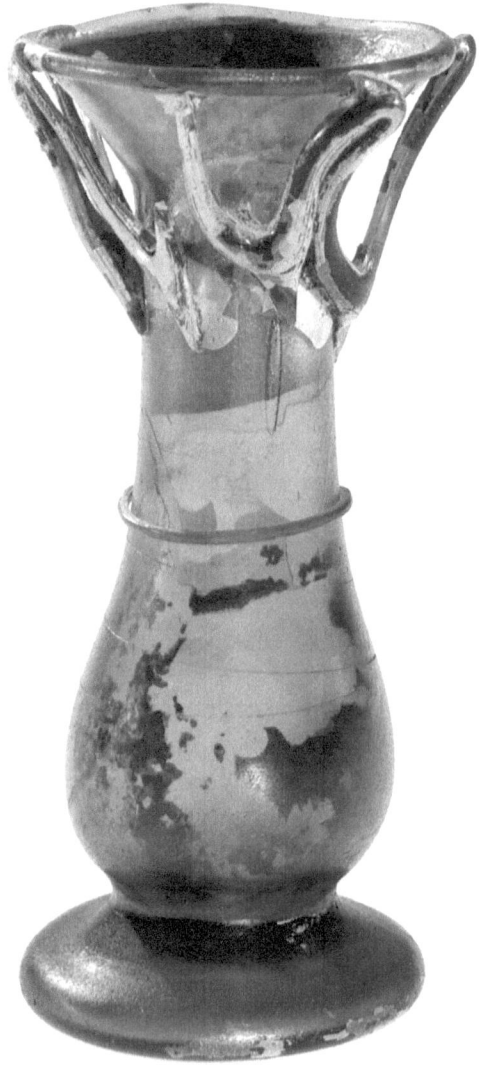

Figure 11 Cosmetic flask, fourth to fifth century C.E. Collection of The Corning Museum of Glass, Corning, New York. 54.1.47. Gift of I. C. Elston Jr.

breaking the Sabbath. These "smelly" women do not wear this jewelry or carry these vials in order to adorn themselves, and they are not likely to take these items off and lay them down; perfume is simply a part of their regular dress.[134]

It is precisely this sense of the ordinary, the familiar, and the commonplace that is so apparent in the rabbinic allusions to spice in the home. Each of these passages exemplifies not only rabbinic knowledge of spices, perfume, and incense but also an intimate acquaintance with the use and enjoyment of aromatics. For example, the Tosefta includes an allowance on the Sabbath for the person who brings fragrant wood (עצי בשמים) to another who is sick. The wood may be waved in front of the person or crushed, but it should not be broken.[135] While the distinction between crushing and breaking may be significant for the rabbis, the importance for us lies in the medicinal use of fragrance. Likewise, we don't know whether any woman actually obeyed the rabbinic regulations concerning perfume, but we may surmise that enough women wore perfume on the Sabbath that the rabbis not only debated the issue but felt some need to attempt to regulate it. Like their counterparts throughout the empire, the rabbis used fragrance in almost every area of daily life. They applied fragrance to their bodies, wafted it throughout their homes, and even inhaled it in order to cure certain ailments. And these practices did not end with death, for spices also played an important role in burial.

At the Time of Burial

While we lack archaeological evidence for funerary activities such as preparation of the body and procession to the burial site, the rabbinic literature does describe and refer to burial practices.[136] According to the texts, upon death, the corpse was anointed with oil, rinsed, and wrapped in a linen shroud or other type of linen garment.[137] As part of this dressing process, the chin was tied, the eyes closed, and the orifices stopped up.[138] The body was placed in a bier or coffin or on some type of wooden structure, often referred to as a "bed" (מטה). The bed was then carried in a funeral procession from the home of the deceased through the community to the outskirts of town and then to the burial site.[139] During the procession, stops might be made for the hired wailers, often women, to sing or lament and clap their hands loudly.[140] Located outside the city limits, the burial sites were frequently man-made caves into which were carved deep recesses for the burial.¹⁴¹ The rabbinic term for such a recess is a *kokh* (כוך).¹⁴² In the late Second Temple and early rabbinic periods, a second form of burial, known as the "collection of bones,"¹⁴³ often took place approximately one year after the initial burial. The archaeological evidence confirms this activity, as many ossuaries have been discovered with bones inside.¹⁴⁴ For the most part, ossuaries were phased out after the destruction of the Second Temple in 70 C.E., although evidence of ossuary use exists through the third century C.E.¹⁴⁵ Scholars have conjectured as to the meaning and significance of the collection of bones in ossuaries, but no surviving primary text explains plainly why Jews performed such a rite.¹⁴⁶

It is likely that spices were used in each of the three phases of burial—corpse preparation, funeral procession, and interment—but it is sometimes quite difficult to discern to which mortuary practice the rabbinic literature points.¹⁴⁷ For example, in the Mishnaic passage concerning the lamps and spices of the dead (*m. Ber.* 8.6), it is impossible to know which phase of burial the rabbis had in mind. Fortunately, this is not the case everywhere, and the washing, anointing, and wrapping of the body is clearly mentioned in a discussion of the types of work one is allowed to perform on the Sabbath:

> They may make ready [on the Sabbath] all the needs of the dead, anoint and rinse it,¹⁴⁸ only [provided that] they do not move any of its limbs.¹⁴⁹ They may draw the mattress away from beneath it and let it lie on sand that it may be the longer preserved; they may bind up the chin . . . they may not close a corpse's eyes on the Sabbath.¹⁵⁰

The first part of the passage refers directly to the first step of the burial: washing and anointing the body. Death is a dirty business, and a corpse needs to be washed or rinsed soon after death, as the orifices may leak before, during, or just afterward.¹⁵¹ It is likely that the anointing of the corpse was a long-standing tradition that mirrored typical bathing practices, even though, in the case of death, rinsing occurred after anointment. This difference in the order of activities makes sense, though, if the goal was to clean the body respectfully and with as little disruption to it as possible. An oily surface would be much more difficult to handle. It is also worth noting that it is unlikely that this scented oil was used to mask the stench of decomposition. If the oil was needed to cover the odor, the body would not be rinsed after application. In addition, while it is possible that particular diseases may have caused the early onset of decomposition, for the most part, in temperate climes, the odor of decomposition is not detectible by the human nose until the second or third day—particularly if the body is shaded, unexposed to direct heat, etc.[152]

The second phase of burial, the procession, or the period of time just before the procession, also provided an opportunity for the employment of incense or perfume. Evidence of the funeral procession is found in several places throughout the Mishnah, and it is clear from these passages that the funeral procession involved the sense of sight, as people could see the procession and the bier, and the sense of hearing, as the wailers chanted and clapped.[153] Several passages throughout the literature allude to the possibility that spices were employed as well. Two examples appear in the Tosefta; the first concerns funds collected for express purposes but found to be surpluses: "Rabbi Meir says, 'The surplus for a [particular] dead person will be left until Elijah will come.' Rabbi Nathan says, '[With] the surplus for a [particular] dead person, they build a structure over his tomb, or he may sprinkle perfume[154] for him before[155] his bier.'"[156] Rabbi Meir insists that the surplus money from burials should be kept until the prophet Elijah comes to decide what shall be done with it. Rabbi Nathan disagrees and mentions two appropriate uses: erection of a marker or some other structure over the gravesite or the purchase of perfumed oil to sprinkle before the bier. This passage indicates that spices were used in connection either with the procession ("before the bier") or with the burial (left at the grave).

The next passage, from t. Nid. 9:16, also mentions spices, possibly in association with the funeral procession: "At first they brought out incense (מוגמר) before those [who died] of sickness of the bowels.[157] Subsequently, they brought out [incense] before every one of them on account of the honor of the dead." The focus here is on the change in burial customs over time. At one time, incense was lit only for those who died of stomach ailments—and this seems to imply the masking of odor—but at a later period, incense was lit for everyone.[158] This passage is part of a list that describes changes in burial practices and how these practices went from being so expensive that people could barely afford to bury their dead to being more economical. However, the word "subsequently" (חזרו) is translated literally as "they returned" and may imply either that the custom changed or that the rabbis "returned" to the issue and changed their earlier ruling. One might reasonably infer that the rabbis changed their earlier ruling to align their law with widespread practice. More important, the passage imparts valuable information with respect to spices—namely, that their use was widespread as part of the burial process in the early centuries C.E. Further, the phrases "they brought out incense" (מוצאין מוגמר) and "before every one of them" (לפני כל אחת ואחת) imply the lighting of incense during the funeral procession.¹⁵⁹

The Yerushalmi also uses this expression with reference to spices. In its exposition of the Mishnah's ruling that one does not say a blessing "over the lamps or spices of the dead" (*m. Ber.* 8.6), we read:

> Rabbi Ḥizkiyah and Rabbi Jacob bar Aḥa in the name of Rabbi Yossi son of Rabbi Ḥaninah, "This is [to say] they are put above the bier of the dead person." "But if they are placed before the bier of the dead person, they bless. I say they are used for the honor of the living."¹⁶⁰

R. Ḥizkiyah and R. Jacob bar Aḥa point to the differences in placement of the spices in relation to the bier in order to clarify their respective opinions on blessing. R. Ḥizkiyah seems to indicate that spices placed above the bier are not to be blessed,¹⁶¹ whereas R. Jacob bar Aḥa asserts that if the spices are placed "before" (לפני) the bier, they are blessed because they "honor the living." Although the text is vague, we may reasonably infer that the spices in front of the bier are there for the "enjoyment" (or use) of the mourners or others who may witness the procession; that is to say, they are akin to the wailers' calling and clapping, alerting those in the street that a funeral procession is coming. When one smells the incense, one blesses the fragrance, stops to see who the mourners are, and shows respect, thereby "honoring" the living.¹⁶²

Other issues surrounding death, burial, and fragrance appear throughout the rabbinic corpus. Many of these appear in the tractate *Semaḥot*, generally dated to the eighth or ninth century C.E.¹⁶³ Although the tractate quotes early tradents on issues and decisions regarding death, burial customs, and other postburial events and questions, it is difficult to know whether the customs described therein reflect accurately this much earlier stratum of rabbinic practice in Palestine. A few practices are notable, however, as they seem to align with those customs described thus far. One such convention appears in a list of practices for which the rabbis continually intone the refrain that such practices are "not considered the ways of the Amorites";¹⁶⁴ that is, these behaviors may appear to be in opposition to rabbinically acceptable praxis (i.e., they could be seen as idolatry or witchcraft), but they are not. Among the listed activities is the erection of a wedding canopy over the graves of brides and bridegrooms (i.e., those who die prematurely) and the suspension of various articles from it.¹⁶⁵ Among the many fruits, breads, and other effects allowed to be hung from such a canopy are "vials of pleasing oil" (צלוחית של שמן ערב).¹⁶⁶

The repetition of the claim that such practices are not superstitious may reveal deep anxiety on the part of some rabbis or later redactors about this and other mortuary practices of their fellow Jews. It is also possible that these explanations express self-consciousness on the part of these rabbis over earlier rabbinic rituals and beliefs; if so, the defensive claim may suggest later redaction. Either way, it is difficult to discern whether the rabbis are trying to mitigate their own seemingly "heathen" traditions, moderate the activities of their fellow Jews, justify earlier rabbinic customs, or simply state that these practices are in line with their own beliefs.

David Kraemer has demonstrated that the Mishnah and Tosefta share many "rituals and sensibilities with 'primitive' funerals in other societies distant from Palestine."¹⁶⁷ He remarks that these funerals were as much "human" as they were "Jewish." It seems reasonable to assume, therefore, that the traditions surrounding how to care for and bury the dead would have significant similarities to the practices of other societies. Following Saul Lieberman, Kraemer sees within the texts a strand of rabbinic belief that views the dead as sensate beings who are aware of what goes on "above ground" and who actually feel pain as their flesh decays.¹⁶⁸ The use of perfume and incense in death would thus be as important as it was in life (if not more so). And the texts seem to support this claim, as bodies were anointed, biers were sprinkled, and incense was lit. Likewise, the archaeological evidence points strongly in this direction, as the greatest number of intact unguentaria have been found at burial sites—perhaps as a symbolic gesture or a desire to bury one's loved ones with their personal effects.

It is important to stress that the burial caves that have been excavated account for only a small percentage of the buried populace; most burial caves have not been found or excavated and of those that have been, only the richest members of these communities were likely to have been buried there.¹⁶⁹ There is no method to determine how or in what manner the majority of the population was buried. Of the burial evidence we do have, some of the best is from Beit She'arim, where the tombs are quite large, were in use for several centuries (making the dating of individual burials difficult), and include burials of both local Jews, including the family of the patriarch,¹⁷⁰ and diasporic Jews.¹⁷¹ However, because of either changes in style or variations in tradition possibly related to the different cities of origin of the mourners, the evidence in the caves suggests a wide variety of burial practices. Two distinct types of burial niches were employed at Beit She'arim: the *kokh* (a burial niche usually dug perpendicularly to the tomb wall) and the *loculus* or *arcosolium* (a rectangular niche dug horizontally or parallel to the wall; an *arcosolium* also has an arched top).[172] Different types of sarcophagi and some ossuaries are also present, the former becoming more prevalent during the third century C.E. (the period of greatest expansion of the tombs) and the latter becoming less common. The decorations and epigraphy on the tomb walls, markers, and sarcophagi are quite varied. Some of these differences may be the result of changing practices, but others may simply reflect differences in custom (local versus foreign, familial, or fashion).

Unguentaria, common in Second Temple burials like those at Jericho and Jerusalem,[173] remain so in the Roman and Byzantine periods.[174] These bottles are often associated with other "grave goods." Grave goods may be household items, such as storage jars, cooking pots, bowls, jugs, and lamps; or they may be of a more personal nature, such as hairpins, jewelry, spindle whorls, and cosmetic bottles. It can be difficult to decide whether a perfume bottle should be considered a household item (because it is made of the same materials as other common utensils) or a personal item (because of its close association with cosmetics and adornment). In many instances the bottles are of poor quality,[175] and this has led some archaeologists to conclude that the bottles were produced specifically for burial. As a result, these archaeologists do not consider the bottles personal items.[176]

There is some disagreement on the typical locations of grave goods and unguentaria within the burial complexes. With respect to the Second Temple period, Rachel Hachlili has identified storage jars as being located most often at the entrance to tombs, whereas cooking pots may be found inside tombs on shelves, in pits, or even in *kokhim*.[177] Amos Kloner, by contrast, argues that cooking pots are not usually found in *kokhim*. Of the perfume bottles, Kloner indicates that they may be sealed in the *kokhim* or deposited in ossuaries.[178] In the Akeldama tombs, the perfume bottles are all found near and around the coffins and bones—particularly those burials of the later Roman period—while the cooking pots and other jars are found in other areas of the larger chambers.[179] A definite connection between the placement of perfume bottles and cooking pots has yet to be determined. Unfortunately, some archaeologists do not record the precise placement of such items, and there is ample evidence of tomb robbing and secondary use of tombs, which makes placement of the items suspect in any case. We may never gain a precise understanding of the relationships, if any, among the placement of unguentaria, cooking pots, and other grave goods. And although several scholars have speculated on the meaning of cooking pots—as vestiges of the rites of meal offerings or as symbols of the commemorative meals celebrated in the Greco-Roman world—they have not tied the significance of the unguentaria to these food-oriented theories. Rabbinic textual evidence is also sparse, as in the case of the perfume to adorn wedding canopies or the mention of other types of personal effects that were buried with people (e.g., the key and writing tablet of Samuel the Small).[180]

The pottery evidence of unguentaria from the late Hellenistic and early Roman periods, combined with the glass evidence from the late Roman and early Byzantine periods, is somewhat overwhelming, not only for burials that may be distinctively Jewish but for all the burials in Palestine. This is particularly true in the Galilee,[181] where burials are more likely to be Jewish in the later periods, and in environs farther north (e.g., Ḥanita).[182] The best example of glass bottles in definitively Jewish burials is again from Beit She'arim, where perfume bottles were found undisturbed (*in situ*) in two locations: catacombs 12 and 15. In catacomb 12, an unguentarium, a mother-of-pearl necklace, a bronze spatula, and five clay lamps were found concealed in a depression in the floor. Naḥman Avigad suspects that this small depression escaped the notice of tomb robbers.[183] Catacomb 15 also contained unguentaria *in situ*, in an *arcosolium*. Evidently the ceiling of hall B of catacomb 15 collapsed in antiquity, making the hall impenetrable to robbers.[184] With respect to the glass vessels at Beit She'arim, Barag points out:

> It seems very reasonable to conjecture that these vessels were produced by Jewish craftsmen; at any rate, they were used by Jews. The vessels from catacomb 15 are doubtlessly funerary gifts. As to the rest of the vessels, it is difficult to determine their exact function, i.e., whether they were burial articles or not. The fact remains that almost all of them are small or medium-sized closed receptacles, radically different in character from the rich group of vessels characteristic of several tombs discovered in Northern Palestine (e.g., el-Manawat, el-Maker, Nahariya, Yeḥiam, Ḥanita), which contained open vessels mostly, such as cups, plates, and bowls.[185]

Barag implies that most of the glass vessels at Beit She'arim, unlike the majority of those of northern Palestine, were used to hold perfumed oil. In addition, a small jar of the type usually associated with ointments was found in catacomb 20. While it is impossible to prove that all the vessels should be considered personal effects, the only two groups found *in situ* would indicate just that—in one instance having been sealed with the body and in the other case found among other personal items.

While the bottles of Beit She'arim are not surprising in light of the long history of Jews burying their dead with unguentaria and other household and personal grave goods, the continuation of this practice into the third and possibly fourth centuries C.E. at a place in which either rabbis or members of the patriarch's family were buried[186] may be significant in light of the fact that no rabbinic literature deals with the perfume bottles, either directly or in passing. The presence of the bottles themselves suggests the rabbis' tacit approval of the custom. It seems that Jews, like their neighbors around the Mediterranean and their fellow citizens in the Roman Empire, used perfume as part of their daily routine and ritual—for both the living and the dead. In fact, as Dan Barag pointed out years ago and as Yael Israeli has reiterated more recently, the surfeit of glass bottles found in burial sites from the late Roman and early Byzantine periods not only reflects the persistence of ancient burial customs but also demonstrates the employment and importance of these items among the living in these settlements.[187]

Conclusion

The rabbinic texts refer to perfume, incense, and spices in a variety of contexts, and in almost all of these discussions the references appear without caveat. The rabbis buy spices in the market, anoint themselves with oil, and light incense at the end of the meal. They discuss these activities without any indication that they are adjusting their daily regimen in accordance with the practices of other Jews, and they do not appear to consider the use of these products to be Roman or foreign. Whether in the market, in the bathhouse, or at home, fragrances were wafting in the air and were enjoyed by these men. Even the one area of possible rabbinic ambiguity, perfume for the dead, does not point to unfamiliarity. On the contrary, as we will see in the interpretative texts, the rabbis forge a deep link between death and aroma.

Assessment of the material remains and the literature of the wider Roman culture in concert with the rabbinic texts demonstrates how strong the presence of aromatics must have been in Palestine. But the texts also reveal the subtle observations of the rabbis on the subject of olfaction, and their understanding—conscious and otherwise—of the operation of scent. Detectible between the lines of the rabbinic references to perfume and incense are the cultural qualities the rabbis assigned to these fragrances, and these valuations are both negative and positive. The scent of perfume carries with it associations of pleasure, which in turn evoke conflicting feelings of excitement, anxiety, arousal, bliss, and powerlessness. In the case of Rabbi Ḥiyya, the transport from the mundane to the sublime effected by perfume is at once appreciated and considered suspect because of its setting in the bathhouse. Similarly, the scent of burning incense gives rise to feelings of contentment, satisfaction, and delight. But these instinctively expressed emotions must be checked when comparable scents related to idolatry are encountered. As we will see, when perfume and incense are interpreted or employed as analogies, these subtle valences are also deployed as part of the interpretive process.

However, the rabbinic midrashim do not rely entirely on personal experience with aroma for their interpretive force. They are also products of a creative effort that weaves this personal experience with theology and strands of tradition and imagery already present in the biblical texts. We thus turn now to the biblical texts in which aroma plays a key role and so influences rabbinic interpretation, as well as to those passages most often cited by the rabbis in connection with interpretations of fragrance.

3

Election and the Erotic:
Biblical Portrayals of Perfume and Incense

Just as rabbinic experience and cultural familiarity with aroma find their way into rabbinic interpretation, so too do the images and valences of aroma drawn from Scripture. Indeed, it is these images, ideas, and representations that become the primary metaphors of interpretation. For example, in the Song of Songs (the Songs), the lover describes his beloved as a locked garden filled with exotic spices, whose scent wafts out to him and draws him ever nearer. In the midrashim based on these verses, the rabbinic voices employ these thematic details by piling up metaphors until one midrash portrays the sealed garden as God's abode, another describes the exotic spices as manna with which the Israelite women perfume themselves during forty years of wandering in the wilderness, and yet another imagines the scent of Israel's righteousness as wafting up to the Divine. Each of these midrashim preserves the original valences that attach to the female as the "garden of spicy delights," including the suggestions of wafting aroma, emotional arousal, and the allure of the exotic. This chapter, therefore, seeks to isolate the contexts of these biblical images of aroma, to explain them, and to unpack the valences that attach to them. The ensuing chapters investigate how these images and valences, along with rabbinic experience, migrate into the midrashim and are transformed there.

Close scrutiny of the Hebrew Bible demonstrates the importance of aroma in the Israelite cult as well as in almost every other area of Israelite life and culture depicted therein. Important references, both literal and metaphorical, appear in all three sections of the Scriptures (the Torah, the Prophets, and the Writings). Notably, these descriptions, allusions, and passing comments parallel, in many respects, the divergent opinions expressed in the rabbinic and wider Roman literature. For example, the Bible suggests that women, and in some cases men, fumigated their garments, anointed themselves with perfumed oil, and lit incense at festive meals.[1] Some passages describe these customs neutrally or positively, while others, particularly those that are erotic, carry negative overtones. Although many of the practices and much of the scent terminology found in the Bible are similar to those in the rabbinic literature, two issues account for some of the dramatic differences in perception. The first is that the Bible refers to an active cult whose members are anointed and light incense twice daily and whose high priest brings incense into the innermost sanctum of the Temple on the Day of Atonement. As such, the priestly literature goes to great lengths to stress that this perfume and incense are categorically different from other scented oils and fumigants and must remain solely under the purview of the priestly caste. The second issue, related to the first, presents a cultural distinction. While the rabbis view themselves as direct descendants of an already ancient Israelite culture, they nevertheless live in a much later period and are surrounded by cultures different from those of the biblical period. As a result, their "aromatic lexicon" and, more significantly, the cultural valences that accompany these words, are quite similar in some respects but dramatically different in others.[2] For example, except for a few very early tradents who were active when the Second Temple was still standing, none of the later rabbis (after 70 C.E.) could have smelled the priestly or royal anointing oils or cultic incense. And it is doubtful that even these "early" rabbis would have experienced firsthand the aroma of the incense lit in the inner confines of the Temple. The rabbis must therefore interpret these scents on the basis of their own experience with perfumed oils, unguents, and fumigants. In fact, it is likely that their understanding of Temple incense is drawn in some measure from their experience of idolatrous incense or fumigatory practices.

In light of these differences and the Hebrew Bible's focus on sacrifice, the cult, and communication with the Divine through burning, it is evident that the texts have their own unique cultural constructions of aroma and olfaction. The books of Exodus, Leviticus, Numbers, and Chronicles refer to incense and perfume as an integral part of their descriptions of the priesthood and the various issues surrounding election, duty, and the interactions of the priests with other Israelites. Therefore, the valences that attach to the priestly imagery of aroma include exclusivity, atonement, and tranquility. On the other hand, the poetry of *eros* and the idyll found in the Songs also employs images of incense, perfume, and specific spices to describe yearning and the memory of deeply intimate encounters between an anonymous lover and his beloved. Here the fragrances suggest arousal, seduction, and impulsivity. Different still are the prophetic books of Isaiah, Ezekiel, and Malachi, in which the odors of Temple rites are commingled with more sensual and exotic metaphors in order to chastise or rebuke. Consequently, this portion of the study endeavors to catalogue and assess the contexts in which these references appear in the Hebrew Bible and to uncover the more subtle attributes that adhere to these terms and contexts. We begin with a brief review of the salient terms and their meanings. The inquiry then examines the settings in which the terms are used, including some specific examples of how these terms operate in the texts and an evaluation of the nuances and meanings that adhere to these often clustered images.

Terms

Each of the terms related to perfume and incense, and even to the activities of breathing and anointing, has a close semantic relationship with terms in other languages of the ancient Near East, such as Akkadian and Ugaritic. Given that the peoples of these regions, from Egypt to Mesopotamia, had a long history of using and trading spices before the Israelites ever came onto the scene, this is not surprising.[3] Biblical scholars and historians suppose that the Israelites adopted practices already common among the Canaanites, but no written record exists for these Canaanite peoples, and so it is impossible to specify the similarities and differences in languages or practices. Nevertheless, it is reasonable to assume that just as the words, phrases, and descriptions of spices in the surrounding cultures had subtle nuances in meaning, so too did the Hebrew expressions and Israelite practices.[4]

This type of nuance can be seen in the term *qetoreth* (קטורת), which is used to identify the incense lit in the Temple. Closely related to *qetoreth* are the verbs for the act of sacrifice or turning something into smoke: *hiqtir* and *qitter* (הקטיר, קטר).[5] Because sacrificing anything (a ram, a bird, grain, etc.) requires one of these two verbs, there is an automatic subtle association between incense and the general act of sacrifice through the common root *q-t-r* (קטר).[6] In addition to *qetoreth*, the priestly texts also employ two related terms, *qetoreth sammim* (קטורת סמים), "perfumed" or "spiced incense," and *qetoreth sammim daqqah* (קטורת סמים דקה), "finely ground perfumed incense."[7] *Sammim* is difficult to translate precisely and may have resonances with medicinal herbs and plants, as does its Akkadian relative, šammu. Of note, unlike the rabbinic texts, the biblical text does not have a term for noncultic incense, although it alludes to such fumigants.

The biblical literature does, however, use two different terms for the two kinds of anointment. The anointment of God's elect (priests and kings) is described by the term *mashaḥ* (משח).[8] But for those who anoint themselves after bathing, the text employs the root *sukh* (סוך).[9] As for the oil itself, the text may use the simple term "oil" (*shemen*, שמן) and make clear by description that this oil is perfumed, or, as seen in the rabbinic texts, the term *shemen tov* (שמן טוב), or "good oil," may be employed. Other terms for "perfume" or "perfumed oil" include *merqaḥ* and *roqaḥ* (רקח, מרקח), which, deriving from the root "to mix" (רקח), can also mean the person who mixes spices (i.e., the perfumer or apothecary) or a mixture of ointments, spices, or oils. Another prevalent term for perfume is *bosem* (בשם)—the same term so common to the rabbinic literature. As in that corpus, the biblical texts also have a wide lexical spectrum for this word, including "to be sweet," "balsam," "perfume," and "spice." And, as in the rabbinic literature, *bosem* is paired from time to time with specific spices or appears as the "chief of spices" (*ra'shei besamim*, ראשי בשמים). In these contexts, *bosem* appears to mean "balsam."

The two spices that most often appear together in the text are frankincense (*levonah*, לבונה) and myrrh (*mor*, מור). Widespread use of these spices is well attested in the ancient world and long predates the Israelites. Egyptians used myrrh extensively for perfuming and embalming, while other civilizations, such as Mesopotamia, used myrrh for incense in cultic rituals, as a medicine, and as an ingredient in perfume. Frankincense was also commonly used as an ingredient in incense. The two spices are mentioned together in almost every source from the ancient Near East, not only because they are so fragrant but also because they derive from the same region of southern Arabia and Somaliland and therefore were imported together.[10]

Frankincense and myrrh both have lexical similarities to other words in Hebrew and other languages. While these similarities do not play a significant role in inner-biblical interpretation, they are occasionally important in later interpretation and so worth noting here. The term for frankincense, or *levonah*, is associated with the word *laban* (לבן), meaning "white." Pliny describes the frankincense from the summer crop, harvested in the autumn, as white in color.[11] Myrrh, which derives from the root *m-r-r* (מרר), has similar forms in Ugaritic (*mr*) and in Akkadian (*murru*). In Akkadian, *murru* also serves as a substantive meaning "bitter taste."[12] Similarly, a close semantic relationship exists in Hebrew between *mor*, the term for "myrrh," and *mar*, the term for "bitter." Later rabbinic literature also associates the verb *hithmarer* (התמרר), "to embitter oneself" and "to burn," with the same root. Pliny stresses that the best kind of myrrh, stacte, is that which flows on its own without need of incision into the branch, and he finds an association between the spice stacte (στακτή) and the Greek verb "to drip" (στάζω). Similarly, the Septuagint translates the substantive of *nataf* (נטף), which means "to drip" or "to flow," as stacte (Exod 30:34).[13]

The Hebrew term for "fragrance" or "odor" in the Bible is *reah* (ריח). In the priestly literature this term is often paired with *nihoah* (ניחח), which can mean "quieting," "soothing," or "tranquil." The phrase *reah nihoah* (ריח ניחח), therefore, is often translated as "soothing odor" and is used to describe the competent completion of a sacrifice, that is, God's acceptance of the sacrifice. In more ancient traditions such terminology expressed the appeasement of the gods through sacrifice, since they breathed the wafting smoke and were calmed. Nuances of this notion are clearly carried over into the Hebrew text, which employs this term after the description of every type of sacrifice except that of incense.[14] The semantic relationship between *reah* (ריח), "fragrance," and *hariah* (הריח), "to breathe," may also be indicative of the strong connection between the act of sacrifice and divine reception of this gift.[15] The word most closely associated with this root, *ruah* (רוח), is also highly suggestive of the Bible's conceptual connection between humans and the Divine, as the expression means "breath," "wind," and "spirit." As in other ancient and modern languages, the biblical terms for scent express the subtle interplay among the ideas of smelling, breathing, and the ephemeral nature of fragrance and of life itself. Fragrance cannot be seen, heard, or touched, and it does not last, but one can be aware of its existence. So, too, wind and spirit can be described as transitory and elusive, discernable only through an inner sense.

Priestly Contexts and Concerns

In the Hebrew Bible, the most important communication with the deity occurs through sacrifice, and, as mentioned above, the acceptance of that sacrifice occurs through God's smelling it. When completed, the sacrifice is pronounced a "soothing odor." Even communication through prayer, as articulated in the Psalms, most often occurred at the Temple, which must have been redolent with the odors of blood, smoke, and burning flesh. The environs of the Temple itself were gradated in terms of holiness, and this meant that incense sacrifice, which took place in the inner regions of the Temple, represented a higher level of holiness than or distinct purpose from other sacrifices that took place in the outer regions. The acts of lighting incense and the anointment of the priests are also depicted through highly evocative images of distinction and exclusivity. All of these require elucidation if we are to fully understand the operation of fragrance in the Bible and, more important, the relationship between aroma and theology.

But the rabbis did not adopt these thematic concerns as their own. To the contrary, as is evident in much of the late Roman and early Byzantine rabbinic literature, various rabbis clearly did not hold the priesthood in particularly high esteem.[16] This may have had to do in part with the priests' caste system, which was, at least on the surface, antithetical to the rabbinic conception of authority based upon scholarship (and yet which had its own elite hierarchy based on "schools" and "teachers and students"). The rabbis may also have viewed the priesthood or the priestly families, in a theoretical sense, as a threat to their own authority—even though many who were designated "rabbi" were also priests.[17] Rabbinic authority, if there was such a thing, is difficult to prove and must have been a late development.[18] But the priesthood at least had a *history* of authority and influence over a large percentage of the Jewish population, and thus there may have been a tradition about that history. Indeed, the importance of priestly material to rabbinic interpretation has little to do with the priests or their interests or spheres of control. Rather, it is the connective tissue surrounding sacrifice, communication with the Divine, and the significance of atonement that are so thoroughly embedded in rabbinic theology. Still, in order to understand the rabbinic metaphors of aroma, the relevant priestly passages must first be dissected and then readdressed in their larger frameworks. To that end, the passages presented below are organized according to the categories that can be derived from the biblical texts. These categories include prescription, atonement, and assertion of authority/suppression of rebellion.

Prescription and Aroma

Many of the fragrance terms found in the priestly material (e.g., Exod 30 and the books of Leviticus and Numbers) are prescriptive in nature; that is, they give instructions to the priests about what should be sacrificed, the operations involved (slaughter, sprinkling of blood, etc.), the utensils to be used, and the occasions for sacrifice. For example, directives for incense include the recipe for the holy incense, the lighting of incense by the priests twice each day and on the Day of Atonement, and the prohibition on lighting "foreign" incense on the holy incense altar.[19] Reference to incense also appears in the description of the construction of the incense altar, its appearance, and its location.[20] Exodus 25–31 describes the construction of the ark, the menorah, the table, and several other priestly appurtenances. These chapters begin with a list of primary materials an Israelite shall bring "as his heart moves him" (25:2); included in this list are "oil for lighting, [and] spices for the anointing oil and for the aromatic incense" (25:6).[21]

Prescription for the priests and proscription for regular Israelites are concepts that are often tied together—as in this description of the anointing oil:

> Take fine spices: flowing myrrh—five hundred weight—fragrant cinnamon, half as much—two hundred and fifty—and fragrant cane—two hundred and fifty—and cassia—five hundred [as measured] by the Sanctuary shekel and a hin of olive oil. You will make it into a holy anointing oil, a skillful mixture of ointments, the work of a perfumer. It will be a holy anointing oil. And you will anoint (ומשחת) the tent of meeting with it, the ark of the pact, and the table, and all its utensils. . . . And you will anoint (תמשח) Aaron and his sons and you will make them holy in order for them to serve me as priests. And you will speak to the Israelites saying, "This will be a holy anointing oil for me for all your generations. No man should anoint (ייסך) his flesh [with it] and you shall not make anything like it in composition. It is holy and it will be holy to you. Any man that will compound [anything] like it or that puts it on [something] foreign will be cut off from his people."[22]

The passage begins with the recipe for the anointing oil and continues with a long list of what is to be anointed and thereby consecrated (made "holy"). This list includes every item in the Tabernacle, as well as the priests themselves.[23] Finally, Moses is to tell the Israelites that anyone who uses this oil for regular anointing of his or her body or who compounds anything that smells like it will be expelled from the congregation.

Translations of the specific spice terms are made difficult by the large number of terms, the fluidity of their definitions, and the historical problem of concrete identification. These issues aside, the passage is thick with information. For example, the prohibition against Israelite employment of this particular perfumed oil assumes that Israelites regularly anoint their bodies. The use of anointing oil in general is not prohibited; the text merely restricts one particular concoction. Most important, the proscription of this perfume in concert with the presentation of the precise recipe and the exhaustive list of cultic furniture and implements further distinguishes the priests as the only authority over the cult, once they are anointed by Moses. After their initial induction, the priests will anoint others, thereby segregating the group. And because the priests are the only people allowed to wear this fragrance, their election and holiness are actually identifiable by their scent—if not to the "outside" world, then at least to each other.

A corollary to the anointment passage appears just after it, in Exodus 30:34–36. There God specifies the ingredients and measurements for the incense. Spices such as stacte, onycha, galbanum, and frankincense are mentioned.[24] Like the oil, Temple incense is off limits to regular Israelites: "The incense that you make in this measurement, you must not make for yourselves; it will be sacred to you for the Lord. A man that will make any like it to smell it, will be cut off from his people" (30:37–38). As with the anointing oil, the passage assumes Israelite employment of incense; otherwise, there would be no need to regulate it.

The use of perfume and incense by Israelites and priests implies a professional role for the perfumer or apothecary, and such a person is mentioned in each of the descriptions. No other profession may be as elusive to characterize in the biblical text, however. Two intriguing references to perfumers indicate that they belong to priestly families. The first (1 Chr 9:30) attests, "and from the (sons of) the priests were mixers of the mixture of spices."[25] The reasonable assumption would be that the role of these priests was to mix both the anointing oil and the special incense, although the specifics of the job are not included in the description. In Nehemiah 3:8 we find a description of those who helped to rebuild the wall around the newly rebuilt Temple in Jerusalem, along with their family or guild designation and place of assignment.[26] Of one Hananiah, the text states that he was the "son of," or possibly "of the guild of," perfumers. It is doubtful that priests were the only perfumers. A reference to the perfumer in Ecclesiastes 10:1, while not negating a priestly connection, does not endorse one either. And the priestly connection is quite suspect in 1 Samuel 8:13; there the prophet includes the profession of "perfumer" among the many jobs to which the daughters of Israel will be subjected if a king is appointed by God to lead the people. Historical progression, centralization of the cult, or a thriving spice trade may all serve as possible explanations for the displacement of female perfumers and the ascendancy of priestly ones. That is, the role may have become so specialized or economically advantageous that a specific (male) priestly guild took over this lucrative position.[27] But it is also probable that priestly texts are more likely to mention priests involved in the perfume industry, suggesting that both priests and regular Israelites served as perfumers. At a literary level, priestly references to priests as perfumers indicate the segregation of cultic oil and incense even in their original spice form. Such separation adds to the relative importance, rarity, and sense of exclusivity surrounding the spices, the oil and incense, and even the fragrances that waft through the air of the Temple.[28]

Although never used in reference to the incense sacrifice, the term "soothing odor" is employed throughout the prescriptive literature to indicate God's acceptance of sacrifices.[29] It is often clustered with other technical cult terms, such as specific types of sacrifice (whole burnt offering, grain offering, etc.) or more descriptive terms (e.g., "an offering made by fire" or "gift" in Exod 29:18).[30] In all these cases, some portion of the sacrifice is burned on the altar and "consumed" by fire there. While the word "soothing" implies that God's anger is assuaged by sacrifices—that they have a calming effect on the Divine—the term "soothing odor" also operates as a reified legal or ritualistic statement within the priestly operational system.[31]

In line with ancient tradition that considers sacrifices food for the gods, another technical term, leḥem (לחם), "food," also appears in connection with these sacrifices.[32] For example, God commands, "You will make sure to bring to me at the appointed times my offering, my food, my offering by fire of soothing odor to me" (Num 28:2). While it may appear from this example that the human's job is to prepare "food," in the form of sacrifices, for the deity at regular intervals, the implications of "soothing odor," whether literal or metaphorical, extend the trajectory of meaning beyond food or physical sustenance. Within the metaphorical frame rests the idea of a human-divine relationship that observes regular ritual and therefore regular interaction and communication. On a literal level, the term implies that sacrifices performed by humans affect God's mood or judgment and thereby effect a change in the rapport between humans and God. As we will see, the rabbis openly express this desire to change God's disposition through sacrifice in descriptions of atoning sacrifices, and these too are drawn from the biblical text.

Incense and Atonement

The priestly source views incense as a unique type of sacrifice.³³ In this system, laden with signs and symbols, incense has a special status in terms of its geography, form, function, holiness, and effectual purpose. One of the primary differences between incense and other sacrifices is that incense is lit on a separate altar and in a distinct location. The Temple may be considered to have three spheres of holiness.³⁴ The outer court, which contains the altar for burnt offerings and in which regular Israelites may be present, is the least holy space. Sarna comments that "from the altar of sacrifice, the Israelites reach out to God."³⁵ As one moves toward the inner area—toward the Holy of Holies—one enters the zone of the menorah, the table, and the incense altar, and holiness increases. Of the three items found in this area, the incense altar is the closest to the Holy of Holies and is the only one of the three objects situated directly in front of it.³⁶ Only priests may enter this inner area. Finally, the area of the Holy of Holies, the innermost area of the Temple, which contains the ark and the veil and into which only the high priest may enter, is the most holy. Of this orientation, Sarna comments, "From the Ark and the Holy of Holies, God reaches out to Israel."³⁷

What, then, are we to make of the space that surrounds the Holy of Holies (the adytum) or that lies just outside it? This area seems to contain more holiness than the outer court but is less holy than the adytum itself.³⁸ Unlike the other spheres, this intermediate space is not well defined but is marked by its liminality. The priests have access to the area and may carry out their duties there, but they must do so with great caution, for God's "anger" (i.e., his holiness or power) may erupt at any time from the innermost sanctum.³⁹ Perhaps as a further protection, the incense sacrificed in this zone was even more distinct than the regular incense (*qetoreth,* קטורת). This extra-special incense is described as "aromatic incense" or an "incense of spices" (*qetoreth sammim,* קטורת סמים),⁴⁰ and its pleasant fragrance would have wafted around this inner area, creating a cloudy, somewhat opaque or hazy environment. As a result, not only the geographic space, with its dangerous proximity to the physical manifestation of the Divine's glory, but also the air in the space obtained a status of higher holiness and exclusivity.

Incense, however, plays more than a supporting role in the priestly scene. On the Day of Atonement, the incense cloud is mentioned prominently as part of the ritual performance:

> [The high priest] shall take a panful of glowing coals from on the altar before the Lord, and two handfuls of finely ground aromatic incense, and bring [it] behind the curtain. He shall place the incense on the fire before the Lord, and the cloud of incense will cover the veil[41] that is over the Pact, so he will not die (Lev 16:12–13).

Interpreters, both ancient and modern, have argued at length over the ritual minutiae involved in this passage. The Sadducees and Pharisees disagreed over whether the high priest lit the incense before he entered the Holy of Holies (as the Sadducees maintained) or after he was already inside the area (the Pharisees' position).[42] Contemporary scholars continue to debate whether the purpose of covering the veil is to ensure the invisibility of the ark, to hide the divine glory that is present and also described as a cloud, or to assuage the wrath of God.[43] The text indicates that the purpose of the cloud is to cover the ark, but it is likely that the cloud had a dual function: to screen the high priest from the divine presence and to remind him of it—akin to the pillars of fire and smoke that accompanied the Israelites in the wilderness and the cloud that rested over the Tabernacle during the wandering (Exod 40:34–38).[44] None of these reasons addresses the requirement for incense, however; many substances could have produced this cloud—from burning wood or leaves to flesh or grain. Why incense? And why does the high priest bring it into the adytum with him? He could just as easily have closed his eyes as he entered. To answer these questions, we must return to the purposes of sacrifice and priestly interests.

Most of the sacrifices appear to celebrate holiness, to rectify violations of purity, or to acknowledge God. For example, the *tamid* (תמיד), or "regular" sacrifices, were a twice daily acknowledgment of God, while the *'olah* (עולה), or "whole burnt offering," served to garner the attention of the Divine—either by making expiation for oneself or by gaining redemption from divine wrath. Levine, therefore, translates Leviticus 1:4: "He [the presenter] shall lay his hand upon the head of the burnt offering, by its acceptance on his behalf it serves as redemption (כפר) for him."[45] Further, although incense sacrifice occurs in the inner portion of the Temple and therefore is in the area in which Sarna envisions God reaching out to Israel,

Paul Heger reads the lighting of incense twice a day on the special incense altar as implying that sacrifice is "going up" to God. He notes that every reference to offering incense, save the one that discusses the incense altar, uses some form of the root *q-t-r* (קטר), "to turn to smoke." However, when Exodus 30:7–9 refers to the incense on the special incense altar, it uses the term *'olah* (עולה), "to offer up"; like other sacrifices, the purpose of incense is also to get God's attention.[46] Therefore, this sphere is one of reciprocal communication.

If Sarna is correct that the priests considered the presence of God to be present always, then the incense sacrifice may be an attention-getting device in line with Levine's reading of the *'olah*. The twice daily incense sacrifice communicates to God that the priests are present and in his service. Or perhaps God's presence is in the vicinity but not immediate. The incense sacrifice would both encourage God's attention as well as lure the deity down toward the adytum.[47] In this fashion, the aroma of the special incense works analogously to noncultic incense or perfume. It changes the "mood" of the area by literally creating a new atmosphere in which the deity desires to be present.[48]

The intent, though, may not be to change the ambiance of the area but rather to have a direct effect on God—to change God's mood. As Levine has stated, the wrath (or holiness) of God can be unleashed at any time, and, as we have seen, the area closest to the innermost sanctum was considered more dangerous than others. If so, incense might serve as a more effective method than a regular *'olah* offering of preventing an eruption. Its aroma would calm the deity and change his mood. Quite literally, incense is a "soothing odor"—it has the power to lure and to calm and thereby to restrain or appease God's anger. Oddly enough, this may be why the term "soothing odor" is applied to other daily sacrifices but not to the incense offering. Unlike the other sacrifices performed by the priests on behalf of the Israelite community, incense sacrifice does not celebrate holiness, or rectify impurity, or even acknowledge God. Rather, the priests light incense on their own behalf in a restricted location. The incense sacrifice is for God to smell and to enjoy just as humans smell and enjoy incense and perfume. However, while the effects on humans and the Divine are the same, ritual incense is highly restricted: it is made of different spices or in different measurements, has a different scent, and may be employed only by the priests.

Considered another way, incense sacrifice does not symbolize a single idea. Rather, it represents two conceptions in a single process: the incense sacrifice is used twice daily to get God's attention, wherever he may be, by way of creating a pleasant and calm environment for him, and it serves as protection for the priests from God's holiness or wrath. The twice-a-day sacrifice is a "communication with God" in the sense that it calls God to be present and in a "good mood." It is lit on a special altar in one of the holiest areas (just outside the adytum). In addition, the incense smoke and scent are produced in a liminal area. Whereas the outer area of the Temple represents people reaching up to God and the innermost area represents God reaching down to humans, this in-between space is an area of two-way communication and reciprocal activity: the priest initiates the scent and smoke that ascends to God, and God's presence descends on the ark. This space and the activities that go on there serve as the trigger point for the human-divine relationship.

Returning to the incense ritual surrounding the Day of Atonement, we see both a heightened process and the full symbolic power of the cloud and the aroma. Distinct from any sacrifice or offering, the incense moves with the high priest into the inner sanctum of absolute holiness; it is directly in front of God's presence (and may commingle with it) and is taken as far inside the Temple precinct as one can go. The incense cloud protects the high priest both from seeing what he is not supposed to see and from divine wrath.[49] This protection is effected not only by the cloud screen but also by the suffusion of the entire area with pleasant aroma. Surely the pleasant scent is not for the enjoyment of the high priest; rather, its purpose must be to effect some change in God's temperament by means of his smelling it. The purpose of the Day of Atonement is for the high priest to make expiation (atonement) for all the Israelite people, and the act of bringing incense into the Holy of Holies accords well with this purpose. The superficial justification for the cloud is protection for the high priest; the more profound reason for incense in particular is communication with God—a desire to get God's attention and to bring about a favorable demeanor in the deity. Concurrently, as the priest moves to the most dangerous position within the Temple—as far inside as possible—the incense itself becomes his protective agent against divine wrath.[50]

As we have seen, many of the attributes of the incense lit on the Day of Atonement also apply, albeit less intensely, to the incense used in the daily sacrifice. We may thus conclude that cultic incense is encoded in the priestly prescriptive literature with some basic representational characteristics. In terms of space, incense is closely associated with interiority, as it is lit deep inside a building and then carried to its innermost recess. Incense also entails elements of restriction and exclusivity, both as part of its spatial issues and as outlined in the recipe and rituals that attend it. The authority of the priesthood and its holiness or purity are also represented in this incense by virtue of who may handle it and where it is lit. Finally, as for its effects: on God, this includes a sense of calm or serenity, and for humans it includes expiation or atonement. The confluence of these characteristics and their clustering around cultic incense seem to initiate unspoken associations at each mention of the word "incense" in the biblical texts, and several more examples of this effect are given below. In addition, a similar clustering effect is evidenced in the rabbinic literature, particularly around the sacrifice of incense, its influence on the Divine, and atonement; this phenomenon is discussed in chapter 5.

Authority and the Suppression of Rebellion

If cultic incense does in fact attract a set of traits as outlined so far, then it stands to reason that these "incense valences" would appear in other passages within the corpus—at least in those passages where priestly concerns are paramount. Nowhere is this more evident than in the narratives that concern priestly authority or reassertion of power after insurrection. Four such narratives on priestly authority are reviewed here: the incident of Nadab and Abihu (Lev 10), the rebellion of Koraḥ (Num 16), the plague narrative that follows the Koraḥ incident (Num 17), and the encroachment upon the Temple by King Uzziah (2 Chr 26). Each of these episodes is discussed with special emphasis on its role in asserting the authority of the priesthood and the other associations with cultic incense.

Leviticus 10 portrays the events surrounding the deaths of Nadab and Abihu, the sons of Aaron (the first high priest and Moses' brother). The two men offer incense using "foreign fire" (i.e., the coals under the incense). As a result, a "fire came out from before the Lord and consumed them, and they died before the Lord" (10:2). After the incident, God tells Aaron not to drink wine or other intoxicating beverages when he or his sons enter the Tent of Meeting because they will die (10:9). Regardless of the cause of death (alien fire or intoxication), the punishment for breaking the rules is swift and severe.[51]

Although the entire Israelite community appears to be the audience for the incident, a closer reading reveals the episode to be a guide primarily for the priestly circle. Moses interprets the event as relative to a statement made by God, and so recalls it to Aaron: "Through those near to me (בקרבי) I show myself holy, and gain glory before all the people" (10:3). The term *qarov* (קרוב), "to be near," "to draw near," refers directly to the priesthood, as priests are the only ones allowed to draw close to the Lord and to be near him.[52] All of the directions and actions that follow involve only the priesthood: the brothers are dragged by their cousins (other priests but not immediate relatives) outside the camp by their tunics; the immediate family of priests, Aaron and his two sons, Eleazar and Ithamar, are told not to dishevel their hair (or bare their heads) and not to tear their garments in mourning; and they are not to leave the area of the Tent of Meeting because they have been anointed with the holy perfumed oil. These instructions are followed by Moses' delineation of the role, responsibilities, and rights associated with the priesthood. These instructions are given only to the priests and are motivated by the actions of Nadab and Abihu—priests whose guilt lies in failing to follow proper procedures in the first place. In the case of Nadab and Abihu, priestly authority over lighting incense is assumed at the outset and provides the basis for further instruction and clarification to the priests.

The episode thus puts the role of the priests in perspective, not necessarily for the community at large but for the priestly circle itself. By placing the incense ritual at the center of the narrative, the lens focuses on the inner workings of the priestly system. As discussed above, the location of the incense altar indicates that the common Israelite is not present to witness these rituals. Therefore, among the symbolic affinities that adhere to incense (instruction, proper procedures, ritual precision), the narrative also includes the themes of exclusivity and restriction. The narrative is about priests, involves priestly rituals only, is intended for an audience of priests, and reminds priests that their duties are not to be taken lightly. The message is that every detail must be observed closely and each ritual law followed scrupulously, or tragedy may result—not only for the priests themselves, as evidenced by the deaths of Nadab and Abihu, but for the entire community as well, which may be struck by the wrath of God (10:6). The narrative also serves as a subtle reminder to the community of the unique role of the priests and the imminent dangers to which they are regularly exposed. The employment of the incense ritual is a further reminder of the priesthood's exclusive position within the community and the role of priests as representatives to God.

Whereas the Nadab and Abihu narrative is directed toward priests related to Aaron, the Koraḥ rebellion narrative is addressed to the Levites (a lower caste of priests) and Israelites. Koraḥ, a Levite, rallies the community against Moses and Aaron, declaring that the entire community is holy.[53] Moses frames his response with respect to the priesthood. He reminds Koraḥ that the Levites are already set apart from the rest of the community and that their role is to serve in the Tabernacle. Moses then asks Koraḥ whether he seeks the priesthood as well. Most scholars agree that the text as it appears in its final redaction comprises at least two separate events that have been joined together: that of the rebellion of Koraḥ against the Aaronide priesthood and that of Dathan and Abiram, probably against the leadership of Moses.[54] However, as the narrative stands, Dathan and Abiram (regular Israelites but descendants of Jacob's firstborn son, Reuben) support Koraḥ's rebellion along with the tribal chieftains. Moses designs the ordeal of incense to prove the legitimacy of the Aaronides. First, the earth swallows the rebel leaders and their families, and then a fire consumes 250 of the rebellious followers (Num 16:32, 35).[55]

The Koraḥ rebellion dramatically asserts the authority and power of the Aaronide priesthood through the essential action of the ordeal (the lighting of incense) and the destruction of Koraḥ's band. The reader knows before the contest begins, however, that common Israelites and Levitical priests have no prerogative in the incense ritual. This knowledge adds to the tension of the narrative, for the reader knows that no good can come of this insurrection. Aaron's sons have already died through incense sacrifice, and they were of the proper caste. The tension escalates through repetition of key words and concepts. For example, as in the Nadab and Abihu narrative, the term "to be near," "to draw near," "to have access" (קרב) appears no less than four times in the Koraḥ narrative.[56] Most significantly, Moses declares to Koraḥ, "[In the] morning, the Lord will make known who is his and who is holy and who are close to him. And he whom he will choose, will have access to him" (יקריב) (Num 16:5). The last part of this verse can also be understood as "will offer sacrifice to him," as the various forms of this root can mean "to make an offering," in the sense that one draws near to God to offer sacrifices. Although there can be no doubt that God will choose Aaron as the one close to him, Moses tries to placate Koraḥ by intimating that the Levites are special to God and chosen by him: "the God of Israel set you aside from the company of Israel to be close (להקריב) to him" (16:9). Moses uses the same language of nearness to God to express exclusivity; but this time he draws a comparison between the Levites and regular Israelites. Like the priests, the Levites too are able to draw near and have access to God.⁵⁷ In the second half of the verse, though, Moses clarifies that the role of the Levites is to serve in the Tabernacle and to serve the community—he makes no mention of offering sacrifices.

The similar punishments of Nadab and Abihu and Koraḥ and his followers draw stark antinomies with the daily and special rites of Aaron's properly performed incense rituals, thereby reinforcing Aaronide authority and the dire consequences of sedition or infraction. In the narrative of Nadab and Abihu, the two brothers are "consumed" or "eaten" (*tokhal,* תאכל) by fire (Lev 10:2). During the Koraḥ episode, God requests that Moses and Aaron separate themselves from the congregation so that he may "consume" (*akhaleh,* אכלה) the rebels (Num 16:20–21). After the ordeal, the earth opens its mouth and swallows (*tivla',* תבלע) Koraḥ, his family, and several of his followers and their families (Num 16:32). And at the end of the Koraḥ incident we are told, "And fire went out from the Lord and consumed (*tokhal,* תאכל) 250 of those offering the incense" (16:35).⁵⁸

These themes are repeated, but with different emphasis, in the general rebellion that takes place just after the Koraḥ episode. In the opening verses, Koraḥ's fire pans are made into plating for the altar so that all who see them will remember that only the descendants of Aaron are permitted to offer incense (Num 17:1–5). This is followed by the statement that the entire Israelite community rebelled against Moses and Aaron, complaining that the two leaders had caused the death of God's people (17:6). Moses and Aaron turn toward the Tabernacle and realize that God's cloud of glory has descended upon it (17:7). As in the Koraḥ narrative, when Moses and Aaron reach the Tabernacle, God asks that Moses and Aaron separate themselves from the community so that he may "consume" (*akhaleh,* אכלה) it in an instant (17:10). As in the earlier sequence, Moses and Aaron fall on their faces.⁵⁹ This time, however, rather than attempt to reason with God, Moses instructs Aaron to "take the [fire] pan and place on it fire from the altar. And put incense [on it] and go quickly to the community and make expiation (*vekhapper,* וכפר) for them. For wrath (*qetsef,* קצף) has gone forth from the Lord; the plague has begun" (17:11). Aaron stops this plague of uncontrollable wrath by wafting incense among the people.⁶⁰ In stark contrast to the catastrophic results of incense lighting in the Koraḥ episode, Aaron's expiation by incense works. The plague is stopped.

In each of these examples, proper or authoritative incense offering is contrasted with the severest punishment—death—either by consumption by the deity or by annihilation by plague. This retribution is driven by the unpredictable element of God's wrath (*qetsef*, קֶצֶף).[61] Issues of authority, exclusivity, and restriction are communicated both by the narratives themselves and by theme words (i.e., "to be near," קרב, and "to consume," אכל). In two of the narratives, the Koraḥ rebellion and the plague incident, Moses and Aaron fall on their faces in utter submission to YHWH, but this action does not resolve the crisis. Rather, as we see in the Day of Atonement example, only the wafting of incense by the proper authority, the high priest Aaron, can bring about the necessary appeasement to pacify or soothe divine wrath.[62] Once the wrath of the deity is calm, expiation can occur and atonement can be made.

So far we have seen the priests ensure that members of their own caste do not deviate from precise incense protocol. We have also seen them assert their authority, by means of incense, over the Levites and other Israelites. In the next example, the priests assert their authority once more, but this time over a king who encroaches upon the sancta of the Temple, thereby provoking the priesthood.[63] After becoming king of Judah at the age of sixteen, Uzziah is described optimistically as following in his father Amaziah's footsteps (2 Chr 26:3–4). What he does is "pleasing to the Lord." Among other deeds, he worships God, erects buildings, and spreads farming through his "love of the land." After completing these good works, however, in which he is assisted by the Divine, King Uzziah becomes arrogant and thence corrupt; specifically, "he trespasses against the Lord, his God. He comes into the Temple of the Lord to make an offering on the altar of the incense" (2 Chr 26:16). Azariah, the high priest, and eighty other priests confront the king and warn him that he has overstepped his bounds. Azariah further reminds the king that only Aaronide priests may offer incense. But King Uzziah, who is already holding the censer in his hand, becomes angry and refuses to back down. The result is that God plagues Uzziah until his death with leprosy (26:19–21).

As with the Koraḥ rebellion, the authority and power of the priesthood is threatened, this time by a king.[64] The designation of the Aaronide priests as the rightful officiants of incense is made in two ways. First, the insurgent king is punished. While he does not suffer death immediately, as the rebels of the other narratives do, he is afflicted with a disease that consumes his flesh for the remainder of his life. The narrative relates that King Uzziah is no longer able to come to the Temple (his skin affliction renders him impure), and his son must see to the royal duties (2 Chr 26:21). Priestly authority is also asserted through direct communication. Unlike the contest designed by Moses in the Koraḥ incident, here Azariah declares outright, "It is not for you, Uzziah, to light [incense] to the Lord. Rather it is for the priests, the descendants of Aaron, the consecrated ones, to light [incense]. Leave the sanctuary because you have trespassed.[65] There is no glory for you from the Lord God" (26:18). The high priest does not address Uzziah as "king," and he uses an imperative form of speech to order the king from the premises. There can be no confusion about who is considered sovereign in the realm of the Temple. By entering and attempting to light incense, Uzziah has encroached, trespassed (ma'al, מעל) in the holy territory, where only priests may interact with God.[66]

In addition to the issues of authority and power that are raised here, as in the other biblical accounts, the issue of being "inside"—of drawing close to God—is also apparent in this episode. The king is trying to light incense on the incense altar, which means that he is deep inside the Temple precinct, near the adytum, where God's presence abides. While various passages in the Scriptures tell us that kings occasionally offered sacrifices upon the outer altar, encroachment of this type cannot be tolerated. As in the other narratives, God punishes Uzziah directly—regardless of whatever previous relationship the king may have had with YHWH.

It is evident that in the priestly literature incense is treated as a symbol that is bound up with important themes of authority and election, nearness and accessibility to God, and the desire to attract God's presence down toward earth as well as to contain, soothe, and pacify the unbridled power of God's anger. As the pivotal force in each of these narratives that pits the priests and proper incense sacrifice against pretenders to the office and improper officiation, incense is identified with the priesthood itself and is intimately associated with the primary purpose of the priestly office: communication with God. This communication is both effectuated through sacrifice and is the soothing odor that sacrifice produces. As such, incense is also a synecdoche for sacrifice as a whole. This can be seen in the role of incense on the Day of Atonement, when Aaron sacrifices one animal and sends another (the scapegoat) away as a prelude to the climax of the event—his entrance, incense in hand, into the holiest of places, where he will sprinkle blood to purge the adytum. Incense mingles with the divine presence, protects the high priest, and thereby ensures that proper expiation and atonement can occur. Similarly, escape from the plague in Numbers 17 is brought about entirely through the burning of incense. When words or other sacrifices will not work, incense serves as the most powerful form of apology and appeasement. Although not all of these images are used in the rabbinic literature, many of them are taken up by the rabbinic voices and transformed into multilayered tapestries of interpretation in that literature. Added to these are the erotic images found in the biblical text, to which we now turn.

Erotic Descriptions

The priestly biblical literature presents a unified, if not quite singular, view of aroma. It is concerned with ritual and religious performance, and its actors are exclusively male. The erotic images of fragrance found in the Bible, by contrast, are various and often contradictory. Here we find ourselves gazing on the natural world, the idyll—a world that is unordered in the sense of being unrestricted. It is openly erotic. Its language, while not written by women, focuses on the woman's body, her beauty, and her seductive qualities. Men's bodies also play a role in this world, but to a lesser degree. In contrast to the priestly literature, which often adopts the imperative voice, the literary images of the natural world are expressed in metaphor, simile, and metonymy.[67] Although much of this imagery, most of which carries either neutral or positive associations, appears in Song of Songs, language about the body and aroma also appears in the works of the Deuteronomist and Proverbs. In these books, ordered culture, rather than ungoverned nature, is the focus, and most if not all of the images of women and aroma are negative. In Proverbs, for example, the scent terms and literary devices are comparable to those found in the poetry of the Songs, but the woman is presented in an entirely negative light.

While rabbinic midrash employs some of the imagery and valences from Proverbs, it draws much more extensively upon the Songs for its creative force. Midrash not only employs the broad motifs of the Songs but also quotes extensively from the poetry and reinterprets the verses time and again, layer upon layer, thus embedding the midrashim with such deep and diverse meanings that some scholars argue that the erotic elements disappear. I take issue with that assertion and contend that the rabbis adopt most if not all of the inherent imagery and valences already present in the Songs, and that they redeploy those images within their layers of interpretation. In essence, the rabbinic voices hold the erotic in tension so as to expound more fully upon the verses and to imbue their theological points with an underlying sensuality.

Because these "secular" images of fragrance are so important to the rabbinic midrashim, I explore three categories of erotic aroma imagery here: the evocation of memory, the woman as garden, and the aroma of the "other."[68] Once again, the types are sketched discretely but, like the groups in the priestly source, they constitute an intricate weave of images, motifs, and tropes. Because the quintessential location of perfume and its attendant images in the Bible are all to be found in the Songs, the first two topics, memory and the garden, are roughly organized around the narrative structure of the Songs but include other clustered scent references from the Hebrew Bible as well.

Evocation of Memory

Most commentators choose to focus on the language, visual images, and cultural elements displayed in the Songs.[69] While these are important, to be sure, our concern is with the multitude of olfactory stimuli, their purpose, and their result within the poems. The "aromatic" terms in the Songs include bundles of words such as those discussed earlier in this chapter—for example, "scent" (*reaḥ*, ריח), "fumigated" (*mequtereth*, מקטרת), and "spice" or "balsam" (*bosem*, בשם).[70] Many other fragrant spices and fruits also appear in the Songs, including the apricot, the fig, the lily, and cinnamon, to name only a few. In fact, aroma pervades almost every line and scene in the Songs—often explicitly, but sometimes suggestively—from beginning to end. This is, in part, a natural result of the Songs' subject matter. Descriptions of the pastoral or idyll tend to require strong scent imagery because of their natural reference points.

But the heavy use of comparisons (metaphors, similes, and metonymy) in the depiction of scent is curious. As discussed in chapter 1, the reliance on the language of comparison in this respect may result from the weak language pathways that connect the olfactory bulb with the limbic system (the seat of human emotion and the repository for some of our longest-term memories). Humans seem almost incapable of explaining what something smells like without naming the thing ("a rose smells like a rose"); and yet the human capacity for scent recognition and memory is astounding. The storage facility itself, the limbic system, may account for the strong links among scent, emotion, and memory in humans.

While the method of describing different aromas (i.e., metaphor, etc.) may be similar among cultures, the referents in those descriptions, the points of comparison (or qualities being compared), and the value attributed to the scent (i.e., whether something smells good or bad) differ. These three points of comparison—the referent (that which is being compared), the aspect of comparison (the *tertium comparationis*), and the scent itself—are both singly and jointly culturally defined.[71] In addition, as Othmar Keel explains, "One must also recognize that a simile or metaphor, functioning as a model, can evoke several aspects at the same time."[72] Therefore, as we study the Songs, we must assess the scent comparisons and even the emotions they may evoke, completely and on their own terms, however difficult this may be.

Scent appears at the outset of the Songs, as the female says of the male, "The fragrance of your oils is pleasing, flowing oil,[73] your name; therefore, the maidens love you" (Song 1:3). The names of both the fragrance and the lover are missing, but the metaphor at work is a comparison of the lover's name to flowing oil that smells good. The metaphor suggests that just as the fragrance of the perfume is pleasing to the beloved, so is the lover's name. A metonymy is also suggested here, for the name, which would have stood for the person, is now oil; the lover is called oil rather than by his name. The use of this naming device establishes at once the motif that will develop, the connection between oil standing for the name as a name stands for a person. Later, the oil, or scent, will stand for the lover.

The metonymy of oil for the name and person is further supported by the auditory similarity of *shemen* (שמן), "oil," and *shem* (שם), "name," and the assonance of the "sh" sound, which is repeated three times in the span of six words.[74] The repetition of the sound causes the words to flow like oil, itself a sleek and sensual substance. That the woman can smell her lover's oil indicates physical intimacy. Their bodies are not close together at this moment, however,[75] as the preceding verse—"Let him kiss me with the kisses of his mouth" (1:2)—strongly suggests that the female is remembering her lover. He is not present; she yearns for him. Even the recollection of his scent, which evidently others (the maidens) can also smell, seduces her.

The term *reaḥ* (ריח)—"fragrance," "aroma," or "odor"—appears seven times in the Songs. In three of those instances (1:12, 2:13, and 7:14), something is said to "give forth" (נתן) fragrance, and in three cases (4:10, 4:11, 7:9), the fragrance is compared to something else.[76] The instances in which something "gives forth" its fragrance are significant. These moments connect fragrance, natural substances, and the lovers (the beloved in particular) and move the images toward a climactic metaphor in which fragrance stands for the bodily fluids and scents that flow out of the lovers.

The first instance of "giving forth" appears in the first chapter, in the voice of the beloved:

> 1:12 While the king was in his enclosure,[77] my nard[78] gave forth its fragrance.
> 1:13 My beloved is to me a sachet of myrrh lodged between my breasts.
> 1:14 My beloved is to me a bundle of henna from the vineyards of Ein Gedi.

In verse 12, the woman speaks of her nard wafting fragrance through the air that her lover, who is described as a king, will smell and be enticed by. Fragrance functions on two levels in this verse. The tactile sense of the verse triggers an image in the listener's mind of instances in which the listener may have smelled the aroma of nard. And although the listener is unable to reexperience the scent olfactorily, the person will recall instantly the visual image associated with the aroma, provided he or she has smelled it before. Because nard was used in perfume, it is not unlikely that men and women would have recalled nard in tandem with love or marriage scenes of their own. In this way, just as images of lovemaking and the male lover were evoked in the woman in verse 1:3 (by her memory of his name as oil), so too the listener's memory is triggered by the mention of the spice nard (or spikenard).

On a literary level, the phrasing of the verse is as erotic in English as it is in Hebrew. We are inclined to read the woman's "nard" as her body, which emits a fragrance that draws in her lover. She is either the "nard," as he is the "sachet of myrrh" or "bundle of henna," or she is referring to her own vagina as the nard and her secretions of arousal as the fragrant oil. Again, because she is only able to recall her lover in his absence, the mention of the spices as a perfume of arousal adds to this distinctive self-eroticism. A very subtle horizontal spatial sense is also implied in the initial verse, as the beloved is in one room, and her scent wafts to the room next door. This horizontal position of the beloved is continued in the next image of the beloved lying on her back as the male lover rests between her breasts. As in verse 1:3, the link between memory and love is forged by the scent image. If the woman is present only through her fragrance, then the king recalls her aroma and thereby remembers her. Conversely, if the woman is the person who is remembering, then it is her own arousal and her own scent that cause her to remember her lover and their lovemaking. In light of the physiological evidence for the connections between scent and memory and scent and erotic arousal, the images portrayed in such an ancient source are intriguing.

Furthermore, the entire scene (the king in his enclosure or on his couch) serves as a metaphor for the male lover. In his role as king, the lover represents masculine prowess and political and military power. The connections between spices and royalty are extensive in the biblical literature. This is particularly true for King Solomon, whose name appears seven times in the Songs and who is visited by the queen of Sheba and is presented with a large quantity of spices (1 Kgs 10:2, 10; 2 Chr 9:1, 9). The tribute foreign leaders pay to Solomon also includes spices (1 Kgs 10:25; 2 Chr 9:24). The relationship between royalty and spices extends to other Israelite kings as well. In 2 Kings 20:13 and Isaiah 39:2, King Hezekiah shows his visitors his treasure house, which includes "spices and good oil." In 2 Chronicles 32:27, Hezekiah is described as having many riches, among them "precious stones, spices, and shields." King Asa of Judah is buried with "all kinds of spices mixed in an ointment pot" (2 Chr 16:14). Kings were also anointed both as part of their investiture and probably also in association with regular bathing practices. Psalm 45:9 presents either a description of royal anointing oil or of the fumigation of clothing, probably for the king's wedding day: "All your clothing [is fragrant with] myrrh and aloes[79] [and] cassia."[80] Spices are thus tied to the political realities of trade, the exoticism of foreign courts, the wealth of and respect for Israelite royalty, and the transformative events of marriage and death. In each case there is a subtle assertion of sensuality and a hint of the erotic. Less camouflaged is the openly erotic image of Esther bathing "for six months in oil of myrrh and six months in spices," before her eventful night with the king (Esth 2:12). The audience of the Songs undoubtedly recalled images like these at the mention of the lover as king. The combination of the wafting aromas, the imagery of lying down, the intimacy of the lovers, the invocation of royalty, and the spices and fragrances themselves enhance the perception of sexual anticipation.[81]

The second example of "giving forth" fragrance appears to be less clearly connected to the motifs of memory, scent, and love, and focuses entirely on nature: "The fig tree spices its figs; the vines, in bloom, give forth fragrance" (2:13).[82] As an uncomplicated pastoral image, the verse may trigger only a memory of early springtime,[83] but this verse also resonates with and echoes the beloved. In the verses before and after it, the male lover describes the beloved in terms of animals of the pastoral scene. "The song of the turtle dove is heard in our land" (2:12), he declares. And he asks, "My dove, in the clefts of the rock, in the recesses of the cliff, let me see your face" (2:14). She is the turtle dove; she is the dove.[84] Similarly, she is cultivated nature (the fig tree, the grapevine), and she is in bloom, giving forth her fragrance.[85] The relationship between nature and the lovers appears throughout the Songs, particularly in the description of the woman as garden (on which more below) and elements of the garden: "My lover has gone down to his garden, to the beds of spice; to browse in the gardens and to gather lilies. I am my lover's, and he is mine; he browses among the lilies" (6:2–3). The vines in bloom in 2:13 also hint at the opening of flowers, as the woman herself opens to her lover (5:2, 5, 6).[86]

The theme of the woman opening up to the man also applies to the last instance of "giving forth" fragrance:

> 7:13 Let us be off early to the vineyards
> Let us see if the vines have budded;
> If the blossoms have opened
> If the pomegranates are in bloom.
> There I will give you my love.
> 7:14 The mandrakes give forth fragrance
> And at our door are all choice fruits
> New with the old, my lover,
> have I stored up for you.

All manner of budding, blossoming, and blooming are taking place. References to "early morning" and "blossoming" point toward springtime. And, as with the spicy scent of the fig trees in 2:13, here the mere suggestion of the fragrance of vineyards and pomegranate trees, both indigenous to Israel, would be familiar to the audience each spring.

The woman promises the male lover that she will "give" (*natan*, נתן) her love to him, just as the mandrakes "give forth" or "waft" their fragrance (נתנו־ריח). If the flowers are open, she too will open her buds and give herself over to her lover. But it is not only the mandrakes, whose human shape made them appropriate for use in fertility rites, that give forth fragrance; the beloved does as well. She has stored up the natural fruits of spring as well as her own fruit, which now she will give to him.

These three instances of "giving forth fragrance" resonate throughout the Songs. Different aromas waft through the air in a geographically horizontal direction and are catalogued in several places until they begin to recall each other. Nard is mentioned three times in the Songs; vines are mentioned four times; blossom or bloom, three times; pomegranate, three times; and vineyard, no less than eight times. Their repetition and appearance in clusters (for example, in 7:13–14, quoted above) create a certain coherence within the Songs. At a deeper level, the scents themselves allude to the erotic. Spices, flowers, and vines are all part and parcel of love—whether they are used in perfume or occur in springtime in the garden. In the Songs, they most often refer to the woman (e.g., "my own vineyard I have not kept," 1:6). In addition, these images depict the strong link between aroma and memory. Throughout the Songs, one of the lovers is always absent—even in places where direct speech occurs—but in each of these examples, the expression of longing for the other is described by recalling the perfume of the lover, whether by smelling the nard of the beloved or by inhaling the fragrance of the fig, the vines, and the trees. In each of these examples, moreover, fragrance pours forth and is emitted into the air as the woman "opens up" to the man in her arousal.

The Woman as Garden

The comparison of the female lover to nature is fully realized in chapter 4, wherein the metaphor of the beloved as garden is sustained for five verses. Also in this chapter, the motif of the aroma as the exudate of the female's arousal is fully developed.[87] Scent images are presented in metonymic lists whose exotic and erotic features mingle to represent both the woman herself and her bodily emissions. These scent images, heaped one on top of the other, are so overwhelming as to practically crowd out every other image. The scene ends with a strong focus on the associations of wafting and flowing aroma to effect a state of heightened arousal or anticipatory climax. A somewhat different translation of these verses is presented below, with a short review of the images themselves, how they operate together in the passage, and a comparison of some of them with other clustered images in the Songs:

4:10 How beautiful is your love, my sister, bride.
How much more pleasing is your love than wine,
and the fragrance of your oils than all spices.
4:11 Your lips drip honey, O bride;
Honey and milk are under your tongue.
The fragrance of your garments
is like the fragrance of Lebanon.
4:12 A garden locked my sister, bride,
A [garden][88] locked, a fountain sealed,
4:13 Your sprouts, an orchard of pomegranates with excellent fruits
Hennas with nards,
4:14 Nard and saffron
Cane and cinnamon, with all trees of frankincense
Myrrh and aloes, with all choicest spices
4:15 A garden fountain, a well of living water,
flowing from Lebanon
4:16 Arise north wind, and come south wind.
Blow upon my garden, that its spice may flow.

Let my lover come to his garden and eat its excellent fruits.

The first lines of this passage recall 1:2–3, in which the man's "love is more pleasing than wine" and "the fragrance of [his] oils is pleasing." However, the metonymy in 1:3 of oil standing for the man and his name is absent here. Instead, the scent of the woman's oils is considered better "than all spices" (*mikkol-besamim*, מכל בשמים), and she is "all the choicest spices" (*kol-ra'shei besamim*, כל ראשי בשמים).[89]

As with the flowing oil in 1:3, a heady and erotic scene is created as the natural elements of the garden flow out of the beloved. The first allusion to flowing appears in 4:10, in which wine, an intoxicant and one of the primary accoutrements of love, is mentioned. In verse 11, the female lover's lips, which drip sweet and sticky honey, also become a locus of flowing and sexual excitement. In addition, as with the striking alliteration we saw in 1:3, verse 4:11 also contains heavy alliteration on the sounds of "n," "t," "ph," and "o" (*nopheth titophnah siphtotaiyikh kalah*, נפת תטפנה שפתותיך כלה). Pronunciation of these words involves the tongue and lips and so adds to the sense of flowing. Roland Murphy points out that "lips dripping honey" can be "kisses as well as words," and he draws a connection between this verse and 5:13, in which the man's lips are lilies "that drip flowing myrrh."[90] Although the two verses are connected by the words "lips" and "dripping," a much stronger tie connects 5:13 and 5:5: "I got up to open to my lover and my hands dripped myrrh, my fingers flowing myrrh on the handles of the lock." Dripping, flowing myrrh, first on her hands then on his mouth, create a strong bond between the verses and simultaneously imply some sexual act. The "flowing" spices beginning in chapter 4 and continuing with the two verses in chapter 5 tie the chapters together and continue to build the theme of arousal.

The second half of 4:11 leaves off describing the woman's lips and resumes the theme of "fragrance" (*reaḥ*, ריח). Whereas the couple had been so intimate that the lover knew what lay under the beloved's tongue, with the comparison of the woman's garments to the fragrance of Lebanon,[91] there seems to be a shift in the positions of the lovers. The male is distant from his beloved, and so rather than continue to describe her lips and tongue, he can now only describe her robes and the aroma that lingers and wafts from them.

Verses 4:12–16 depict both tangible items that emit fragrant odors and the vehicles by which fragrances are transmitted to the nose. In verse 12, the woman is described as a locked or barred garden and a locked or sealed fountain. While the man cannot gain entrance to her, both the scent of her garden and the waters of her fountain waft and flow out to him and attract him to her. He calls on the winds to assist in making the scents flow from her garden: "Arise north wind, and come south wind. Blow upon my garden, that its spices may flow." The image alludes to the early stages of sexual arousal in many ways. First, several of the scents described were either used in scented oils (perfumes) or known to have seductive qualities. The flowing of these fragrances points toward the flowing of the woman's sexual fluids as she becomes aroused.[92] Further, the narrative of these lines pushes toward the climax of the woman's response to the man: "Let my lover come to his garden and eat its excellent fruits." Structurally, the climax occurs as a resolution of opposites held in tension. The woman as the garden is barred and then flows. She is closed and then opens. In the last line, the lovers have progressed from smelling to eating—from experiencing each other passively to experiencing each other actively. The tension of arousal builds toward its resolution in fulfillment.

J. Cheryl Exum also draws an interesting corollary between 4:12 and the preceding verse: "The woman is both a גן נעול [locked garden] and a גל נעול [locked fountain], a מעין חתום [a sealed fountain] and a מעין גנים

[garden fountain]. She is a cistern of living water flowing (נזלים) from Lebanon, and her spices are wafted abroad (יזלו). The odor of spices pervades the poem. In fact, the ריח [fragrance] of the woman's oils is sweeter than all spices (4:10). The ריח [fragrance] of her garments is like the ריח [fragrance] of Lebanon (v. 11), from which her living water flows."[93] Exum views the woman as both the garden and the fountain and connects the spices flowing in the air with the water flowing from the fountain or spring through the repetition of the words "to flow" (*nazal*, נזל) and "Lebanon" (*levanon*, לבנון).[94] Lebanon is important in this sequence for another reason as well. While the alliteration in verses 12 and 13 revolves around the sounds of "g," "n," and "ḥ," the mention of *levonah* (לבונה, "frankincense") in verse 14 creates continuity between the two citations of Lebanon in verses 11 and 15 that frame this section.

As with the other examples of "aromatic" imagery in the Songs, the scent terms in chapter 4 are clustered and echoed throughout the poems. Frankincense, for example, appears two more times in the Songs, and, as in 4:11, both include myrrh: "What is this coming up from the desert, like a column of smoke? Fumigated with myrrh and frankincense, from all the powders of a merchant" (3:6), and "Until the day breathes and the shadows flee, I shall go to the mountain of myrrh and the hill of frankincense" (4:6). Rather than oil ingredients, as listed in the majority of the garden images in 4:10–16 (nard, cane, etc.), these verses allude to incense and use it as the metaphoric tool. The imagery in 3:6 describes the female lover as "fumigated" (*mequtereth*, מקטרת);[95] this word is drawn from the same root as cultic incense and the verbs used to convey turning something into smoke, *q-t-r* (קטר). In this simile, the beloved is the column of smoke. As discussed above, the process of scenting garments involved either waving incense or placing the incense burner under the garments as a means of perfuming them. In 3:6, the woman is prepared for the lovemaking that is to come in chapter 4. The reference in 4:6 also alludes to incense, as the lover goes to a "hardened mountain" and "hill." In this passage, the natural images of hill and mountain stand both for incense and for the woman's breasts.

As for the mention of "myrrh" in Songs 4:14 and the other spices of the garden, all of these together are understood as the ingredients in the woman's oil. As the blossoms and other natural vegetation of the garden burst forth and the fragrances begin to flow, so too the woman's oils (her natural exudates) begin to flow out toward the man. In 5:1 the man comes to his garden and harvests or gathers his myrrh with his spice. He then eats his honeycomb with his honey. As we have seen, in 5:5 and 5:13 myrrh flows from the woman's hands and drips from the man's lips—both highly evocative images of the bodily fluids flowing out of the woman. By clustering the images and then moving the myrrh from her hands to his lips, an allusion is drawn to sexual intimacy, and the disparate parts of the Songs are tied together to produce a rough narrative. On another level, the poems move from enticement, through the passive act of olfaction, to action, as depicted first by blowing (4:16) and then by eating (5:1). That is, the movement of myrrh from the garden-woman's body to her hands and then to the male lover's lips also suggests the movement in the garden from fragrant blossoming, to ripening, to harvesting, to eating.

Returning to the other spices mentioned in verses 13 and 14, it is important to note that while many of these are mentioned in other places in the Hebrew Scriptures and other literature of the ancient Near East, most of them are not found in ancient Israel.[96] The man describes his beloved through the many spices and wonderfully scented items that come from faraway places. In this way the woman is associated with the "powders of the merchant" (3:6); just as the spices are exotic and come from foreign lands, so too does the woman become all the more exciting as she takes on the exotic qualities of the spices. The garden thus belies the pastoral scene evidenced elsewhere in the Songs. No such garden could have existed in Israel. But this, in part, is the point. As Gillis Gereleman observes, this is a "utopian, fantasy-garden," and in that respect it is, in its entirety, a metaphor for the woman—and possibly for any woman.[97] Certainly the garden is unreal, because it is her. The author is not trying to create a garden per se; rather, his aim is to flood the mind with as many fragrant images as possible. The terms are seemingly ordered for their sound quality, but they are also chosen for their aromatic qualities and the memories those scents evoke in the mind of the listener. The exotic spices enhance the exotic image of the woman. The fragrance of any one of these spices reminds the lover of the woman and creates a yearning in him that can only be sated by his entering the sealed garden and eating: "I have come to my garden, my sister, bride! I gather my myrrh with my spices. I eat my honeycomb with my honey; I drink my wine with my milk" (5:1).

Repetition, alliteration, and the clustering of images throughout the poems tie the pieces together and create an outline or form.[98] In addition, the garden stands as the metaphor for the woman, and the oil for the secretions of her arousal. The wafting of fragrance portrays and builds a sexual tension that climaxes in eating. As gardens are open to the air but can be closed to people, so too the woman as garden is both in the open air (so that her scent may flow) but also closed and sealed. Similarly, as the smell of food can remind one that he or she is hungry, the scent of the woman's oils lures the man. Finally, as one may eat many of the fruits that grow in a garden, so too the couple is sated by eating of each other.

The words "fragrance," "garden," "oil," and the many individual spices mentioned in the Songs carry with them several associations. Among the most important are the woman, who is described as the fragrant garden; attraction, as scent works on both lovers to lure and attract them to each other; wafting, as the scent of the woman wafts into the male's enclosure and out of her garden, and as the oil of the male lover may be smelled by the female even when he is absent; flowing, as the scents of the female are compared to a fountain, as the male's name flows like oil, and as myrrh is said to drip from hands and lips; royalty, as the male lover is described as a king and as many references are made to Solomon, royal weddings, and the accouterments of royalty; sensuality, as all these metaphors and scenes of springtime's budding, opening, and blossoming allude to sexual intimacy and tactile arousal; and a sense of the exotic, as displayed by the references to the spices themselves (which come from faraway lands) and the traveling merchant and his wares. In comparison with the priestly literature, the act of eating or consumption takes on a completely different tone in this poetry. There, consumption by God meant punishment and annihilation. Here, eating alludes to sexual intimacy. In addition, rather than the upward and downward geography of sacrifice, the Songs present a horizontal direction for the wafting of fragrance from room to room and from lover to lover.

While no value judgment seems to adhere to the sexual enticements we encounter in the Songs (both lovers take on the roles of seducer and seduced), one should not expect such neutrality in the rest of the biblical corpus. The next section uncovers the motif of the "other" in the Hebrew Bible as expressed through terms related to scent. For woman, "otherness" is intrinsically tied to her role as seductress and sexual being. Rarely does a similar value judgment pertain to the man as sexual seducer, but nevertheless several men are considered "others," either as individuals or as a group.

The Aroma of the "Other"

Foul odor is regularly used in the Hebrew Scriptures to describe the "other." This "other" may be a person, a group of people, or an entire gender, depicted as outcasts, foreigners, or even enemies.[99] They may be physically located within a larger group but objectified as a means of being metaphorically pushed out. Or they may actually reside outside the community, having been either located there already or expelled on purpose. When referring to such people, the Hebrew Bible commonly employs the term *ba'ash* (באש), meaning to have a "bad smell" or "to stink."[100] As such, the term becomes a colloquialism; that is, the people do not actually reek or have a malodorous scent, but references to them employ such figurative speech to objectify them, implying that they are in some way odious, bad, decaying, even dead to the rest of the population. These senses are drawn from the literal meaning of the word, which almost always refers to some animal that is dying, dead, or rotting.[101] The substitution of people as the direct object or subject of the verb "to stink" (באש) conveys that these people engender disgust among the majority, ruling class, or leadership. In this sense, the idea of "stinking" has a political connotation.

For instance, 1 Samuel 13:4 describes the Israelites as stinking: "All Israel heard that Saul had struck the prefect[102] of the Philistines, and also that Israel stank to the Philistines. Then the people were summoned to Saul at Gilgal."[103] The intent is not to convey that Israel "smells bad" in a literal sense, or even that the Israelites are the "other," in the sense of being outcasts. In this instance, it appears that Israel has severely angered the Philistines, whom it will soon meet in battle. Israel is odious or repugnant to the Philistines. However, the colloquialism also implies some of the glaring cowardice of the Israelites. As they wait for Samuel to arrive at Gilgal, they hide in caves, tunnels, cisterns, or wherever they can find cover. And when Samuel is late, the people begin to scatter.

Similarly, in 2 Samuel 10:6, the Ammonites stink: "And the people of Ammon realized they stank to David."[104] In this case, the text plainly discloses that the Ammonites insulted King David by humiliating his messengers. As a result, David is angry. As in the example above, the Hebrew Bible expresses this type of anger as repugnance or odiousness. Like the Israelites in the first passage, the Ammonites are presented as the military enemy.[105]

Two more examples of *ba'ash* (באש) appear in the books of Samuel, and while both are political, it is the individual person who is considered an outcast or the "other" by the leadership. In 1 Samuel 27:12, David is working as a mercenary for Achish. Achish surmises that he can trust David because "surely he has made himself stink to his people, Israel."[106] David is the consummate outcast, or "other," having to fend for himself and serve another king as mercenary. In this role he is a foreigner with respect to both the people he serves and the people he battles. In 2 Samuel 16:21, Absalom listens to the advice of Ahitophel, who instructs Absalom to have sexual intercourse with David's concubines. The adviser tells Absalom, "Then all Israel will hear that you stink to your father and everyone on your side will gain strength."[107] While the two examples, David's mercenary work for Achish and Absalom's sleeping with his father's concubines, display what appear to be two very different metaphorical uses of the verb "to stink," there are several thematic similarities between the two that demonstrate some of the term's connotations. As noted, both stories depict the main characters as odious outcasts in the opinion of the leadership. In the case of David, Achish believes that David will be rejected by Israel, his own people. In the case of Absalom, the leader is King David, the father. As such, the two stories raise issues of disloyalty. In the case of David, disloyalty is raised both by Achish's belief that David will attack Judah and by the nature of David's role as a mercenary. In the case of Absalom, who sleeps with his father's concubines, no single act could be considered more disloyal on the part of a royal subject or a son. An affinity with the term "shame" (בוש) also appears in both these narratives.[108] While David does not actually perform disloyal or shameful acts in his military efforts with Achish, on the surface he would be considered shameful by his people. Conversely, Absalom's actions are quintessentially shameful.[109]

In one of the oldest uses of this colloquialism, Exodus 5:21, issues of shame, the outcast, and leadership also play a part. The Israelites, already "other" because of their position as foreigners and slaves, become furious with Moses and Aaron after the two approach Pharaoh for the first time. Pharaoh has responded to the request of the two leaders to let the Israelites leave Egypt by increasing the workload of the Israelite slaves. The foremen of the Israelites approach Pharaoh in person to ask about the situation. On their way back from their meeting with Pharaoh, the foremen encounter Moses and Aaron. "And they (the foremen) said to them, 'The Lord will see you and judge you because you have made our scent stink in the eyes of Pharaoh and in the eyes of his servants, by putting a sword in their hand to kill us.'" While the verse is syntactically clear, it is completely illogical and mixes metaphors. One cannot stink in the eyes of someone. It is likely that two colloquialisms, both referring to the "other," one that was scent-centered and another that was vision-centered, have been conflated over time.

Even with the mixed metaphor, however, the audience easily comprehends the intent of the verse. The readers (and the actors as well) assume that because the Israelites are both slaves and foreigners (are "other" twice over), they can sink no lower. But this is proved false. Now the Egyptians hate, loathe, and detest the Israelite slaves. They are disgusted by them as one would be by a foul odor. The term "scent" (*reaḥ*, ריח) takes on its own figurative meaning. It is not that the people actually "stink" but that the Egyptians now regard their "scent" as stinking. Even a whiff of the Israelites, even the thought of them, is now odious to the Egyptians. In addition, the themes of battle, cowardice, and fear are undercurrents: a sword has been put into the Egyptians' hands. Stripped of any social status or power and metaphorically stinking, the Israelites may be slaughtered at the whim of the Egyptians.

Each of these examples is a useful indicator of the odious person or community. Israel as a foreign, enslaved, weak people, David as the outcast and foreigner, Absalom as the disloyal insider and soon-to-be outcast—all of these representations are tied to images of the "other." And all of the passages foreshadow imminent conflict, positioning for power, and issues of authority. These conflicts of authority may be conceived narrowly, as within families, particularly between sons and fathers,[110] or they may be perceived more broadly in terms of the old yielding to the young or the supersession of God's elect over the current leadership.[111] In each case the elect of God experience "otherness" for a specified duration. Antinomies related to this concept of the outcast include insider-outsider, foreigner-citizen, and weak-strong. The relationships between David and Achish and between Absalom and David also raise issues of loyalty and disloyalty, and in the latter case the notion of sexual perfidy is attached to the concept of the other.

In each case the focus is on the individual male or the predominantly male group (military corps, delegation of foremen, community).[112] This presents us with a puzzle. Why are women, whom some would consider the classic "others" of the Hebrew Bible, absent?[113] In all of these examples the "other" is male (or the male-dominated community) and has a bad smell; in essence, *he stinks*. Nowhere in the Hebrew Bible does the term "stink" (*ba'ash*, באש) pertain specifically to women or the female gender.[114] One of the reasons for this may lie in the close identification of women with gardens, spices, and pleasant scents.

As we saw in the Songs, the woman is identified both with nature, in the form of a garden, and with culture, in terms of perfumed oil (royalty) and incense (foreign trade). Often these identifications occur through the use of scent clusters or lists of specific spices. However, some of the scent clusters used to describe the female in a positive light in the Songs are redeployed in Proverbs with the opposite intention. In Proverbs, the sensuality of the woman is altogether unfavorable: "For the lips of the strange woman drip flowing honey, and her mouth is smoother than oil. But her end is bitter like wormwood and sharp as a sword of mouths" (Prov 5:3–4).[115] While this image employs language similar to that of Songs 4:11 ("Your lips drip honey, O bride; honey and milk are under your tongue"), the import is thoroughly negative. This woman is the "other" because she is the foreigner, the stranger—not in the sense of her being Ammonite, Philistine, or Egyptian, but because she is the wife of another man.[116] Like David and Absalom, she is also an insider in the sense that she belongs to the community.[117] As such, this woman is the "inside other"; she is a part of the community but off limits to this man. It is likely that this insider status makes her all the more dangerous. Unlike Absalom, who makes himself odious (literally, "stinking") by his sexual sin and therefore recognizable, the woman of Proverbs is desirable; her offensiveness and repulsive characteristics are hidden.[118] The desirability that was such a positive attribute in the Songs becomes completely negative in Proverbs. The woman in Proverbs 5 is the "other" precisely because of her sensual desirability, seductive power, and sexual appetite. But this depiction of women is not the only one in Proverbs. Proverbs 1–7 shifts between two archetypes: woman as valorous wife, or Wisdom, and woman as seductress, temptress, adulteress.[119] The second type, the disturbing "other" who resides within the congregation, leads the unsuspecting male to death and Sheol (Prov 5:5–9), as her honey seduces him into sexual perfidy.

Although the language echoes that of the Songs, the aspect of comparison in the metaphor is altered. Fox clarifies: "The adulteress works her wiles more by speech than by beauty (though she may be beautiful; see 6:25) or by physical stimulation (she begins with just a hug and a kiss; see 7:13). Her honeyed words are described in a lovely assonance, which intimates the dripping of the honey by its very sound. . . . Presumably, the felicitous wording [in Song of Songs 4:11] originated as praise of a beloved woman rather than as a description of decadent lures."[120] Proverbs 5:3 employs the metaphor of Songs 4:11 (the scent or sweetness of the woman's lips and tongue) to describe the "smooth tongue" of the seductress, that is, her rhetorical skill at seduction rather than her beauty. But the use of the Songs' language recollects the woman from the Songs and telegraphs an image of her beauty here. As a result, the physical beauty of the adulteress is subtly implied in this passage.[121] In the same way, the beauty of the wife is also implied. The student is told to "drink the water from your cistern and flowing from your well." The beloved as a well of living and flowing water from Songs 4:15 is echoed here. The male should drink from the well that is open to him and refuse water from the fountain that should be sealed but is not. In Proverbs 6:24–25, the rhetorical skill and beauty of the adulteress as metaphors of seduction are brought together again, with reference to how Torah or commandment may protect the man: "[It will] guard you against an evil woman, from the smooth tongue of the alien.[122] Do not desire her beauty in your heart or let her take you in with her glances." Here the judgment of the woman is taken one step further—not only is she beautiful and able to seduce the man with her eloquent and convincing language; she is also evil.

As the Proverbs passages build one upon the other, they present interesting contrasts with the passages from the Songs. In chapter 4 of the Songs, the woman as the garden embodies nature and is geographically outside, sexually out of reach, and closed. The seductress in Proverbs, who lives in the city, should be inside (in terms of her geography) and sexually out of reach, but she is not. Instead, she is out of the house and walking toward the young man as he approaches her home: "a woman comes to greet him, in harlot's garb, her intent hidden . . . her feet stay not at home" (Prov 7:10–11).[123] She is "now outside, now in the street. She lies in wait near every corner" (7:12). This woman is outside her home, where she should not be, walking in the streets of the city.[124]

The narrative continues to build toward its destructive climax as the woman invites the man into her home. The geography shifts to an inside location, but it also implies that she is entirely accessible. She declares, "I have waved myrrh, aloes and cinnamon [over] my bed. Let us drink our fill of love until morning. Let us rejoice in love" (Prov 7:17–18). By inviting the male into her husband's home and into her bed, she moves as far inside as possible. Ironically, this inside space is even worse than her location outside, because now she is concealed from public gaze. Likewise, she is completely open to the male and inappropriately within reach. She is the antithesis of the woman in chapter 4 of Songs and of the valorous woman with whom she is juxtaposed in Proverbs.

The images of the spices that we saw in the male's description of the beloved as garden in chapter 4 of Songs reappear in the woman's speech in this passage from Proverbs. This woman seduces the innocent male by describing her bed as a locus of perfume and exotic attraction. Further, she blatantly expresses her desire for lovemaking by reiterating the images of "drinking" found in the Songs (5:1). The metaphor shifts from the woman as garden to the woman as bed. No longer is the sexual arousal held in an unrequited tension. She is not the sealed garden, which is outside and in public view but at the same time retains its propriety in its state of closure. Rather, through allusions to fumigation, the scented woman of Proverbs is the bed—inside—hidden from public scrutiny. And she is utterly open to the lover, inviting him and encouraging him to commit adultery with her. The seductress of Proverbs is presented as unfettered by society's rules and mores. She rebels against proper conduct. She not only breaks the commandments by committing adultery (Prov 7:19–20); she perverts them by using the sacrifice of well-being as part of her seduction (7:14–15). Unlike the male "other" who is defined by his odious stench,[125] the female "other" of Proverbs is defined by her beauty, her skillful speech, and her exotic and erotic fragrance.

In contrast to the beloved of the Songs, who is also beautiful, speaks poetically, and possesses many of the same exotic and erotic qualities, the female of Proverbs has been judged by the mentor and society. She is open when she should be closed, inside when she should be outside and vice versa; she is evil. Much of the imagery of fragrance and clustered spices is the same, but the intent of the metaphors is completely opposite in result. The confluence of images in the Songs produces a character who is nubile and alluring but also vulnerable and somewhat naïve. As a locked garden and sealed fountain, she appears to be still *virgo intacta*. Her nard wafts into the room of the king, and myrrh drips from her fingers as she tries to open the door to her lover, who calls from the other side; the audience knows that the male is absent. She is alone and must call on her memories in order to stimulate herself. In contrast, the narrator of Proverbs presents the "strange" woman as older, sophisticated, adept at deception. She seeks out sexual companionship when she should not. There is no sense that she may be vulnerable to seduction. She is the alluring temptress who will ensure a man's downfall, desolation, and death. In the Prophets, as well as in the rabbinic literature, we see these two sets of images come together in new formulations. The Prophets assuredly draw more heavily on the images from Proverbs, while the rabbinic voices are more focused on the Songs.

Prophetic Formulations

In the Hebrew Bible, the prophet speaks the words of God; he or she is a messenger who may be sought out for information, whether current or predictive. Ordinary Israelites may have turned to a prophet to find out when the rain would come, how the crops would fare, or, as in the case of Saul, where the lost sheep were (1 Sam 9). Some prophets are considered "court prophets." Their role may be described as "speaking truth to power," as in the case of Nathan to King David or Elijah to King Ahab (2 Sam 12; 1 Kgs 21). In some cases the prophets traveled in bands, speaking in tongues and making their predictions (1 Sam 10:10; 2 Kgs 2:3). Some of the best-known prophets were those to whom books have been attributed. Most of these messengers describe a state of affairs in Israel or Judah that is in violation of the original Sinaitic covenant and its higher aspirations. These prophets often predict God's imminent desolation of the land, the destruction of the city by a more dominant outside power, and even exile as punishment for the sins of the people. Such predictions are usually followed by the announcement or promise of redemption—sometimes in universalistic or utopian language.

While the basic framework of the message of the prophets is succinct, the messages themselves are multivalent and multilayered. These messengers yearn for a return to former times, when the newly freed Israelites gladly took on the covenant of God's commandments in the wilderness. In exchange, God promised to keep them safe in their land and to provide an abundance of food, water, and all the bounty the land had to offer. But the people have not kept their part of the covenant. They are guilty of idolatry—either literally, through sacrifice to iconic images of deities, or metaphorically, by belief in, or sacrifice to, other gods. Or they are guilty of self-worship, by putting self-reliance, self-interest, or political exigencies before reliance on God. Other prophets express anger at the Israelites for their desertion of sacrificial practice or for sacrificing ailing or old animals. For many, the issue is not sacrifice itself but the motivations behind it. The people have failed to protect and care for the most vulnerable of society: the poor, the widow, the orphan. Some of the literature says that the day of reckoning has not yet come—God has not yet repaid the Israelites for their neglect and abandonment of their duties. In this case, the role of the prophet is to warn that the reckoning is imminent and to exhort the people to return to the Lord and repent. In other cases, however, the day of reckoning has arrived, and the prophet either laments or consoles the people, telling them that at some future date the Lord will remedy their plight and put things right again. One of the exceptional features of this highly poetic language is the sustained image of Israel as the wife or consort of God. The prophets who employ this metaphor idealize the Sinai event as Israel's betrothal, during which she entered into a covenant of marriage with God. But she has made her husband a cuckold and run after other gods and nations as her lovers.

We find both priestly and erotic imagery of perfume and incense throughout the prophetic poetry. Whether in discussion of sacrifice, economics, politics, agriculture, or marriage, spices, such as frankincense and cane, and descriptions of perfume and cultic incense are employed to drive home the images, various points of reference, and new theological formulas. We will look now at a small number of these images and at how they operate in the prophetic literature. Again, the images have been grouped into three categories that are distinct but also often overlap. The first group includes prophecies that critique sacrifice or use priestly terminology to make a case for valuing right conduct over worship. While some prophets are directly concerned with sacrifice and the cult, others are more interested in the wider representation of sacrifice and motivation with respect to the covenant at large. The second category involves fragrance images of Israel as the adulterous wife. In these instances both cultic and more "secular" images are employed to paint the scene of a long marriage gone terribly wrong. The final group is made up of descriptions of God's "anointed one" (*mashiaḥ*, משיח), or messiah.

The selection of material presented here provides a necessary backdrop to the rabbinic material. In many ways the rabbis are similar to the prophets and, more important, see themselves as the inheritors of the prophetic legacy. After all, according to rabbinic legend, the oral Torah is passed down through the prophets—not through the priests or kings.[126] Although they may desire it, the rabbis do not carry the power of the kings (or even of the patriarchate in their own time). Likewise, although they have a certain interest in the now defunct Temple, if a third Temple were to arise, it is unlikely that the rabbis would have any authority in its operation. But, like the prophets, they see themselves to varying degrees as both victimized outcasts and as the "true" leadership of Judaism. Also, it would seem that the prophetic messages of proper motivation toward fulfilling the law, doing justice, and caring for the lowly of society are precepts that often guide rabbinic interpretation. More important for the purposes of this study, however, is the similar style of layered metaphors and other imagery used to stake out new theological territories and to insert other key messages along the way. As we will see, the rabbis not only quote Scripture and use it to buttress their points; in many instances they also employ the Bible's own didactic methods to accomplish similar work.

Critique of Sacrifice

In the prophetic literature, Israel is often castigated or rebuked for its lack of sacrificial observance, its improper motivation for sacrifice, or its idolatrous practices as a way of demonstrating how the people have abandoned the covenant or perverted its core messages. Scent-related priestly terms, such as "frankincense" (*levonah*, לבונה), "incense" (*qetoreth*, קטרת), and "to turn to smoke" (*qitter*, קטר), often appear in these contexts. In addition, these terms are often clustered with other priestly terms to heighten the emotional pitch of the oratory. The prophet may also use groups of priestly terms metaphorically to describe abominable practices or Israel's sins and iniquities more generally. Likewise, this literature sometimes engages clusters of "secular" scent metaphors, employing them as symbols of political power or the cult, or to describe Israelite redemption.

Issues surrounding the failure to sacrifice properly are well illustrated in Isaiah 1:13.[127] In this passage, God asks the Israelites to stop bringing meaningless offerings: "Bring no more offering of emptiness; incense is offensive to me." Here, "incense" is paralleled with the "offering of emptiness."[128] The deity is not angered by cultic practice per se[129] but by the improper motives behind sacrifice. Cultic terminology is used both literally and metaphorically here and no doubt implies a criticism of the cult as well. The offerings are offensive to God because the people commit so many other sins, and by sacrificing the offerings of the people the priesthood is also complicit.

In Isaiah 43:22–24, God complains that the Israelites have left off sacrificing completely and instead burden him with their sins:

> 43:22 You have not called upon me, Jacob
> That you should be weary of me, Israel.
> 43:23 You did not bring me sheep for your whole burnt offerings
> And you have not honored me with your sacrifices;
> I have not burdened you with grain offerings
> And I have not wearied you with frankincense.
> 43:24 You did not buy cane for me with silver
> And [with] the fat of your sacrifices you have not sated me;
> Instead, you have burdened me with your sins
> You have wearied me with your iniquities.

Because this passage uses Israel's neglect of sacrifice as a metaphorical image for her sin and iniquity, the verses are replete with key priestly terms. These include "frankincense"; two of the major types of sacrifice, "grain offering" and "whole burnt offering"; the word "sacrifice"; and two of the objects of sacrifice, "sheep" and "fat." The mention of the spice "cane" (*qanah*, קנה) in verse 24 is a play on the verb "to buy" (*qanah*, קנה). More significantly, cane stands as a synecdoche for holy incense—even though this spice is not included in the recipe for the sacred incense (Exod 30:34–37).[130] In this passage, as in others in which this spice appears (e.g., Jer 6:20 and Ezek 27:19), the implication is that cane is a somewhat rare or expensive commodity. Here, the prophet refers to its expense by mentioning "silver" (כסף). We can be almost certain that the spice was not indigenous to Israel, for it is described twice (in Jeremiah and Ezekiel) as coming from distant lands, and it seems to be expensive.[131]

The message of the passage is underscored by the repetition of two key terms, "to burden" and "to weary"; both God and Israel are described as burdened and weary.[132] The people are weary of bringing sacrifices, although God avows that he has not burdened them. God, on the other hand, is burdened with their sins. The essential meaning of the passage, therefore, is not about sacrifice; rather, it concerns Israel's sin of ignoring God generally and exhibiting weariness of the relationship by leaving off sacrifice. God then becomes the wearied partner, burdened with the sins of the people. The language of sacrifice is used to demonstrate Israel's neglect of God—not only in the area of sacrifice but broadly in terms of sin and iniquity. Sacrifice and the priestly terms associated with it are employed as a metaphor for the deterioration of Israel's relationship with the Divine.[133]

A cluster of priestly sacrificial language appears again in Isaiah 66:3.[134] In this instance the prophet's derision is expressed in a description of regular Israelite rituals mixed with abominable practices: "Slaughtering the ox, slaying a man, sacrificing the sheep, breaking the neck of a dog, offering up a [grain] offering, blood of a pig,[135] giving the token portion of frankincense, blessing an idol. So[136] they have chosen their pathways and their soul delights in their abominations." In this passage the clustered terms include slaughtering, sacrificing, offering up, grain offering, the giving of the token portion, and frankincense. These cultic terms for legitimate practices are interspersed with—and so literally juxtaposed against—the many references to illicit practices: slaying a man, breaking the neck of a dog, offering up the blood of a pig, and blessing an idol.[137] A literal reading of this verse implies condemnation of priestly practices and officiates, as God will "choose to mock them" (66:4).[138] It would seem that God's affection is for "the poor and broken in spirit," who "tremble" at God's word (66:2). However, this negative reading of cultic practice disregards the several other places in this chapter in which descriptions of the cult are either neutral or positive.[139] It is more likely that the prophet is expressing sentiments similar to those described in Isaiah 1:13, in which the prophet desires proper motivation for cultic practice along with a cessation of other sinful practices.

In the opening to Isaiah 66, the metaphor of legitimate and illicit cultic practices is juxtaposed against the repetition of God's "word" and those who "trembled for God's word" (66:2, 5).[140] God "calls but none answer; [he] speaks but they do not hear" (66:4). These prophetic concepts of speaking, hearing, and communication through words present a strong contrast to the priestly language in which communication occurs through the physical means of sacrifice and the response of God's glory coming to rest on the Tabernacle. In addition, the poor and broken of spirit as the central recipients of God's care and attention contrast sharply with the priestly perception of the priests themselves as God's elect and chosen and therefore God's partners in dialogue. The consistent focus in Isaiah on the weak, the humble, and the widow and orphan creates an intrinsic antinomy between the downtrodden and those with social power and authority. The positions of the elect and the downtrodden are reversed, so that the downtrodden become the elect of God. Spatial representation is also different in Isaiah. Although similar to the cultic perception of smoke traveling upward and God's response and presence coming downward, a somewhat more ambiguous sense of spatial relations obtains in the Isaiah passage. God describes heaven (upward) as his throne and the earth (downward) as his footstool in 66:1, but his presence with the "poor and broken of spirit" is simultaneously emphasized in 66:2.[141] That is, much more focus is concentrated on downward motion in this prophetic passage than we saw in the priestly literature, in which most sacrifices, or communicative activities with the deity, are described as traveling upward.

In the passages discussed so far, frankincense, grain offering, and other cultic sacrificial terms are used as metaphors and metonyms. As metonymic illustrations of the cult, these clustered terms are employed to portray Israel's sinful practices and the lack of ritual observance as foils against which the prophet pits proper motivation for sacrifice and concern for the poor and humble. However, as we saw with the reference to cane in Isaiah 43:24, some of these priestly terms also possess "secular" connotations and cultural information. Isaiah 60:6 presents such a case, but with a different spice: frankincense. In this passage the prophet describes future redemption in terms of Israel's receiving riches from distant lands: "Dust clouds of camels will cover you; young camels from Midian and Ephah. All will come from Sheba; they will carry gold and frankincense; they will bear tidings [of the] glory of the Lord." The prophet employs a list of riches to amplify his description of the pleasant political, economic, and religious existence after redemption. In the next verse, the scene turns even further toward the cultic with the inclusion of flocks and rams being offered up "with acceptance on [God's] altar" (60:7). The prophet's vision of the future thus encompasses the universal not only in terms of the other nations coming to believe in YHWH as God but in terms of an Israelite political-cultic leadership as well. Here, the more general cultural associations do not work as antinomies against the cult; rather, all the images together form a coherent, all-encompassing picture of the perfected future.

Jeremiah also deftly unites "secular" images with cultic terms but does so to chastise Israel: "Why is this frankincense that comes from Sheba and the fragrant[142] cane from a distant land for me? Your whole burnt offerings are not acceptable and your sacrifices are not pleasing to me" (Jer 6:20).[143] As in Isaiah 43:23–24, Jeremiah alludes to the grain offering and the *minḥah* sacrifice by mentioning frankincense, and he refers to sacrifice of incense through the use of fragrant cane. This specificity delineates two types of sacrifices and forms a parallel structure with whole burnt offerings and sacrifices in the next half of the verse. In addition, the reader is provided with the place of origination for the frankincense: Sheba.

The prophet implies that ritual sacrifice, regardless of its proper conduct, is a vain effort unless the people repent of their sinful ways.[144] The expense of the spices heightens the sense of futility. Unlike other scenarios (e.g., in Isaiah), the Israelites are worshipping the deity in the proper form, and they are expending adequate effort and capital to obtain the requisite sacrificial materials. But the prophet calls for repentance rather than sacrifice. It is the conduct and motivation of the people outside the ritual practices that are displeasing to the Lord (Jer 6:1–19). Without repentance, sacrifice is of no use. The prophecy becomes even more direct in Jeremiah 17:24–27:

> If you obey me, declares the Lord, and you do not bring in burdens through the gates of this city on the Sabbath day, and sanctify the Sabbath day, and do not do any work on it, then through the gates of this city kings and their officers, who sit on the throne of David,

will enter, riding on chariots and horses—they and their officers, the men of Judah and the inhabitants of Jerusalem. The city will be inhabited for all time. . . . They will come from the cities of Judah and from the surrounding areas of Jerusalem and from the land of Benjamin and from the Shephelah and from the mountain and from the Negev bringing whole burnt offering, sacrifice, grain offering, frankincense, and offerings of Thanksgiving to the House of the Lord. But if you will not listen to me to make holy the Sabbath day and not to carry burdens and come in through the gates of Jerusalem, I will set fire to its (Jerusalem's) gates and it (the fire) will consume the fortresses of Jerusalem and it will not be extinguished.[145]

In this instance, the prophet groups the priestly terms, including frankincense, together, to articulate a positive image of sacrifice *if* Israel listens to God and obeys the other commandments. The description of proper cultic performance is part of God's response when the commandments of the Sabbath are followed. In addition, Jerusalem will be inhabited, and she will have political peace and stability (a descendant of David will be king and will ride through the city with his courtiers). Therefore, the reward for proper observance of the covenant is presented as both political ascendancy and cultic acceptance. Here, the entire covenant is represented in terms of Sabbath observance (and its disregard through commercial transactions);[146] the single commandment serves as the example or paradigm for observance of all the commandments. When these commandments are kept, the sacrificial cult prospers. The opposite also obtains: the sacrificial cult is of no consequence if these other commandments are not observed. The prophet thus places more importance on these "other" commandments than on the cult.[147]

As we have seen, the prophetic literature employs many priestly terms, among them the individual spices used in the incense and *minḥah* offerings, to elucidate issues concerning the cult itself, Israelite practice (and ritual negligence), and abominable practices. The prophetic voice also uses clusters of these terms to contrast perceptions of sin and iniquity with new themes of piety, concern for the poor, and the importance of commandment observance (outside that of cultic practice). In this way the prophetic literature often entails a polemic that is either directly critical of the cult or subtly disapproving of it—or at least considers it less important than other realms of Israelite belief and activity. The themes articulated in the priestly literature (e.g., authority, exclusivity, atonement, and appeasement), as attached to incense, are either abandoned in favor of other constructions or completely redefined by the prophets. The elect are the people of Israel writ large or the lowliest of the society who believe in the word of YHWH. Atonement and appeasement are achieved by a turning of the heart, proper observance of all the commandments, and sacrifice made with the proper motives. In addition, the prophetic literature uses "secular" scent metaphors to describe the materials of the cult and to introduce universalist imagery or further the critique of ritual observance. These "secular" images provide cultural information as well as blending and expanding the meaning of the texts.

The combination of royal, economic, and priestly images is not entirely unusual. The prophets often connect Israel's military, economic, and agricultural woes to her religious infidelity, because all aspects of Israel's existence as a polity, a people, and a supplicant to God are interconnected. Ezekiel, for example, says of Israel's economic history, including the spice trade, "The merchants of Sheba and Raamah, they were your merchants. For your wares, they gave of the choicest spices, of every precious stone, and gold" (Ezek 27:22). The term "choicest spices" (*bero'sh kol-bosem,* בראש כל-בשם) recalls the royal visit of the queen of Sheba to Solomon, the priestly terminology, and the spice trade at once.

The author of Malachi also conflates these terms, but in yet another manner. The prophet chastises Israel, and the priests in particular: "A son should honor his father, and a slave his master. Now if I am a father, where is the honor due me? And if I am a master, where is the reverence due me?—said the Lord of Hosts to you, the priests, scorners of my name" (Mal 1:6). The messenger employs the familial metaphor of "sons" and the political metaphor of "slaves" to communicate God's displeasure with the sick and lame animals the priests offer up (1:8). That is, rather than use priestly terminology, the prophet uses other cultural images to describe the relationship of the priesthood to God.[148]

The prophet then illustrates the proper practices of non-Israelites by using priestly terminology: "For from where the sun rises to where it sets, my name is honored among the nations. And in every place incense is brought near for my name, and a pure grain offering, because my name is great among the foreigners—says the Lord of hosts" (Mal 1:11). The foreigners, who are not commanded to bring sacrifices to the Lord, bring "incense" (*muqtar,* מקטר) and "pure grain offerings" (*minḥah tehorah,* מנחה טהורה) to him.[149]

In this verse, cultic terminology is employed to discuss cultic practices. But these are not the practices of the Israelites; the priestly imagery is recontextualized here to describe the sacrifices of the "foreigners."

In the next two lines, the prophet returns to using cultic terms to present both everyday and cultic images simultaneously: "And you profane it (the name of the Lord) when you say, 'The table of my Lord is defiled and its fruit, its food, is despised.' And you say, 'Behold. What weariness,' and you snort at it" (Mal 1:12–13).[150] To drive his point home, the prophet reverses the roles of God and Israel. Instead of God snorting derisively at Israel's sacrifices (as we would expect a master to do to his slaves), Israel snorts at God's table (like an unappreciative or rebellious son).[151] The table represents the altar, and the food, sacrifices. In this example, the terms of the cult are colloquialized to further emphasize Israel's impertinence to God and disrespect for sacrifice. In this sense, the priestly language and its associations are circular. Cultic terms such as "priest," "altar," "incense," "grain offering," and "sacrifice" all appear in this section with reference to the priesthood, but for the purpose of building a noncultic metaphor that compares the priesthood to itself. The text presents two sets of metaphorical antinomies: the master and his slaves and the father and his sons. Connected to these concepts are the oppositional characteristics of "honor" and "reverence" (1:6), contrasted with "scorn" and "curse" (1:12, 14). God expects his people to honor and revere him, but instead they scorn him. As a result, he will not accept their sacrifices, and he will curse their blessings (2:2). However, the prophet does not sustain the metaphor; rather, he creates a new metaphor. He accuses the priesthood (or Israelites) directly of bringing and preparing sick and lame animals for God's table.[152] Correspondingly, the prophet claims that foreigners, who are not a part of Israel, regularly sacrifice properly, for God's name is great among them. The oppositional relationships of master/slave and father/son include the notions of strong and weak, respect and disrespect (or insurrection), and, on a more subtle level, loyalty and disloyalty. These intimate associations also entail a sense of an unbreakable bond: the master owns the slave and the father and son are blood relatives. But their relationships are fractured. God complains that he is not treated the way he deserves to be treated—ostensibly by his own family. Yet he is treated well by the foreigner, who takes the place of the priests and usurps their authority by offering incense. As a result, insiders and outsiders are also an issue in this passage, and their roles are also reversed.

Israel, the Adulterous Wife

No familial relationship is more intimate than that of husband and wife, and probably no relationship entails more "baggage" and dysfunction than a long and problematic marriage. In the books of the Prophets, we find a close analogy between Israel and an adulterous wife. Like the seductress encountered in Proverbs, Hosea depicts a sustained image of Israel as the faithless and philandering wife who cuckolds her "husband," the Divine (e.g., Hos 2:4–7). Similarly, Isaiah 3:16 details the results of the "vanity," "mincing gait," and "roving eyes" of the "daughters of Zion." The daughters are a metaphor for all Israel, who will be stripped of her clothes, jewels, amulets, and other finery, and "instead of perfume (*bosem*, בשם), there will be decay; instead of an apron, a rope" (Isa 3:24).[153] While these descriptions of Israel, the wife of God, can be lengthy and detailed, the prophets rarely draw on the types of scent imagery found in the Songs. One reason for this may be that scent is not the primary focus of the prophets, and so aroma does not regularly appear in their discourse. Or one might speculate that because the images of the woman in the Songs are positive, the prophets have no reason to apply the images from the Songs to their negative depictions of Israel. However, the images in Proverbs 7, which draw heavily on many images found throughout the Bible, including Songs, suggest otherwise.

One prophet, Ezekiel, does employ scent images in his representation of the adulterous wife, although he does not take imagery directly from the Songs. Rather, the prophet combines typical scent terms of the priesthood and the regular prophetic descriptions of the wanton woman to convey the metaphor of Israel as the fornicating wife.[154] In Ezekiel 16:16, beautiful Israel, consort of God and fit for royalty (Ezek 16:9–13), becomes a harlot: "You took some of your clothes and made gaily colored shrines and harloted on them—such things will never be."[155] Israel lusts after other lovers and uses the implements of the priesthood for other gods: "You took your embroidered clothes and covered them. My oil and my incense you placed before them. My food that I gave to you—choice flour, oil, and honey—that I fed you, you placed it before them as a soothing odor" (16:18–19). Many of the priestly terms are clustered and reused in this scene to describe the table set by Israel.[156] She uses the anointing oil of the priesthood and the incense used near the Holy of Holies as tools for her seduction. Terms such as the "choice flour" and "my food" are redeployed from the priestly literature to describe the food the lovers feast upon. And, to leave no doubt that the elements cited are cultic items perverted for carnal use, they are collectively referred to as a "soothing odor" (*reah niḥoaḥ*, ריח ניחח) for the male lovers. In this manner, Ezekiel ensures that the audience perceives the other lovers not only as foreign countries but as other gods.[157] As the chapter unfolds, Ezekiel points to the ultimate abomination: Israel's sacrifice of her children to these gods (16:20). The soothing odor at once becomes the sacrificed children, as they are the food for these gods (16:20–21).

The new bundle of phrases, which include the priestly terminology, the descriptions of the harlot, and images of feasting and lovemaking, appear again in Ezekiel 23:40–41, where the prophet describes the adultery committed by the two sisters Oholah (Samaria) and Oholibah (Jerusalem): "And behold, they (the men) came, for whom you bathed and colored your eyes and donned your ornaments. And you sat on a fine couch and set a table before it. And my incense and my oil you placed on it."[158] Ezekiel points to the image of the women setting the feast table for the men as indicated by "the couch." As in the earlier example, royalty is suggested, as the men adorn the women with jewelry and a crown: "they put bracelets on their hands and a beautiful crown on their head" (23:42).[159] The oil and incense are portrayed both as holy (as God says, "my oil and my incense") and as "social" (the women set the table with them).

While there are several surface similarities between Ezekiel 16:18–19 and 23:41, this passage presents the sexual seduction much more graphically—all manner of touching, fondling, grabbing, and handling occurs from the outset—and the priestly oil and incense emerge less as priestly terms and more as tools of seduction. That said, both passages use much of the same priestly and "secular" terminology already discussed, but in novel ways. Rather than employ cultic terminology to launch a polemic against the cult or improper motivation for sacrifice, the prophet uses the terminology to describe both Israel's worshipping of idols and her foreign diplomacy. He creates a double metaphor by employing a neutral social setting (the feast table) and incorporating an illicit seduction (Israel or the sisters and their lovers). Images from the Songs (the king sitting at his table) and Proverbs (the woman seducing and having intercourse with the man) are recollected in the metaphor. Incense and oil become the integral ingredients in the metaphor, because they are located in both the "sacred" and "secular" realms. This new metaphor, Israel as the adulterous wife, thus combines some of the terms from the priesthood (choice flour, incense, soothing odor) with other cultural associations: royalty, now applied to God, Israel, and the lovers (other gods); seduction and sexual perfidy, as Israel seduces the other gods at her husband's table, using the gifts from her husband; a sense of horizontal wafting, as the scent of incense, now located on the table, wafts about the room; and the concept of inside, as the lovers sit at a table (possibly leaning on a couch or bed) in a room.[160]

As we will see, the rabbis accomplished a similar layering of metaphors to heighten the overall effect and enlarge the scope of their didactic purpose. And, like their perceived forebears, the rabbis employed images from daily life and their own experience. But the rabbis were much less concerned than the prophets with priestly endeavors. In part this was because the Temple no longer existed, and so the priests no longer had formal authority or power over Jewish communities. It is thus unlikely that the rabbis viewed themselves as direct competitors with the remaining priestly families and doubtful that the rabbis saw the priests as an embodied leadership to whom the rabbis had to "speak truth." When using the "prophetic voice," the rabbis were more likely to speak consolingly to Israel of her future redemption and salvation.

The Anointed One of God

Redemptive speech and figuration necessarily include the redeemer, and while this most often meant God, both in the prophetic works and in the rabbinic texts, there is also evidence of a human who either helps the process along or reigns after the fact. From the late biblical period onward, this person is considered the "anointed one," or messiah (*mashiaḥ*, משיח), of God. At first this appellation derived from the messiah's status as a descendant of the Davidic royal line. In later Hellenistic and rabbinic Judaism, however, it becomes increasingly clear that the messiah is so called for his special qualities and abilities.[161]

The last example of prophecy that includes a reference to aroma comes from one of the most famous passages in the Hebrew Bible. The opening verses of Isaiah 11 describe the abilities of the "shoot [that] shall grow out of the stump of Jesse."[162] Here, the messiah's talents and capabilities are listed:

> 11:2   A spirit of the Lord shall alight upon him,
>   A spirit of wisdom and understanding,
>   A spirit of counsel and valor,
>   A spirit of knowledge and awe of the Lord.

11:3   And by his smelling in awe of the Lord,
And not by [what] his eyes see, will he judge,
And not by [what] his ears hear, will he will decide.
(Isa 11:2–3)

God's chosen one will not be fooled by his eyes or his ears. He will be able to see past and hear through lies and deception and will know the truth. In the overall context of the passage, the idea of this chosen person "smelling" (*hariḥo*, הריחו) the truth means that he will sense it, discern it, or otherwise feel it in some manner.[163] This deep level of perception is communicated by the several phrases leading up to the verse that detail the personality traits of this person. He is wise, understanding, of good counsel, and valorous.[164] Most important, he has the spirit of the Lord (*ruaḥ YHWH*, רוח יהוה). The term *ruaḥ* (רוח), meaning "breath," "wind," or "spirit," occurs four times in verse 2 and is used with each of the character traits. The tonal similarities between the words *hariḥo* (הריחו, "his smelling") and *ruaḥ* (רוח, "spirit") cause the idea of "smelling" (i.e., breathing or inhaling) to acquire aspects of the idea of "spirit"—that is, something already residing within this man. Today we might call such uncanny knowledge "intuition."

The syntax of the passage is quite difficult, and many scholars believe that the phrase "and by his smelling in awe of the Lord" is simply a dittography of "a spirit of knowledge and awe of the Lord," because the Hebrew characters of the two passages are quite similar.[165] As in other biblical passages, however, the senses here are ordered: olfaction, sight, and hearing.[166] This list of the human senses strongly suggests that the phrase in question is not a dittography, for the list would be incomplete without it, and the means by which this man gains insight into the truth of things would also be missing.[167]

This passage is unique in many ways. For one thing, it demonstrates that the concept of "smelling" as a form of intuition or acquiring knowledge is of ancient pedigree. It also confounds the approach of Western philosophy and psychology, which devalue this sense in comparison with the "higher" senses of sight and hearing. For our purposes, however, the passage is important primarily because it articulates something specific about the "anointed one": he is not an ordinary man but derives his "super sense" directly from God. He thus represents the pinnacle of authority and power and yet is completely distinct from those who typically hold power in society.

Conclusion

The prophetic voices carve out a particular theological space that can be viewed either as new or, better yet, as conveying a hyperliteral understanding of the original covenant. The belief that each person has an ethical imperative, that society has a moral obligation to all its members, particularly those who are most vulnerable, and that motivation toward covenant observance is more important than strict adherence to ritualistic behaviors is not *sui generis* but is innovative in the extreme. As discussed above, one motif at work here is that of an anointed one who, although he may be of the royal line, possesses qualities that set him apart from all other leaders and authorities (priest, king, or prophet). Another motif is that of Israel as the adulterous wife. At one time she was radiant, stood freely, and betrothed herself to the Divine, but now her licentiousness has sullied her. This genre of exhortation also demonstrates an interpretative technique in which analogies are woven together to convey primary and subordinate messages. This involves, among other things, the mixing and matching of fragrance terms from various parts of the cultural milieu: cult, royalty, daily life.

In the erotic descriptions of fragrance from the Songs and Proverbs, we see a close association between perfume and the feminine. The female is variously depicted as the garden and locus of fertility (though unattainable) and as the seductress, whose conduct leads to banishment and death. Whereas the biblical texts describe male "otherness" as "stinking," the female "other" is alluring in her fragrance. Like the perfume she wears and waves about, her aroma wafts toward the male and draws him toward her, shutting off his rational mind and better judgment. Surprisingly, the priestly literature makes a similar analogy about the relationship between God and sacrifice, particularly the sacrifice of incense. God inhales the smoke that floats upward, experiences its "soothing odor," and is drawn down toward earth, making the transcendent imminent. Like perfume, incense encourages the Divine to be appeased to allow room for human atonement, and to be quieted in his judgment.

Many of these ideas resurface in the rabbinic interpretations of the Bible. The midrashim employ a comparable mixing and matching of "aromatic" metaphors, a similar layering of images, the idealization of another messianic figure, "the righteous man," as well as the overarching metaphor of Israel as the wife of God.[168] Using many of the representations from the Songs, the rabbis too portray Israel as the beloved, as garden, and as the pastoral idyll. The rabbinic voices equate the Jewish woman with the wanton woman of Proverbs. And just as fragrance provides a lens through which to view hierarchy, social constructions, and theological motifs of the Bible, it affords the same lens for viewing these aspects of the religion as conceived by the rabbis. Just as we have teased out the associations and affinities of fragrance, spice, perfume, and incense in the biblical texts, so too will we be able to see how aroma, its constituent parts, and its echoes operate within rabbinic midrash.

Spicy Ideologies: Fragrance and Rabbinic Beliefs

The recontextualization of perfume and incense that begins in the prophetic texts is fully realized in the rabbinic interpretative literature. The rabbinic voices pick up the imagery of aroma, laden with all manner of erotic and priestly associations, as they analyze and interpret nearly every verse from the narrative and poetic sections of the Hebrew Bible—particularly the Song of Songs. In so doing, the rabbis transform the images of the garden, the beloved, and mutual love into thickly layered teachings on such subjects as virtue, righteousness, and scholarship. The most erotic of these passages maintain their intimate and sensual electricity while they are overlaid with religious claims about piety and devotion. Likewise, the structural antinomies of scent (inside/outside, up/down, pleasing aroma/stench, arousal/calm) are not only brought to bear in the rabbinic interpretations; they are also transformed in order to express new trajectories of thought and ideology. This chapter and the next explore the ways in which the rabbinic literature reworks and redeploys the concept of aroma, in all of its literary, structural, and cultural complexity. These chapters also peek behind the metaphor as they show that daily experience with aromatics "infuses" rabbinic interpretation. The rabbis' personal experience with fragrance—in the bathhouse, the home, and the market—along with other cultural standards and traditions enables the deep reflections on olfaction evident in many of the rabbinic midrashim.

The rabbis are clearly intrigued with scent and how it operates. Wherever they can, they address the biblical images of aroma. They interpret every verse from the Songs, layering one interpretation upon another in an effort to expound the text fully. Along the way, the rabbis take up and recouple the erotic and sacred scents in the Bible, as well as the attendant meanings and associations, as they reframe the biblical passages. But this is not all. The rabbis are so preoccupied with fragrance, and it so fills their daily existence, that they find ways to introduce aromatic images into biblical texts that have nothing to do with smell. Scent therefore migrates within rabbinic literature in much the same way that perfume migrates throughout the rooms of a house. For the rabbis, fragrance becomes another interpretive tool with which to express the love and sacredness of the relationship between Israel and God—often in the most ephemeral of ways. In midrash, the relationship between rabbi and student is likened to the pouring of perfumed oil. Israel's acceptance of the commandments produces the "soothing odor" of sacrifice. And the "smell" of circumcision wafts up to God and arouses in him feelings of mercy and love. Aroma enjoys a primacy in the rabbinic texts not only because some of the Bible's most beautiful images incorporate pleasing odor but also because, by its very nature, its porosity and ephemerality, fragrance becomes a powerful interpretive instrument.

This chapter is organized around four themes. Two of them derive directly from the erotic motifs of the Bible and two are new rabbinic formulations. The first theme, the garden, concentrates on the "reassociation" of the garden with other locations, spaces, and even motion between places. Such places and spaces include the tent, the world, Eden, and heaven. The second theme involves shifting and ambivalent rabbinic attitudes toward the "other" (usually the female) as depicted by pleasurable and arousing fragrances. The other two motif themes, unique to the rabbis, are rabbinic values and historical moments. By "rabbinic values" I mean concepts considered paradigmatic in rabbinic thought, such as the importance of study, good deeds, and righteousness. The midrashim link these values to fragrance and then compare, rank, and argue them. The last theme, historical moments, is the alignment of biblical images of aroma with the historical events and moments depicted in the Bible, among them the exodus from Egypt, the building of the golden calf, and the bestowal of the Ten Commandments. Like the biblical themes addressed in the previous chapter, these midrashic categories are admittedly somewhat arbitrary, and in several instances they overlap. Nevertheless, this arrangement is helpful in organizing such a vast array of intricate texts and in demonstrating the subtlety of the material.

This chapter and the next address midrashim primarily but not exclusively from *Song of Songs Rabbah* (*Songs Rabbah*), an exegetical work of interpretation (midrash) based on the biblical book of Song of Songs.[1] Because the Songs contain an abundance of "aromatic" images and the midrash is *lemmatic* (i.e., its interpretations correspond closely to the verse structure of the Songs), *Songs Rabbah* constitutes the largest single collection of these midrashim. Where appropriate, the investigation includes examples from other rabbinic texts, primarily *Genesis Rabbah*. This text, dated earlier than *Songs Rabbah*, employs many verses from the Songs either as prooftexts or as metaphorical comparisons.[2] As a result, *Genesis Rabbah* often provides much earlier parallel sources for the midrashim from *Songs Rabbah*, making it worthy of examination for nuances in language, emphasis, meaning, and the use of tradents. Most important, *Genesis Rabbah* offers evidence of an early tradition of several midrashic formulations. These rather concise units appear as fuller and more expanded expositions in *Songs Rabbah*.[3] Parallel sources are most often discussed in the notes. Other sources, such as *Leviticus Rabbah*, the Tosefta, and the Talmud Bavli are also occasionally employed as points of comparison or to fill in gaps.

In addition to the profusion of "aromatic" images, the biblical Song of Songs is also unique for its depiction of the relationship between the male and female lovers. As we saw in the previous chapter, this relationship provides one of the most intriguing and fruitful metaphors of Jewish interpretation: that of God as the male lover and Israel as his beloved.[4] Gerson Cohen has noted that the role of Israel as the beloved may not only predate rabbinic interpretation but may also explain the inclusion of the Songs in the Hebrew Bible.[5] Cohen argues that the Songs offer a counterpoint to the Prophets. In answer to the portrayal of Israel as the sullied, adulterous wife who ruins her marriage, the poetry of the Songs recalls a time of courtship between Israel and YHWH, when their relationship was new and filled with mutual ardor.[6] In the midrashim that we examine in this chapter, one cannot help but concur with Cohen's observation, as we see the rabbis repeatedly turning the verses to their own ends, heaping one metaphor upon another, yet all the while holding their message and the erotic imagery in tension.

Theological Geography

In the analysis of the Songs in chapter 3, we saw that several of the pastoral environments associated with indigenous aromas are further imbued with metaphorical images of spices, blossoms, or other fragrance producers not found in Israel; for example, the garden is filled with all kinds of exotic spices, and the male lover goes to the mountain of myrrh (Song 4:12–16, 4:6). In each verse in which a geographical place is mentioned, a fragrance image is either implied or explicitly articulated, and in most instances these places in the natural world are compared to the female lover by means of an encoded scent image. The male lover wants to enter the garden, which is the female, because her scent, the spice that flows out to him, attracts him; and the mountain of myrrh to which he travels is the female.

As *Songs Rabbah* picks up the garden image, it multiplies these referents almost exponentially. Through constant shifting and realignment of these images, the rabbinic voices render entire series of interpretations on wide-ranging subjects. Sometimes the rabbis also use the vineyard, field, orchard, or other natural setting to highlight some facet of the female Israel that cannot be described adequately by the garden reference alone. In some cases they employ these other pastoral locales to introduce new referents or to underscore specific aspects of the interpretation. For instance, *Songs Rabbah* 8:9 describes the Sanhedrin, or rabbinic court, as being like a vineyard because it is arranged in rows and divisions.[7]

In the examples that follow, the rabbis reinterpret the geographical setting to represent a place or a space in order to elucidate key theological points. In each case, experience with aroma plays a central role in the interpretation. The "aromatic experience," however, is not necessarily that of the garden or other natural element. On the contrary, what makes these particular midrashim so captivating is that the intimate experience of fumigation and anointment lies at their crux, and an understanding of the relationship between the garden images and olfaction thickens the exegetical points.

The Garden as Eden and God's Abode

One of the earliest examples of the conflation of the garden of the Songs with some other place occurs in the travel visions in *1 Enoch*. There, the pleasing scents and sensual spices that appear in the Songs become enticing trees encountered on the way to Eden from God's abode in Jerusalem. In Eden, the righteous are able to eat from the tree of life forever—an intimation of the fusion of the garden image with heaven.[8] In the rabbinic midrashim, these symbols are stretched even further. In one midrash, Eden serves as the bridal chamber of the Shekhinah (*Songs Rab.* 5:1).[9] In another, Eden becomes the dwelling place of the Shekhinah on earth (*Gen. Rab.* 3:9). In yet another midrash, the blending of images of Eden, the Shekhinah, and the garden of the Songs renders the place "God's garden" and thus serves as the basis for an extended interpretation of Eden, or Paradise (*pardes*, פרדס),[10] as God's heavenly chamber.[11]

The midrash examined below presents a similar case; the spices of the garden in Songs are transported to the trees of Eden; the two gardens are thus melded together.[12] Notably, the verse upon which the midrash is based contains no scent image at all: "Behold, you are beautiful, my companion. Behold, you are beautiful; your eyes are doves" (Song 1:15). The male speaker compares the beauty of his beloved to that of the dove.[13] The midrash is stimulated by reference to the dove, which is considered to be the dove that Noah sent from the ark at the end of the flood. The rabbis disagree on where the dove got the olive branch that she carried back to Noah:

> From where did she bring it? R. Levi said, "She brought it from the young shoots of Israel." This is according to what people say, "The land of Israel was not stricken by the waters of the flood." As it is said by Ezekiel, *Son of man, say to her, "You are an impure land, not rained upon in the day of indignation"* (Ezek 22:24). R. Yoḥanan said, "Even the lower millstones of the mill were dissolved in the water."[14] R. Taryi said, "The gates of the garden of Eden were opened to her and from there she brought it [the leaf]." R. Aibu said to him, "If she had brought it from the garden of Eden, wouldn't she have brought something prominent like cinnamon or balsam?" Rather, she gave Noah a hint. She said to him, "My master Noah, [I would rather have something] as bitter as this from the hand of the Holy One, blessed be He, and not something sweet from your hand." (*Songs Rab.* 1:15)

The midrash is structured as two propositions, proofs, and refutations. The first assertion, that the dove flew to Israel and plucked the olive branch from there is bolstered by a prooftext from Ezekiel. However, this theory is quickly refuted in a thoroughly mundane manner—namely, if all the lower millstones were dissolved in the flood, then everything, even Israel, must have been under water. Evidently, though, Eden is not, as R. Taryi proposes, the source of the olive branch. He argues that the dove flies to Eden and receives an olive branch from God.[15] R. Aibu counters that had the dove flown to Eden, she would have plucked a leaf from some spicy tree.

The connecting link between the Songs and the flood story is the dove, but the bond between the dove and Eden is the garden of the Songs. Like the dove in the Songs, the garden is an analogy for the beloved. The two geographical spaces, the garden of the Songs and the Garden of Eden, are linked through fragrant spices. R. Aibu assumes that because the garden of the Songs mentions aromatic spices, the very special Garden of Eden must contain aromatic spices as well. Thus all of the associations that the garden of the Songs entails, including the wafting of fragrance, arousal, and attraction, are inscribed onto the Garden of Eden. In addition, both gardens are closed to those (males) who desire admission; in fact, this closure seems to heighten the sense of arousal. In the Songs, the female is described as a locked garden and a sealed fountain that the lover wants to enter. Eden must also be sealed, since it is not inundated with water during the flood; the dove can enter only when the "gates are opened" for her.[16] This jibes with the biblical text, wherein God closes Eden as part of his punishment of Adam and Eve for the sin of eating from the Tree of Knowledge (Gen 3:23–24).

This passage imparts important information about spices and tells us what spices R. Aibu values.[17] By specifying cinnamon and balsam, the rabbi intimates that these spices were held in "high esteem" and considered "praiseworthy" (*me'ulah,* מעולה). But if one has no knowledge or experience of these spices, then the rabbi's comment is meaningless. The entire point of the midrash—that the dove would rather receive something bitter from God than stay safely in the ark with Noah—is lost unless the rabbi's comment is fully understood.

One could reasonably argue that the Bible itself uses these terms and that the rabbi is simply drawing on the Song of Songs. For the term "balsam," this argument might make sense. However, as discussed in chapter 2, not only was balsam the only spice actually produced in Israel and thus held in high esteem by the rabbis, many in the Roman Empire also thought it had the best fragrance; it was therefore highly valued by Jew and non-Jew alike. There is even less reason to associate the fragrance of cinnamon with the Bible. Cinnamon is mentioned in the Bible only three times (Prov 7:17; Song 4:14; and Exod 30:23), and never in reference to the Garden of Eden. It is thus unlikely that R. Aibu takes his cue directly from the biblical text. Rather, his association and its meaning are drawn from his cultural understanding and valuation of these spices.[18]

Eden and Hell: Jacob and Esau

In the next example, the rabbis invert the biblical technique of using a place to represent a person. Whereas the garden stands for the beloved in the Songs, here the person takes on the characteristics of the place and in a sense symbolizes it. Because the locations involved are Eden and Gehenna (hell),[19] both places and people represent polarities of theological justification.

The midrash is based on Songs 4:11 ("The fragrance of your garments is like the fragrance of Lebanon"), which the male lover says to the female in the context of his description of her as a garden. Here the rabbis reinterpret the verse as Isaac's words to Jacob on the occasion of Jacob's receiving his father's blessing (Gen 27):

> It is written, *And he came near, and kissed him. And he smelled the smell of his garment* (Gen 27:27). R. Yoḥanan said, "There is nothing more evil[20] and difficult smelling than washed goatskins,[21] and [yet] he says, *He smelled the smell of his garment* [*and blessed him*]. Rather, when Jacob our father entered, the garden of Eden entered with him; and therefore he (Isaac) says to him (Jacob), *See, the scent of my son is like the scent of a field that the Lord has blessed* (Gen 27:27)." [But] when the wicked Esau came near his father, Gehinnom entered with him. What is the sense of this? *When pride comes, then comes shame* (Prov 11:2). Therefore he (Isaac) said to him (Esau), *Who then* (Gen 27:33) [as if to say,] "Who is baked in this oven?" And the Holy Spirit gave answer, *He who has taken venison* (Gen 27:33). (*Songs Rab.* 4:11)[22]

The midrash revisits the biblical passage in which Isaac, who is blind, uses his sense of smell as the final arbiter to determine which son stands before him. Isaac is duped both by his own senses and by his son, as Jacob has dressed himself in goatskins so as to appear as hairy as his older brother, Esau, is. Having smelled the scent of Esau, Isaac gives Jacob the blessing due the eldest son. The midrash completely restructures the biblical scene according to the oppositional relationship between Jacob and Esau already constructed by rabbinic interpretation. Jacob, the Israelite, is considered upright and righteous, while Esau, the Edomite or Roman, is presented as the embodiment of evil.[23] One brother smells good and the other smells bad, a difference that stems from the different "places" in which they reside or that "enter" with them. The Garden of Eden, associated with purity, virtue, and incorruptibility, smells good. *Gehinnom* (Gehenna), or hell, is associated with stench because its inhabitants are wicked, immoral, and malevolent.[24] R. Yoḥanan acknowledges, however, that in fact, "scent-wise," the brothers should smell the same, because Jacob has donned washed goatskins. But they do not. Jacob actually gives off a pleasant aroma because of his virtue, and this aroma overpowers the bad odor of the goatskins.[25] Scent, therefore, becomes part of the oppositional relationship through the association of the two antinomic locations: Eden and Gehenna.

The midrash is triggered by the term "fragrance" or "scent" (*reaḥ*, ריח) and by the reference to "garments" (שלמתיך).[26] The construction is an enjambment, as the two verses are only separated by the words "as it is written." In this way the speech of the male lover to the beloved in Songs 4 is transformed into Isaac's dialogue with Jacob; now it is Isaac who says to his son, "The fragrance of your garments is like the fragrance of Lebanon." By intimating that the fragrance of Eden enters the tent with Jacob, R. Yoḥanan expresses a keen awareness of the operation of scent. In the sense that the fragrance of a place can cling to a person's clothing, Eden does enter with Jacob. As we saw in chapter 2, scenting garments and fumigating rooms involved lighting incense with the express purpose of creating pleasant-smelling clothing and surroundings. In the process, not only the clothing but the hair and perhaps even the bodies of those who performed the fumigation or were exposed to it were also infused. Here, R. Yoḥanan employs knowledge of these fumigatory techniques and their by-products and transposes their results onto Jacob. Similarly, the editor or anonymous author of the Esau example agrees in principle and tenor with R. Yoḥanan, since Esau brings the smell of the hot, baking oven of Gehenna with him.[27]

Geography and the character traits of Jacob and Esau, who are associated with places, are interwoven and then presented as two polarities. In the quotation from Proverbs 11:2, Esau is insolent, presumptuous, and arrogant (*zadon*, זדון/זד), and the results of his character defects are dishonor, humiliation, and shame (*qalon*, קלון). In contrast, Jacob is considered humble, righteous, and virtuous. The burning odor, Gehenna, and Esau are all interpreted negatively, while the scent of the field, Eden, and Jacob are interpreted positively. Like the Bible's descriptions of the "other," the midrashic narrative portrays Esau at once as the "other" and as having a repulsive odor. By this time in the interpretive process, though, Esau has also taken on the qualities of wickedness. The feud between the brothers that begins in the biblical account is extended and greatly amplified in rabbinic interpretation. The two brothers, the eponymous founders of Israel and Edom in the biblical text, come to represent the two antagonistic cultures of Israel and Rome in the rabbinic narratives.[28] As part of this theological geography, Jacob represents the insider and Esau the outsider (even though the sociopolitical reality thoroughly contradicts this construction).

For the Blossom in the Orchard, the World Is Spared

In the Bible, the Garden of Eden is a beautiful but dangerous place. Adam and Eve are tricked into eating from the Tree of Knowledge, with the result that they are cast out and endure hardship for the rest of their lives. It is not surprising, therefore, that other gardens and constructed "natural" spaces in Jewish literature also become locations of extreme beauty and peril.[29] These tropes appear in the next midrash, wherein the orchard symbolizes the world and the topical focus is the sweet-smelling flower of Israel. As in the midrashim discussed above, this passage also seeks to elevate Israel by means of comparison. But this time, rather than compare two brothers, the blossom is contrasted with the chaotic and overgrown orchard.

The verse in question comes from Songs 2:2: "Like a lily among the thorns, so is my companion among the daughters." The male lover of the Songs speaks about the beloved and compares her beauty to the lily that grows among thorns and briars (i.e., other women). The primary human sense perception implied in the verse is vision, as the scene presents a single lily growing among thorns, weeds, and prickly plants. The sense of smell is also encoded within the image, however, as the lily also has a pleasant fragrance. Because the midrash on this verse is a parable, it consists of two basic parts: the *mashal* and the *nimshal*.[30] First, the *mashal*:

> *Like a lily among the thorns, so is my companion among the daughters* (Song 2:2). R. Azariah said in the name of R. Judah: R. Simon said, "It is comparable to a king who had an orchard in which they went and planted a row of fig trees and a row of vines and a row of pomegranates and a row of apples. He handed it over to a keeper[31] and went away. After a time the king came and looked at the orchard to know what was going on. He found it full of thorns and thistles. So he brought wood-cutters to cut it down. He saw in it one blossom[32] of a rose, he took it and smelled it and his soul rested because of it. The king said, 'For the sake of this flower, the orchard shall be saved.'" (*Songs Rab.* 2:2)[33]

Like so many other midrashic parables, this one focuses on a king and relates a brief and seemingly elementary narrative.[34] This *mashal* comprises three segments or scenes. In the first, the king has an orchard planted with several varieties of edible fruits, and he turns over responsibility for the orchard to a field hand. In the second segment, the king returns to his orchard to find that it is full of weeds and thorns, and so he hires woodcutters to chop it down. In the final scene, the king finds a single flower, which he plucks and smells. The act of inhaling (*heriaḥ*, הריח) the fragrance of the flower causes the king to feel a sense of calm and restfulness (*shavath nafsho,* שבת נפשו). As a result of this pleasant experience, the king ceases the destruction of the orchard and announces that he is sparing the entire orchard because of this one flower. The connection of the narrative to the verse seems clear. The verse from Songs ("like a lily among the thorns") has been reread literally, without any metaphorical reference to the female. The king bends down and actually picks a lily from among the thorny overgrowth.

As in many midrashic parables, however, the *nimshal,* or explanation, of this parable is somewhat more difficult and layered than the *mashal* suggests:[35]

> Just so the world was created only for the sake of Israel.[36] After twenty-six generations the Holy One, blessed be He, looked at his world to see what was going on. He found it one mass of water. The generation of Enosh was wiped out with water. The generation of the flood was wiped out with water. The generation of the dispersion [was punished] with water. He brought woodcutters to cut it down, as it says, *The Lord sat [enthroned] at the flood. [The Lord will sit as king forever]* (Ps 29:10). But he saw a blossom[37] of a rose—this is Israel. He took [it] and smelled it at the time when Israel received[38] the Ten Commandments, and his soul rested on account of it. At the time when Israel said, "*We will do and obey*"—The Holy One, blessed be He, said, "For the sake of this rose, the orchard will be spared; for the merit[39] of the Torah and those who study it,[40] the world will be spared." (*Songs Rab.* 2:2)

The purpose of this *nimshal* is to express the notion that the world is saved on account of Israel.[41] As with the plucking and smelling of the flower by the king in the *mashal,* the *nimshal* expresses that God's relationship with Israel spares the world from certain destruction. As is common in rabbinic parables, the king of the *mashal* is replaced by God in the explanation. In addition, the *nimshal* reflects a more complex structure, in which the three segments of the *mashal* are layered and subdivided even further. The first section of the *nimshal* is aligned with the first segment of the *mashal* through key words and events: the orchard is read as the world, and the act of planting the orchard is equated with God's act of creating the world.

God's return to earth to give the law after twenty-six generations have lived and died introduces the second segment of the parable. This description should parallel the king's return to the orchard, but here the structure of the *nimshal* departs from the *mashal*. The *nimshal* presents a threefold structure of rebellion and chaos to represent the thorns and thistles. For each rebellion, God punishes the people with water. As the instrument of divine punishment, "water" forms a parallel with the "woodcutters." God uses water to punish and destroy the inhabitants of earth, much as the woodcutters destroy the orchard. But water takes on a dual representation in the midrash, as it is both God's punishment and the symbol of the sinful and rebellious people. Employment of the phrase "He found it one mass of water" also parallels the "thorns" in the parable. It is the "people" that God finds when he returns after twenty-six generations. The "orchard" is not just the geographical "world" but also the people who are in it. Further, the world as a "mass of water" suggests the opposite of the organized and well-planned orchard. The world has returned to the chaos it was before creation.[42] The end of the second portion of the *nimshal* is indicated by the prooftext of Psalm 29:10: "The Lord sat [enthroned] at the flood." This reference to the flood in Psalms indicates that God reigns supreme despite the threefold challenge.

The final segment of the *nimshal* presents the climax. As the world is about to be destroyed, God inhales the scent of the flower that is Israel and cancels his own decree. The scent of Israel is released in her acceptance of the commandments. As she stands at Sinai and says, "we will do and we will obey," her words act as fragrance that both calms the mood of the Divine and reestablishes world order (against the chaos of water). But the *nimshal* does not end here; it continues and again diverges from the structure of the *mashal* in saying, "for the merit of the Torah and those who study it, the world will be spared." The term "merit" (*zekhut*, זכות) provides the key to this parable, for this term also means "by means of" or "on account of." That is to say, the Torah and those who study it have spiritual credit by means of which they are able to save the world. In this way the Torah and its adherents have salvific powers; by means of study alone, one can save the world.

The scene is one of great intimacy and has embedded within it a deep reflection of the influence of perfume. Combining the erotic image of the garden from Songs and that of the prophets in their depiction of Israel as the consort of the Divine, the rabbis reframe both the Songs and the event at Sinai around God's inhalation of Israel's perfume of compliance and commitment. Here the associations of perfume (attraction, arousal, and the feminine) are combined with ideas of covenant and devotion. The interpretation also recalls the priestly concept of "soothing odor," as it points out that by sniffing Israel herself, God is appeased and calmed.[43] That the author knows how subtly perfume works—that one can completely change his or her mind, attitude, or course of action on the basis of something as simple and ephemeral as a whiff of a beautiful aroma—there can be no doubt. Once again the rabbinic voice demonstrates a familiarity with fragrance that could not be gleaned from the Bible alone. This midrash also displays two characteristics often overlooked by scholars. The first is that any anxieties that the rabbis may have had about perfume, or the women who wore it, are absent here. The second is that the eroticism of the Songs itself informs the midrash, even though the message is about commandments and study. The rabbis in no way diminish or try to suppress the erotic imagery. To the contrary, this midrash depends completely on the erotic for its meaning. The act of sniffing, ingesting what is Israel into God's "body," is completely sensual—that she has a physical and emotional effect on him, that he responds to her, emphasizes the sensuality of their relationship rather than the more legalistic and subservient aspects of their bond.

The images in this midrash seem to have a certain flow that is reminiscent of both perfume and water. It moves from the general to the specific (the orchard to the flower), from down to up (the plucking of the flower), and from fluid to solid mass (from water to Sinai). These entail further oppositional valences, of which most are processes: chaos to order, destruction to salvation, idolatry to monotheism, disobedience to obedience, rebellion to acceptance.

Timelines, time periods, and the erasure of time are all subtly suggested. At the end of the midrash, God does not spare the world only when Israel accepts the Ten Commandments. On the contrary, the Divine continues to spare the world for the sake of the Torah and those who study it. The implication is that God spares the world because of those who consider the study of Torah to be of paramount importance; that is, the rabbis, their students, and their followers. But the *mashal* also points toward a specific time period in its reference to the four types of fruit planted in the orchard. These no doubt stand for the four empires: Babylon, Media, Greece, and Rome.[44]

Some rabbis of the third and early fourth centuries C.E. perceived domination by Rome not only as their current predicament but perhaps also as the last ordeal before the coming of the messiah.[45] Israel's relationship with the empires, particularly with the Roman Empire, is hinted at here. Rome, which at times is referred to as Edom (and at others as Esau), is depicted in stark opposition to the chosen Israel in almost every respect. The illicit acts of Rome and the other nations inspire God to end the world. If not for Israel, according to the midrash, the world would already have ceased to exist.

Each of the midrashim presented here ties the fecund garden of spicy delights from the Songs to other locales: Eden, the orchard, even Israel itself. In this way the rabbinic voices use their experience with aromatics to express their own theological beliefs. In the first midrash, a geographical shift between the garden and Eden blends space imagery to describe God's abode and to embellish and spiritualize the biblical account of Noah and the dove. In the midrash on Jacob and Esau, geographic locations and their attendant scents are injected into the personalities and reshape them into symbols of good and evil, righteous and shameful, virtuous and degraded. In the parable of the king and the orchard, the flower's ability to arouse and attract is combined with priestly imagery ("soothing odor") in order to identify the ability of the Torah and its adherents to save the world from utter destruction and a return to chaos. At the same time, this third midrash delivers a political indictment of Roman rule and makes a self-referential theological claim to rabbinic methods of Torah study. In each of these midrashim, the places of the Songs (the garden, the orchard) are recontextualized and combined with other places or people in order to open up new possibilities of interpretation.

The next section continues in the vein of the Jacob and Esau midrash, as it addresses issues surrounding "the other." Like the biblical material, the Jacob and Esau material links "bad" smells with the male "other." But rabbinic attitudes toward women are much more complex than this.

Perfume and the "Other"

As we saw in the previous chapter, the biblical concept of the "other" includes the other as outsider, as the shameful person or group, as those worthy of scorn, and as the enemy. Scent references that pertain to the other often involve the socially powerless, such as women and Israelite slaves in Egypt. In addition, the two antinomic categories of scent—foul odor and pleasant aroma—correspond in the Bible to the two genders of male and female. The male "other" is described as stinking, while female "others" are commonly associated with the pleasant scents of various spices, such as myrrh and cinnamon, or with the incense used to fumigate garments or lit at festive meals. The negative qualities of women, which have to do almost entirely with their sexuality (unbridled eroticism, cuckolding, leading young men to ruin, sexual aggressiveness), derive from the powers of seduction attributable to perfume and incense.

This section isolates the variety of rabbinic attitudes toward the "other" in order to demonstrate that the rabbis both extend the interpretive trajectories found in the Bible and draw on their own cultural and theological understandings in their interpretations. Two categories of the "other" may be delineated in rabbinic literature. The "inside other" is that person or group who resides within the community—for example, Jewish women and Jews who do not agree with, or do not define their own Jewishness in the same way as, the rabbis. "Outside others" are those whom the rabbis consider completely outside the community; these include "descendants of Esau," or Romans, as in the midrash on Jacob and Esau, and other "idolaters," or non-Jewish men and women. Because the focus here is on perfume, incense, and pleasant aromas, most of the examples refer to the female "other" rather than the male. In the majority of instances, these women are considered part of the Jewish community and therefore the "inside other."

For organizational purposes, this section divides the cases of women and scent into two broad categories: "the conceptualized female" and "real women." The "conceptualized female" is that woman or female character who is not present in the community; this category includes the metaphor of Israel as female, the matriarchs (Sarah, Rebekah, Leah, Rachel, and other Israelite women of the Bible), and formulations of a theoretical female who is most often employed as a pedagogic tool. As for "real women," these are women who would have lived within the rabbinically defined Jewish community; this group includes the mothers, wives, daughters, and female servants of the rabbis.[46] In many instances the associations and affinities of scent attached to these groups overlap or shift back and forth. The boundaries of the groups themselves may also shift, as we will see.

Because so many midrashim from *Songs Rabbah* cast the female lover as Israel, it is necessary to draw from other rabbinic sources as well if we are to do justice to the variety of representations of women and scent. This section thus includes some selections from the Tosefta and Talmud Bavli.

The Conceptualized Female

The "conceptualized female" is a paradigmatic construct or teaching tool of the rabbis. She may resemble real women, but she is a figurative construction. Whether she is a biblical character or a representation of Israel, this female is a type. Let us turn now to a few examples of how the rabbinic midrashim use this "female type."

The first example presents a potential rift in the attitudes of the rabbinic interpreters with respect to the idealized female, in this case used to represent Israel. The midrash is based on Songs 1:12: "While the king was in his enclosure, my spikenard gave forth its fragrance." The midrashim on this verse present several metaphorical representations for both the subjects of the verse (the king and the female lover) and the fragrance (the spikenard). In the opening sequence, two rabbis dispute the depiction of Israel as the ideal female:

> *While the king was in his enclosure,*[47] *my spikenard gave forth its fragrance* (Song 1:12). R. Meir and R. Judah [disagreed]. R. Meir says, "*While the king,* the king of kings, the Holy One blessed be He, *was in his enclosure,* in the firmament, Israel gave forth an evil[48] scent. And they said to the calf, *This is your God, Israel* (Exod 32:4)." R. Judah said to him, "Enough, Meir! There is no interpreting Song of Songs for [the purpose of] shame; rather [it is] for praise. Song of Songs was given only for the praise of Israel. And what is, *While the king was in his enclosure?* While the king of kings, the Holy One blessed be He, was in his enclosure in the firmament, Israel gave forth a good fragrance before Mount Sinai. And they said, *All that you have spoken God, we will do and obey* (Exod 24:7)." It is the opinion of R. Meir to say, "My refuse gave forth its odor." Only a tradition was brought by Israel from the Babylonian captivity which they transmitted,[49] that God leapt over the deed of the calf and established [first] for them the deed of the Tabernacle. (*Songs Rab.* 1:12)

The midrash is structured around a debate between Rabbis Meir and Judah.[50] Both rabbis take the Songs' metaphor of the king as the male lover and apply it to God; they assign the role of the beloved to Israel. Their argument centers on the question of whether the verse from Songs refers to Israel's episode with the golden calf or the acceptance of the law at Sinai. The subtext of the argument is whether the Songs may be interpreted to disparage Israel or only to highlight her merit. The last section of the midrash resolves the dispute by infusing a sense of authority into the discussion and subtly supporting R. Judah's interpretation.

R. Meir's negative portrayal of Israel and R. Judah's positive one both hinge on the interpretation of the scent of spikenard that wafts up to God. In the first part of the midrash, R. Meir asserts that while God was in the firmament, Israel gave forth an "evil scent" (*reaḥ raʻ,* ריח רע) as she erected and worshipped the golden calf.[51] While it is possible that R. Meir thinks that spikenard smells bad, it is more likely that he employs the ambiguity of the term "evil smell," or "bad smell," on purpose; as Israel practices idolatry in worshipping the calf, she emits an evil-smelling fragrance. Since the biblical scene is laced with sexual innuendo (Exod 32:6, 18), R. Meir appears to associate Israel's "perfume" with licentiousness and idol worship. Biblical images of the woman in Proverbs 7, the woman who personifies Israel in Ezekiel 16, and the sisters who personify Israel in Ezekiel 23 also come to mind. This is the Israel who is the unfaithful wife and uses aroma as a tool to cuckold her husband with other gods and men. This female is seductive, alluring, rebellious, and brazenly sexual. She breaks the Lord's commandments and may lead others into transgression as well. In this way, R. Meir's reading of the verse fits well with at least one of the female types in the Bible. R. Judah counters that Israel gives forth the scent of pleasant-smelling spikenard when she accepts the yoke of the commandments at Mount Sinai.[52] This female Israel is faithful and obedient to God; she is compliant and fully accepting of God's law. Not only is the female Israel viewed favorably, but "spikenard" also takes on positive meaning in its association with the giving of the commandments. Perfume retains its pleasant qualities but reverses its charge from negative to positive. Both interpretations, however, change the direction of the flow of fragrance. In the Songs, the perfume of the beloved wafts horizontally toward the king in the next room. In the midrashim, because God is in the firmament, the scent wafts upward, recalling the wafting smoke of sacrifice.

The final sentences of the midrash subtly favor R. Judah's opinion. In the biblical text, the golden calf episode (Exod 32) appears out of chronological order. The incident should appear earlier, before the building of the

Tabernacle, while Moses was on top of the mountain receiving the commandments. In the midrash, the Babylonian tradition accounts for this anomaly by explaining that God intentionally skips over the calf incident and focuses instead on the building of the Tabernacle. The Babylonian tradition does not necessarily contradict R. Meir but values Israel's positive actions over her negative ones. The tradition first acknowledges Israel's misdeed (and possibly her evil scent as well), and then subverts this reading by asserting that God deliberately ignores the deed. In its focus on the positive acts of accepting the commandments and building the Tabernacle, the midrash in its final form supports R. Judah's position.

By creating a religious frame for the verse, however, and reading the female of the Songs as an idealized Israel, R. Judah's opinion of actual women remains opaque. The reader does not know whether he views women's use of perfume as positive or negative, only that as Israel, the metaphorical female may be viewed favorably, particularly in interpretations of the Songs. While R. Judah's opinion of women is ambiguous, he does acknowledge R. Meir's viewpoint.[53] Although R. Judah reprimands his colleague for presenting Israel in a detrimental light, he never directly contradicts R. Meir's interpretation. In fact, R. Judah's comparison of Israel to the female whose scent spreads toward God, the king, involves all of the same referents and even the same scent associations as R. Meir's interpretation—only the event, and therefore its placement on the positive-negative axis, has changed.[54] R. Judah's position on Israel as female, though, is articulated more clearly in *Songs Rabbah* 2:4. There, R. Meir interprets Songs 2:4 ("He has brought me to the house of wine") as the "evil inclination" ruling over Israel during her episode with the golden calf. Once again, R. Judah admonishes R. Meir, saying, "Enough, Meir! . . . Song of Songs was given only for the praise of Israel." R. Judah goes on to describe the wine cellar as Sinai. One rabbi interprets wine as a negative influence that "confuses judgment," while the other interprets wine as a symbol of joy.

Although the midrashim are quite similar to each other, one difference stands out: the midrash on spikenard employs fragrance to justify the rabbis' positions on women, while the midrash on the wine cellar employs aspects of wine.[55] In the first midrash, odor's associations are the same, but the interpretation of those associations may be either negative or positive. The corresponding qualities of perfume (seduction, attraction, sensuality) may be perceived as pleasant, and even beneficial, or as malevolent. In the cultural typology of the rabbis, it is evident that perfume can be considered either *shevaḥ* (שבח), to one's "betterment" or "improvement," or *gen'ai* (גנאי), to one's "disgrace" or "shame." In the midrash on wine, by contrast, the associations of wine shift. The two rabbis draw on different qualities associated with wine in their interpretations. R. Meir views wine as an intoxicant that confuses the judgment (*gen'ai*). The result is corruption, moral depravity, and transgression of the commandments. Conversely, R. Judah bases his interpretation on the use of wine as a symbol of celebration, happiness, and love (*shevaḥ*). In this case, two different sets of qualities adhere to the substance. The use of wine at feasts and other joyous events, or for enhancement of feelings of love, is not considered improper or wrong. Therefore, the wine cellar may be used as a metaphor for the Sinai event. Israel consumes wine to celebrate her joyous acceptance of the commandments. R. Judah does not perceive Israel's judgment as impaired at Sinai; instead, he implies, the bride Israel joyfully partakes in the acceptance of the commandments, and joins the groom in imbibing wine at a wedding feast. Read in concert with the succeeding verses of the Songs, Israel is intimately joined with God as he supports her head and covers her with his banner of love (the commandments). The second half of the verse ("his banner of love is over me") works as a prooftext for R. Judah's position. The banner of love is God's, and therefore the verse must be interpreted positively.

Returning to the midrash on perfume, keeping the midrash on wine in mind, it appears that R. Judah and R. Meir do disagree about the characteristics of the conceptualized female. R. Meir's formulation entails one trajectory from the Bible: that of the perfumed, disobedient harlot whose moral depravity leads others to corruption and degeneracy. R. Judah's conception, however, appears to be more in line with the Songs itself: that of the perfumed female who is beautiful, obedient, and ardently in love.

The next example of the conceptualized female has much in common with R. Judah's view; it also assesses the female and fragrance in a positive light. But, rather than depict the beloved in Songs as Israel, this midrash focuses on Israelite women from the time of Israel's forty-year trek in the wilderness. The midrash is based on Songs 4:14: "Nard and saffron, cane and cinnamon, with all trees of frankincense; myrrh and aloes, with all choicest spices." These images are drawn from the garden scene of the Songs, and the male lover compares them with his beloved. As he catalogues the traits of his companion's beauty, he lists several of the spices that waft out to him from the garden and draw him toward her. The scene is one of intensifying attraction, and the male's frustration is expressed in his increasing desire to enter the sealed garden (Song 4:12). But the midrash uses a completely new metaphor, in which the Israelite women use the spices to adorn themselves with perfume or fumigate their clothing in order to please their husbands:

> *And aloes.* R. Yassa said, "This is *filta*.[56] Why is it called aloe?" R. Abba bar Yudan said in the name of R. Judah, "Because it comes [to us] by way of tents." But the rabbis say, "Because it spreads in the tent." And from where did the daughters of Israel obtain [things] to adorn themselves and gladden their husbands all the forty years that Israel was in the wilderness? R. Yoḥanan said, "From the well. As it is written, *A garden fountain, a well of living water* (Song 4:15)." R. Abbahu said, "From the manna, as it is said, *Myrrh and aloes and cassia are your garments from palaces of ivory, stringed (instruments) entertain you* (Ps 45:9). From it the chaste and proper[57] daughters of Israel adorned themselves and gladdened their husbands all the forty years that Israel was in the wilderness." (*Songs Rab.* 4:14)

The midrash is organized around two distinct subjects. The first is a generational disagreement between R. Judah and a group of anonymous rabbis on the etymological significance of the word "aloes" (*'ahalot*, אהלות). The second segment assumes a historicization of Songs, in which the verse is seen as informing the period of Israelite wandering.[58] Also structured as a dispute, this part of the midrash presents two differing views on the source of these spices. The disagreements are prefaced by a clarifying remark from R. Yassa,[59] who explains that aloes are *filta*, a form of perfumed ointment or oil.

In the first segment of the midrash, R. bar Yudan[60] quotes R. Judah, who connects the Hebrew word for "aloes" (*'ahalot*, אהלות) with the word for "tent" (*'ohel*, אהל) by means of a pun.[61] The later rabbis, as indicated by the general formula "but the rabbis say," also employ the pun, but to different effect. As they articulate an etymological connection between "aloes" and "tents," they declare that the spice "spreads in tents." The second half of the midrash incorporates the pun and relates a tradition among the rabbis that for the forty years of wandering in the wilderness, the time when Israel would have lived in tents, Israelite women had some means by which to perfume either their garments or themselves. The two rabbis employ two different proofs for their positions. R. Yoḥanan[62] assumes that the women obtained spices from "the well" (i.e., "Miriam's well"), just as the Israelites did with water and wine.⁶³ He employs as his prooftext the next verse from Songs (4:15): "A garden fountain, a well of living water."

But R. Abbahu, a later student of R. Yoḥanan,⁶⁴ suggests that the spices come from the manna. He cites Psalm 45:9 as a prooftext: "Myrrh and aloes and cassia are your garments from palaces of ivory, stringed (instruments) entertain you." R. Abbahu derives his interpretation primarily from a pun on the word for "kind" (*min*, מין) or "string" (*men*, מן), which he interprets as manna.⁶⁵ He is saying that the women obtained spices from the manna they collected. He introduces another play on words with the word for "ivory" (*shen*, שן), which can also mean "tooth"; that is, the women obtained spices from "things of the tooth" (i.e., the manna they collected and ate). Other word associations are incorporated into the prooftext as well. "Myrrh and aloes" are mentioned in the same order in the psalm as they are in the verse from Songs. The word "garments" links the proof and the interpretation, as it is likely that R. Abbahu's term "adorn" refers to the fumigation of garments with incense rather than perfume or anointing oil.⁶⁶ R. Abbahu's choice for his prooftext, Psalm 45:9, also adds to the overall imagery of the Israelite women accomplishing this act for their husbands, as Psalm 45 may be construed as a wedding psalm.

The most interesting portion of the midrash is not the interpretation itself but the assumptions about women and the use of aromatics that underlie it. Overall, the midrash is quite favorable toward the women's practice of scenting their bodies or garments and toward the women themselves. The Israelite women are described as "chaste" and "proper," and these qualities appear to derive from their motivation for the act—pleasing their husbands. Within the boundaries of marriage, it appears that scenting oneself is perfectly acceptable. Similarly, in *Genesis Rabbah* 71:8, Rachel, one of the four matriarchs, is also described as perfuming herself or her garments on her wedding day. Rachel, like the Israelite women, is viewed with respect. In her case, though, it is not her scenting herself for her husband that garners praise but her obedience to her father and her compliance with his wishes.

The affirmative evaluations of these characters seem to carry over to the aromatics as well. The desert midrash understands the verses from Songs as describing the beloved, and it projects this image directly onto the Israelite women. Though the rabbis may never articulate this view with reference to real women, the distance of the "biblical women" affords them safety in venturing some highly sexualized imagery. As we have seen, the aroma that wafts out from the beloved in the garden has a horizontal valence tied directly to the aroma of the tents. The male lover's attraction, arousal, and desire to enter into the garden are also read onto the interiority of the tents. And while it is not clear in the verses from Songs whether the woman has adorned herself with the spices or simply exudes an erotic aroma, the women of the midrash purposely adorn themselves. There is something forthright, even premeditated, about their actions. The Israelite women use spice to keep their husbands interested during the forty years of wandering. Although the garden and the desert contrast significantly, the presence of the women and the spices make the desert as interesting as the garden. Both images employ water and eating to heighten their erotic effect. In the Songs, the woman is described as "a garden fountain, a well of living water," and R. Abbahu picks up this image when he says that the Israelite women got their spices from a well. Likewise, the lover of the Songs plucks the spices and eats his honey (5:1), just as the Israelites eat the manna from which the spices are derived. In this passage the rabbis give the reader a glance at their cultural context—the regular use of spices in perfume and incense—in order to rewrite the "history," as it were, of the period of Israelite wandering. They thus express all the associations of perfume we have seen (attraction, arousal, inside, horizontal wafting, exoticism) with an explicitly sexual overtone that can be achieved only by employing an idealized construction of these characters.

In both of the midrashim discussed so far, the women are presented as idealized types. In the first, R. Judah conceives of Israel as a female. In the second, Rabbis Yoḥanan and Abbahu discuss women from the period of Israel's forty years in the wilderness. Although each of these examples is positive, this is because the female characters act, or are motivated to act, within the boundaries of rabbinic conceptions of how females should behave.[67] For R. Judah, this entails acceptance of and obedience to the commandments. For Rabbis Yoḥanan and Abbahu (in the desert midrash), it entails directing one's life toward the happiness and well-being of one's husband. Nevertheless, the female as an "ideal type" rather than "idealized construction" is not immune to negative description as the "other," as glimpsed in R. Meir's comments.

In the final example, the woman described is also a theoretical construction, used here as a paradigm or teaching tool. In this midrash R. Joshua points to the female's "otherness" as an endowed trait of her creation:

> They asked R. Joshua, "Why does a man come forth with his face downward, and a woman comes forth with her face upward?" He

said to them, "The man looks toward the place of his creation, while the woman looks toward the place of her creation." "And why does a woman need to perfume herself, but a man does not need to perfume himself?" He said to them, "Adam was created from earth, and earth never decomposes. But Eve was created from bone. For example, if you leave meat three days and it is not salted, it becomes putrid." (*Gen. Rab.* 17:8)[68]

The midrash is presented as an instructive lesson from the Beit Midrash in which certain didactic assertions about women and men are assumed (e.g., that women are born face up and men face down). Only a portion of the midrash is presented here. In its complete form, the midrash explains a wide swath of social disparities, customs, and religious rites assigned to women as the responsibility they bear for corrupting Adam and bringing death into the world.

In terms of odor, the midrash describes women's motive for perfuming themselves as a "need" (*tsrikhah*, צריכה) rather than a "desire." R. Joshua explains this need as the result of woman's (Eve's) creation from bone. As the midrash progresses, so too do the contrasts between men and women—down and up, earth and bone, creation and decay, aroma and stench, positive and negative—until woman is blamed for bringing about man's corruption and death. No wonder she smells bad![69] The comparison to putrefying meat leaves little room for doubt about woman's "otherness." The discussion itself,[70] coupled with the entirely male setting in which it occurs—the Beit Midrash—where those asking the questions are the students of R. Joshua and therefore all males, only adds to the perception of women as "other."

The circular logic of the midrash hints at its careful crafting. At the outset, R. Joshua and his students already perceive woman as bringing corruption and death into the world. Death is associated with various types of decay and putrefaction; woman must also have a bad odor because she is associated with death or putrefying meat; thus she requires perfume.[71] One is reminded of R. Eliezer's comment that women who smell bad are exempt from the proscription of carrying (wearing) perfume on the Sabbath because it is part of their everyday dress.[72]

Notably, aroma itself is not presented negatively—only the women are, and not by virtue of their association with fragrance (as in the case of R. Meir). The issue is not that women give forth a pleasantly erotic scent that is therefore bad or evil, or that their actions are in some way disreputable;

rather, the female here is innately predisposed to smell bad because of the sin and corruption of her female forebear. One surmises that perfume and incense can only help and are not related to the original crime. As such, the midrash presents an inversion of both of the female types presented above. Perfume is viewed as beneficial and therefore it carries a positive value, but the "conceptualized female" is viewed negatively.

This midrash is an outlier; the large majority of interpretations of "female Israel" are positive. Her characteristics, as demonstrated in the few midrashim analyzed so far, include obedience, acceptance of the commandments, and fidelity to God. Likewise, the interpretations involving the matriarchs and other women of the Bible are positive. These characters exhibit proper compliance with rabbinic formulations of the law, chastity, and a focus on pleasing their husbands. Admittedly, though, in the final example, pleasing aroma is separated from the identity of the female; and while the fragrance of perfume remains positive, the female is associated with corruption, destruction, and death. In each of the cases, deeply held cultural beliefs about aroma, as well as the operation of fragrance (how it moves from one place to another, its effect on those who smell it) are employed to describe the scenes, create the comparisons, and inform the ideas. The next section addresses rabbinic attitudes toward "real" women, and there the ambiguity and anxiety rises to the surface.

Real Women

Descriptions of "real women" are difficult to find in midrash because the literature is so often focused on scriptural interpretation. We must turn, therefore, to other types of rabbinic literature for discussions of "real women" (i.e., family members, neighbors, and women of the community) and their aromatic practices. Unlike the midrashim analyzed above, these discussions are of a legal nature. Of the two examples discussed here, one is found in the Talmud Bavli and the other, although it is from *Songs Rabbah*, is described as a *baraita*.

The first discussion is drawn from a familiar passage in the Mishnah that describes the religious practice of blessing a pleasant scent: "No blessing may be said over the lamp or the spices of idolaters, or over a lamp or spices used for the dead, or over a lamp or spices used for idolatry. No blessing may be said over a lamp until one can enjoy its light."[73] By reframing and reorganizing several discrete passages from the Yerushalmi, the Talmud Bavli first addresses the spices of the dead, those of the privy, the oil used to remove residue from the hands after eating, and the spices of the spice shop.⁷⁴ Topics covered in the discussion include the demonstration of appreciation to God for the creation and experience of pleasurable things (*birkhot hanehenin,* ברכות הנהנין), discernment of the utilitarian aspects of aromatics, and the issue of "deriving benefit" from spices and light.

The focus then turns to whether one should say a blessing when one experiences a pleasant scent and is not personally acquainted with the purpose or motivation for the aroma. Two categories of "the other," idolaters and women, are introduced:

> Our rabbis taught: If one is walking outside the town and smells a [pleasant] scent, if the majority of the inhabitants are idolaters, he does not say a blessing. But if the majority are Israelites, he does say a blessing. R. Yossi says, "Even if the majority are Israelites, he does not say a blessing, because the daughters of Israel light incense for witchcraft." Do all of them light incense for witchcraft? A minority was used for witchcraft and so too a minority for scenting garments. Consequently, the majority is not for making scent, and wherever the greater part is not used for making scent a blessing is not said over it. Rab Ḥiyya bar Abba⁷⁵ said, "R. Yoḥanan said, 'If one is walking on the Sabbath evenings in Tiberias or at the end of Sabbaths in Sepphoris and smells a [pleasant] scent, he should not say a blessing because the presumption is that it is only the scenting of garments.'"⁷⁶ Our rabbis taught: if one is walking in a market of idolaters and enjoys smelling [the pleasant scent of spices], this is a sin. (*b. Ber.* 53a)⁷⁷

The argument is structured around three propositions, all based on the circumstance of walking past a town and smelling a pleasing fragrance. The final sentence, which falls outside this structure, seeks to reaffirm the law in the strictest possible sense by introducing a new scene, that of the idolaters' market, and by reminding the reader that to derive benefit from anything of an idolater or idolatry—however remotely connected—is not allowed.

The passage begins with an injunction against blessing the aroma of idolater's incense or spices, regardless of their purpose or function. The speaker supplies the broadest possible context: a situation in which one is not sure whether the pleasing aroma comes from idolater incense. The next ruling specifies that if one is walking by a town in which there is an Israelite majority, one does say a blessing. Taken together, these two rulings reveal that idolaters employ spices and incense in much the same way that Jews do, and so the actual aromas may be quite similar. Therefore, one must know who lives in the town in order to determine whether a blessing should be said. The scent in question must come from incense lit for pure enjoyment, for sacrifice, or for some utilitarian function other than for the dead or for privies because rules governing these scents have already been dictated.

In the second part of the discussion, R. Yossi[78] raises an objection. He insists that a blessing should not be said, even if the town is predominantly Jewish, because so many Jewish women use incense for witchcraft. R. Yossi's comment focuses on the purpose of incense and suggests that one may not base the decision of blessing solely on the identification of the residents of the town. The passerby must also know about the function of the incense. The argument appears to move from the broad to the specific. It begins with the towns of the idolaters and the Jews and moves on to the consideration of Jewish towns only.

On its own terms, R. Yossi's comment clearly identifies the practice of lighting incense by Jewish women as witchcraft. Because this case follows just after the example of idolaters, it appears as though R. Yossi associates the practice of witchcraft with the practice of idolatry and Jewish women with gentiles. R. Yossi's statement is significantly stricter than the previous two. The objection raised to R. Yossi's comment is intriguing, because it suggests that his opinion may be too strident. The objection is made in the form of a rhetorical question: "Do all of them light incense for witchcraft?" The suggestion here is that the questioner knows that this is not the case. The reasoning now moves in a new analytical direction rather than reformulating the foregoing points. The next statement mitigates R. Yossi's ruling by at once upholding it (one does not say a blessing) and undermining it (only some incense is used for witchcraft). The question remains, to which category does the incense of witchcraft belong? Is it utilitarian? It cannot be, because it would have been included in the category of the fumigation of garments. R. Yoḥanan's[79] comment indicates that this fumigation is utilitarian.[80] He clarifies that one does not say a blessing when passing the wealthy cities of Tiberias and Sepphoris before or after the Sabbath, because so many Jewish women are fumigating their garments. Therefore, incense for witchcraft must either belong to the category of idolater incense or represent its own category. In the final comment, the rabbis stipulate that the markets of idolaters, whether in predominantly Jewish towns or not, are dangerous places. If one enjoys a pleasant scent there, let alone says a blessing, this is considered a sin. The function of the aroma is irrelevant. The fragrance could waft from the spice shop (that is, free, as yet, of any utilitarian or sacrificial function), and the enjoyment (benefit) derived from it would still be a violation.

The Talmud presents the fumigation of garments as a problem because the aroma is both pleasing and spreads beyond the confines of the immediate area, which leads to further problems. The person must consider the nature, type, and function of the scent as well as the characteristics of the person producing it before determining whether to say a blessing or not. According to the passage, however, one is inclined to say a blessing immediately upon inhaling the pleasant aroma. The act of discerning who is lighting the incense and for what purpose disrupts and delays the spontaneous reaction. The final comment in the passage—"if one is walking in a market of idolaters and enjoys smelling [the pleasant scent of spices], this is a sin"—moves that reaction one step backward—from the blessing to the experience. One must not reach even the stage *before* blessing, for enjoyment of anything belonging to gentiles is considered a sin. However, it is well nigh impossible to stop breathing or, once a pleasing fragrance has been inhaled, to stop enjoying the aroma. One cannot stop oneself from smelling! The true purpose of the ruling, then, is apparently to discourage forays into the territory of gentiles.

Several legal categories surface in this argument. These may be viewed as oppositional correlatives (in much the same manner that many of the scent midrashim have been dissected). For example, conceptions about insider and outsider are strongly articulated in terms of Jews and idolaters and then, within the Jewish community, in terms of men and women. Both of these sets of categories raise issues of danger and safety in terms of blessing, daily interaction with either gentiles or women, and geographical boundaries. In turn, these subcategories also display oppositional relationships, such as purposeful and accidental olfaction, blessing and sin, and inside and outside in terms of Jewish and gentile towns and markets (i.e., geographically).

The function of aroma is organized around contradictory characteristics as well, such as employing fragrance for utilitarian or pleasurable purposes (i.e., for no other purpose) and its own spatial relationship of inside and outside; that is, spices are lit inside the towns and the scent flows outside the town to the person walking by. But it is both the crossing of spatial boundaries of which fragrance is capable and the similarity in scents employed for widely divergent purposes that create the problems the Talmud seeks to address. It is apparent that these practices, and other scent-related activities among Jews and gentiles (lighting incense for pleasure, visiting the spice shop, etc.), were quite similar in nature. In fact, these practices were so similar, and the scents themselves so alike, that one would need to know the percentages of Jews and gentiles in a given town in order to determine whether to say a blessing. Aroma is not the principal factor; rather, except for R. Yossi's comment, the strictures regarding blessing are primarily concerned with idolaters, and specifically with their scents. The laws are designed to ensure that one does not say a blessing over any fragrance connected with an idolater, as one should not derive any benefit, either pleasurable or material, from idolaters or their practices. As such, idolaters are the "outside-other," and regardless of what their spices smell like, no blessing should ever be said over one of their aromas.

Similarly, R. Yossi's comment reveals a perception among some rabbis that the practices of Jewish women were not so different from the practices of idolaters. These women reside within the Jewish community, and R. Yossi counts them as Jews, but their actions, at least concerning witchcraft, lie outside the bounds of acceptable rabbinic practices for women. His comment suggests either a population of Jewish women who regularly followed a set of practices or participated in activities some rabbis considered sinful, or a distrust of real women in the Jewish community. Either way, this group represents the "inside-other." As Judith Baskin observes, "The rabbinic vision of women as wives is complicated and unresolved, as in any area where ideal norms collide with experienced reality."[81] While most views of the ideal woman are favorable, views of real women can range from suspicious to severely censorious, and this attitude is reflected in R. Yossi's comment. Although his comments are mitigated in the context of the legal discussion, ambivalence about women is still evident.[82]

Uncertainty invades even texts that are otherwise approving of women, as in the next example. This passage, which appears in several sources, is primarily concerned with members of the priestly guilds (males) and not with women. The guild in question is that of the Abtinas family, which rabbinic tradition considered responsible for incense burned in the Temple. The guild is said to deserve merit in large measure because its women refuse to wear perfume. In most instances, the cycle is a response to the following passage from *m. Yoma* 3:11:

> But [the memory of] these [was kept] in dishonor: They of the House of Garmu would not teach [any other] how to prepare the Shewbread.

They of the House of Abtinas would not teach [any other] how to prepare the incense. Hygros b. Levi had a special art in singing but he would not teach it [to any other]. Ben Kamzar would not teach [any other] in [his special] craft of writing. Of the first it is written, *The memory of the just is blessed* (Prov 10:7), and of these [others] it is written, *But the name of the wicked shall rot* (Prov 10:7).

The midrashic cycle that responded to this passage appears in the Tosefta and both Talmuds (Bavli and Yerushalmi).[83] It usually begins with the house of Garmu, continues with Abtinas, and so on. In the cycle, the narratives about Garmu and Abtinas are quite similar, and these two guilds are eventually remembered with praise. Hygros b. Levi's account is ambiguous, and Ben Kamzar is remembered negatively.

In *Songs Rabbah*, the midrashic cycle is driven by Songs 3:6: "What is this coming up from the desert like a column of smoke? Perfumed with myrrh and frankincense, from all the powders of a merchant." In the verse, the male lover alludes to the exotic and seductive qualities of his beloved by comparing her to the caravans of spice merchants. Because the house of Abtinas was considered the guild in charge of the spices for the Temple's sacrificial incense, the connection to the verse relies on the mention of myrrh, frankincense, and the "column of smoke." The midrash is quite long, and only a portion of it is presented here:

> It says in a *baraita*: the House of Abtinas were experts in making the incense, compounding the incense, and [making] its smoke go up. But they did not want to teach [their art to anyone else]. The sages sent and brought from Alexandria skilled workers. They were expert in making the incense but they were not experts in sending the smoke up like that of the House of Abtinas. . . .
>
> And when the sages knew of the matter they said, "Everything that the Holy One, blessed be He, created, He created only for his honor. As it is said, *All that is called by My name, I created for my honor*" (Isa 43:7). And they returned the House of Abtinas to its place. They (the sages) sent after them (the House of Abtinas) but they did not want to come until they (the sages) doubled their wages.
>
> They (the sages) said to them, "What have you seen that you will not teach?" They said, "There is a tradition in our hands from our fathers

that in the future the Temple will be destroyed. We do not want to teach [how to make the incense] so that [people] will not be conducting and making [it] for their idols as in the manner that we do it for the Holy One, blessed be He." And [because of] this matter, they (the sages) remembered them with praise.

And not only this but also a woman and a child from them did not go out perfumed. And when they took a woman from another place, they agreed with her that she will not perfume herself ever so that Israel would not say, "From the spices of the incense they perfume," to establish what is said, *You will be clean*[84] *before the Lord and before Israel* (Num 32:22). And it says, *You will find favor and good approbation in the eyes of God and man* (Prov 3:4). (*Songs Rab.* 3:6)[85]

The midrash is divided broadly into four sections. The first addresses the passage from the Mishnah and explains why the Abtinas family is remembered with disfavor: because of its refusal to teach its special art of making incense. The family appears to be rebellious toward the authority of the sages, as well as being unhelpful and stubborn. In the second section the priests agree to return to Israel, but only if their wages are doubled. The third section focuses on the sages' inquiry into the family's obstinacy about teaching the art of making incense; the sages discover that the house of Abtinas foresees the destruction of the Temple and is concerned that its spices and secret recipe will be used for idolatry.[86] The rabbis then realize that they should praise rather than curse the house of Abtinas. The midrash, therefore, explains the Mishnah's justification "The memory of the just is blessed" (Prov 10:7).

The last section of the midrash describes the Abtinas women and children as never wearing perfume. In this version, this is an additional reason to praise the Abtinas guild, whose humble women and children recognize the need to observe absolute decorum and remain completely beyond reproach. They derive no personal benefit from what is considered "holy." Because the Abtinas women refrain from wearing perfume (or scenting their garments), no Israelite will be inclined to slander them. The issue is not the act of perfuming oneself but the threat of slander or conflict within the community. The guild's attitude toward the sages is markedly different from its view of the larger Jewish community. The guild appears unmoved by the threat of slander by the sages, even to the point of relinquishing its position within the Temple hierarchy. Slander from the community, by contrast, is to be actively avoided.

Curiously, slightly different wording in the earlier version of this story in the Tosefta gives it a markedly different meaning there: "And because of this matter, they were remembered for praise, that a woman of theirs never went out perfumed. And not only this, but also that when they married a woman from another place . . ."[87] The *apodosis* of the phrase that praised the men of Abtinas is applied, in this version, as the *protasis* to the actions of the Abtinas women. And the phrase "And not only this, but also" is placed later in the passage. As a result, the Tosefta version implies that all the praise due the Abtinas family results from the behavior of its women and not because of any meritorious action on the part of the men. The Tosefta version neglects to praise the men for protecting their secret spice recipe or for returning to Israel. Rather, the praise for the house of Abtinas is earned by its women, who do not go out perfumed and who honor the marriage agreement stipulating that they will not wear perfume; that is, the women agree to alter *their* behavior. Notably, the reference to "children" is missing from the older version.[88]

The favorable depiction of women here is somewhat surprising. Often in rabbinic literature, women are described as being frivolous, petty, or worse.[89] One possible reason for the positive emphasis in this midrash is that the women are used as a foil for the men precisely to demonstrate how unappealing the men of the Abtinas guild are. Read closely and in its entirety, the midrash shows that the rabbis praise the Abtinas guild only grudgingly, for the guild does not give the sages the respect they assume as their due. The rabbis may have seen the priestly guilds as another group of the "inside-other."

The connection between the *lemma* and the midrash also presents a contradiction or inversion. The question "What is this coming up from the desert like a column of smoke? Perfumed with myrrh and frankincense from all the powders of the merchant" is answered negatively. The answer is: nothing from Egypt (i.e., the Alexandrians, who are unable to produce the incense properly), and not the women of the House of Abtinas.

This instance of women who are meritorious, worthy, humble, and obedient is reminiscent of the valorous woman of Proverbs 31. Unlike the ideal woman of Proverbs, however, the Abtinas women are the "real"[90] wives of the guild members, that is, members of the community. In addition, the association of these women with perfume is altogether positive—except that the connection stems from their abstinence from perfume. As a result, no strand of rabbinic literature connects "real" women with perfume or incense in a positive way. For both of the passages presented here on "real" women, however, the later sources seem to take a harsher stand toward women than the earlier ones do. In the case of Abtinas, the passage from the Tosefta heaps praise on the women, while the later passage from *Songs Rabbah*, through an admittedly slight change in wording, muffles that praise. Similarly, R. Yossi's comment in the Talmud Bavli on women being witches does not appear in the same discussion in the Yerushalmi.[91] Obviously, one or two cases do not constitute a trend, but these two cases do establish the fact of rabbinic conflict, or at least anxiety, about women and the inherent erotic nature of scented oils, resins, and ointments that were used in everyday life. In the case of the Abtinas guild, that eroticism is assumed as part of the daily activities of the priests and their communication with God. "Holy" perfume and incense must, by necessity of the argument and proscription, smell the same and therefore engender many of the same feelings of well-being and arousal of the senses that everyday perfume does. In any case, this was certainly the perception of the rabbis who transmitted this midrash again and again.

Although the texts analyzed in this section present several conflicting views of women and scent, it is reasonable to postulate that most descriptions of the "conceptualized female" and aroma are positive in nature, while those of "real women" are negative (when the females in question employ perfume or incense). That said, the placement of the Abtinas women in the category of "real women" and the placement of women "needing" to perfume, as discussed by R. Joshua, in the category of the "conceptualized female" are both suspect. Each of these examples could be placed in the opposite category. It is likely that the rabbis saw the Abtinas women as praiseworthy because they wanted to defame the priests of the guild, and so those women are really a "type," while R. Joshua presents a negative view because he is considering "real women." Judith Baskin notes that these texts

> reveal a profound distrust of females, particularly in groups, who appeared to evade the reach of male authority. The resulting association of women with witchcraft is reinforced by parallel discourses framing women as sexually unreliable and potentially dangerous to men. Conversely, aggadic delineations of biblical heroines reveal that God's marvelous purposes can be manifest in the details of women's lives. . . . The glowing portrayals of Sarah, Rachel, and the daughters of Zelophehad

depict women who fulfilled male expectations almost to the utmost degree. In sharp contrast is the antipathy aimed at Leah and Dinah . . . [who] were understood to have breached the boundaries of appropriate female behavior through deception, immodesty, and presumption.[92]

As a purely rabbinic conception, the female may be described in the most erotic of terms and still be considered in a positive light. Thus *Songs Rabbah* utterly transforms the poetry of the Songs into a scene of the female Israel hopelessly in love, and erotically so, with the Divine. Real women, however, and sometimes even their biblical, generalized, or idealized counterparts, as residents of the Jewish community, are the "other" precisely because of their pleasing aroma. The rabbinic commentary thus assumes both the positive and negative perspectives of the female-perfume construction depicted in the books of the Prophets, Proverbs, and Songs. In addition, drawing on the prophetic techniques of layering images, the rabbis' comparisons, critiques, and narrative creations are also multilayered and widely divergent. Although detailed analysis of each midrash reveals an ever-widening framework and deep multivalent nuances in interpretation, the two broad categories of "positive" and "negative" suggest several opposing characteristics of women, including submissive/rebellious, passive/stubborn, modest/brazen, obedient/transgressive, worthy/worthless.

Aroma and its attendant characteristics are somewhat more stable, at least when applied to women. That is, the characteristics of pleasing aroma—that it wafts horizontally, that it awakens erotic impulses, and that it turns off the rational mind and engenders feelings of well-being and calm in those who smell it—are at work in each of the interpretations about women, whether these women are real or typological. In this way, the subsurface categories of perfume and incense are static; it is the women who change. In the next section, as we turn to the subject of rabbinic values, the prophetic technique of layering images and messages becomes even more apparent. We will also see that although the rabbis view themselves as direct descendants of the prophets, their values and messages are as unique as they are self-referential.

Rabbinic Values

In the course of the midrashim, the rabbis reveal the hierarchy of values—the beliefs, ideas, ethical precepts, and religious practices—they hold dear.

These values are too numerous to elucidate completely, and they are also difficult to render in English without the encumbrances of our own cultural predispositions. The concept of "good deeds" (*ma'asim tovim,* מעשים טובים), for example, implies something quite different from our own understanding of the term, "doing something nice for someone." These acts are, for the rabbis, fulfillment of "commandments" (*mitzvot,* מצות), of proper behavior, and may or may not also include "going beyond" the commandment to perform "acts of loving kindness" (*gemiluth ḥasadim,* גמילות חסדים). Similarly, the subtly different words for "purity," "righteousness," and "charity" all derive from the same Hebrew word, *tzedakah* (צדקה). Rather than attempt to define these and other ethically oriented words, this part of the study seeks to present paradigmatic midrashim that demonstrate recurrent themes, primary principles, a variety of interpretive techniques, and some interesting case studies in which the rabbinic interpreters employ aroma in conjunction with one or more of these values. In several cases it appears to be their goal to define or order these values.

The examples are organized in two sections. The first, which I call "Scent, Scholars, and Status," looks at midrashim that use aroma and the sense of smell to assert the value of scholarship and the status of scholars themselves. In the second section, "Mitzvot and Righteousness," I look at two interpretations that use scent imagery to elucidate these key rabbinic values. The emphasis on covenant in the prophetic literature appears again in these midrashim, but with a distinctively rabbinic stamp that explores the issues surrounding suffering, sacrifice, and atonement.

Scent, Scholars, and Status

As we saw in the midrash on the guild of Abtinas, the rabbis did not consider all the men of Israel, or even many of the religiously educated men of Israel, of equal stature with respect to the values or concerns the rabbis themselves considered important. Baskin's assertion that "ideal norms collide with experienced reality" may be applied to rabbinic pronouncements on Jewish men as well as on women.[93] To that end, the midrash below presents a hierarchy of both rabbinic values and the men of Israel. This midrash, from *Pesiqta de-Rab Kahana,* appears in reference to the holiday of Sukkoth.[94] It is based on Leviticus 23:40: "And you will take for yourselves on the first day fruit of the Hadar tree, palms of date palm trees, and boughs of leafy trees and willows of the stream. You will be happy before the Lord your God for seven days."

Another interpretation. *Fruit of the Hadar tree,* this is Israel. Just as the etrog has scent and [it can be] eaten, so too Israel have men who are masters of Torah and doers of good deeds. *Palms of date palm trees,* these are Israel. Just as the date palm can be eaten but has no scent, so too Israel has men who are masters of Torah but are not doers of good deeds. *And boughs of leafy trees,* these are Israel. Just as myrtle has scent but it cannot be eaten, so too Israel has men who are doers of good deeds but are not masters of Torah. *And willows of the stream,* these are Israel. Just as the willow has no taste and no scent, so too Israel has men who are neither masters of Torah nor doers of good deeds. The Holy One said, "To make their destruction impossible, rather they will be made into one bunch and they atone for each other." Accordingly, Moses charged Israel and said to them, "And take for yourselves . . ." (Pesiq. Rab. Kah. 27:9)[95]

This midrash presents a four-tiered classification of Jewish men. Those who both study and do good deeds top the list.[96] The next most important group in the hierarchy comprises those who are masters of Torah but not doers of good deeds, followed by those who do good deeds but have not mastered the Torah; the midrash thus assigns a higher value to those who study than to those who do good deeds. The men who do nothing come last. Although the midrash does not explicitly state that these men are evil, the need for the men to "atone for each other" implicates the fourth group. The inclusion of the phrase "to make their destruction impossible" further suggests that these men at the bottom of the scale are greater in number than those at the top of the hierarchy.

The cataloguing of the different types of men in Israel is accomplished through atomization of the verse. The top rank, the men who are both "masters of Torah" and doers of "good deeds," are compared to the etrog,[97] which can be smelled and eaten. In the first sentence of the midrash, the masters of Torah are aligned with scent or olfaction, and the doers of good deeds are affiliated with eating.[98] In the next examples the order is reversed, and "scent" is aligned with good deeds and "taste" with Torah. The goal is to include all the types of men in Israel in the hierarchy and to make clear that the role of the righteous is to atone for the sinners. The double sensory metaphor of smelling and eating multiplies the "value" categories of Israelite men. Notably, the midrash compares the men along only two axes, scholarship and good deeds, thus demonstrating clearly the values of greatest importance to the rabbinic interpreters.

In comparing themselves to other Jews, the rabbis, not surprisingly, most often view themselves as belonging in the top quadrant. Many midrashim make it possible to distinguish those at the top of the scale from those at the bottom, and several allow discrimination among the upper echelons. As seen in the encounter between R. Joshua and his students (in the previous section), one method of discrimination is to evaluate the questioners and those who answer them. In addition, in the Beit Midrash, the rabbis sit in the order of their rank or status within the school.[99]

These issues surface in the next example, which identifies those at the pinnacle of the hierarchy and raises the issue of the alteration or depletion of the Torah's myriad meanings that result from study and interpretation. The midrash is based on Songs 1:3: "The fragrance of your oils is good; oil poured forth, your name.[100] Therefore the maidens love you." The verse is spoken by the beloved to the absent male as she recalls the scent of her lover's perfumed body. In reference to this verse, Rabbis Eliezer and Joshua each quote, almost identically, a famous midrash usually connected to R. Eliezer's deathbed scene.[101] In the initial comment, the rabbis layer a new metaphor on top of those already present in the verse as they seek to explain the impossibility and futility of trying to learn everything there is to learn from Scripture. Since the comments are so alike, only R. Eliezer's appear here.

> R. Eliezer and R. Joshua and R. Akiba [disagreed]. R. Eliezer says, "If all the seas were ink and all the reeds writing pens and the heaven and the earth scrolls and all the people scribes, they would not be enough to write [the words] of Torah that I have learned. And, I have not extracted [any more] from it than a man who dips the tip of his painting staff into the sea." (*Songs Rab.* 1:3)[102]

The rabbis cue their interpretation to the second half of the verse: "oil poured forth, your name." The rabbis have studied as if pouring oil from one vessel to another. They have "poured" much of the oil of Torah into themselves, but there is still a "sea" to be poured into them. The amount of law and Torah to be learned is infinite. This statement, attributed to two eminent rabbis and the teachers of the most acclaimed rabbi of all, Akiba, is remarkable. They are considered brilliant experts in law but believe they have learned but little compared to what there is to be learned.

At the end of the passage, the rabbis make a pun on the verb "extract" (*ḥiser*, חסר), as they say, "And I have not extracted [any more] from it. . . ."

In a literal sense, the rabbis "extract" meaning from the Torah. But the *pi'el* form of the word can also mean "to lessen" and indicates a "lessening" of the original amount; that is, as one paints, the amount of paint in the original container should diminish. The rabbis are frustrated by their inability to use all the paint. On the surface, the image seems ill suited to the idea of Torah study, as no amount of study should reduce the amount of Torah.

In the next segment of the midrash, R. Akiba compares himself to his teachers:

> I do not have the strength to say as my teachers do. Rather, my teachers extracted from it but I have extracted from it only as one who smells an etrog. The smelling is pleasant but the etrog is not diminished.[103]

R. Akiba appears to be self-effacing; he compares himself to his two great teachers and implies that he is somehow a lesser student than they. He lacks the capacity to make the claims that his teachers make. He appears to think that they actually have been able to extract or learn something from the Torah, but he has been unable to learn anything. The sage says about himself that he has extracted only as one who smells the pleasant scent of an etrog. Akiba's comment is based on the first part of the Songs verse: "The fragrance of your oils is good." Unlike his teachers, who have poured Torah into themselves, R. Akiba has only been able to smell the Torah. It would seem that "oil" is stronger, better, worth more, or more important than "fragrance"; oil, after all, is more substantive than fragrance. But the opposite is in fact the case.

Like his teachers, R. Akiba also manipulates the root *ḥ-s-r* (חסר) to mean "extract" and "to lessen." His initial use of the word is the same as his teachers': "my teachers extracted from it." R. Akiba implies that his teachers have been able to glean meanings from the Torah. But the statement about the etrog—"the smelling is pleasant but the etrog is not diminished"—unequivocally states the opposite. The act of smelling the etrog in no way alters the substance of the scent. What seemed to be Akiba's failure to extract meaning from Torah is in reality his great achievement: to study and obtain knowledge (to extract meaning) without losing any of the Torah's multiple and varied meanings (without diminishing the substance of Torah). The sage learns from Torah without altering its infinitude in any way.[104] Akiba is presented as the ideal sage in terms of his knowledge. At the same time, he is also the model rabbinic student, respectful of his teachers in every way even as he supplants them in the hierarchy of the Beit Midrash.[105]

Returning to the pun "my teachers extracted from it," we see that the teachers have reduced or altered the substance of Torah; they have extracted *from* it or *lessened* it. They have "poured out" from it as oil pours out. In contrast, R. Akiba has merely smelled the good fragrance of the oil of Torah.[106] The focus and weight of the original verse has shifted; the first segment of the verse—"the fragrance of your oils is good"—is stronger than the second. Smelling trumps pouring. An antinomy arises in this midrash between fragrance and oil. Fragrance is insubstantial, without form, ephemeral, while oil has substance. Because it has form, however, oil can be poured out and its amount depleted, while fragrance is unchangeable. The ephemeral nature of fragrance and the fact that it cannot be depleted are the qualities that set it above oil.

With such positive associations between aroma and knowledge, we might assume that the cultural norm of men using scented oils would be uniformly accepted. And yet, as we saw in chapter 2, the later rabbis were ambivalent about scholars being perfumed in public.[107] It would seem, therefore, that the inversions about women wearing perfume are also in play with respect to men. That is to say, a metaphor or interpretation that compares a scholar to a luscious fruit, or learning to sniffing—although erotically charged—does not present the level of threat that the "real" scented man poses in terms of awakening sexual desire. Like the Abtinas women, who are identifiable by their lack of perfume, absence of fragrance helps identify the scholar (*talmid ḥakham*, תלמיד חכם). On this same axis lies the case of R. Eliezer, whose sacrifice in pursuit of scholarship causes him to have bad breath (see chapter 1). His foul odor identifies him as a scholar. As we will see in the next chapter, although odors like R. Eliezer's may be offensive to humans, they are pleasant to God, for they represent the human's commitment to the Divine.

Both of the passages analyzed here, as well as that of R. Eliezer as a young student, identify study or scholarship as one of the rabbis' most prized values. In addition to expressing the importance of study, the midrashim also indicate hierarchies of the rabbis themselves through the metaphorical expression of scent. Aspects of fragrance (inhalation, ephemerality, and nondilution or nondissipation) are contrasted with oil (substance, dissipation). As in the midrashim concerning women, positive attitudes about scent and scholarship become more ambivalent when the focus turns to flesh-and-blood human beings and real-life situations.

The midrashim also portray a deep, almost intuitive understanding of perfume—a familiarity that arguably cannot come from the Bible alone.

R. Akiba's assignment of a higher value to fragrance than to oil reflects an intimate acquaintance with such things, for that appraisal does not appear in the Songs, where fragrance and oil are tied together. Ultimately, though, the point of the midrash is not to reflect on aroma; such reflections are part of the interpretive process and, along with the biblical material, lay the foundation upon which the new metaphoric layers are built.

Mitzvot and Righteousness

The rabbis emphasize the importance of study and the characteristics of the sage through their interpretation of fragrance, and they do the same thing on the subject of the "laws," or "commandments" (*mitzvot*, מצות), and "righteousness" (*tzedakah*, צדקה). In fact, many of their concerns, beliefs, principles, and practices, as expressed in *Songs Rabbah*, are associated with pleasing odors in some form or another. For instance, the redemption of the Israelites from Egypt is described in terms of Israelite "repentance" (*teshuvah*, תשובה), and the penitents are compared to the vines that "give forth their fragrance" (*Songs Rab.* 2:13). Similarly, a verse of Scripture that one "interprets" (*doresh*, דורש) is likened to scented oil and described as having "all manner of excellent thoughts" (4:10). In some cases, the pleasant scent is applied figuratively to a character or actor. In *Songs Rabbah* 2:2, R. Ḥanan of Sepphoris describes the person who performs "acts of loving kindness" (*gemilut ḥasadim*, גמילות חסדים) as a "lily among the thorns." In the same passage, the matriarch Rebekah is described as a lily among the thorns because she is a "righteous one" (*tzadeqet*, צדקת) among many tricksters. Although these concepts come from the Bible, they are also constructions and exertions of rabbinic authority. The rabbis, for example, include those *mitzvot* received at Sinai (for which, as we saw, Israel exudes a pleasing odor) as well as those commandments they perceive as unfolding from their own interpretation of Scripture.

As a window onto this kind of exegetical articulation, this section of the study examines two midrashim in detail. The first concerns itself with the importance of the "commandment" (*mitzvah*, מצוה) as a means by which to know God. The second midrash includes several of the rabbinic values already discussed, but the analysis focuses on the role of the "righteous" (*tzadikim*, צדיקים). As with the other midrashim, experience with aroma underlies the interpretations and serves as a structural component in their meaning.

The first example returns us once again to Songs 1:3: "The fragrance of your oils is good; oil poured forth, your name. Therefore the maidens love you."

> *The fragrance of your oils is good.* R. Yannai, the son of R. Shimon [said]: "All the songs that were said before You by the fathers, they are scents, but ours are *oil poured forth, your name* (Song 1:3)." It is like a man who pours oil from one vessel to another. All the commandments that the fathers did before You, they are scents, but ours are *oil poured forth, your name.* Two hundred and forty-eight commandments are positive and three hundred and sixty-five commandments are negative. (*Songs Rab.* 1:3)

The point of R. Yannai's comment is to stress the importance of the commandments received at Sinai as the means by which to know God ("your name"). To demonstrate his point, the rabbi employs a temporal comparison of the commandments, past and present, by layering another metaphor onto the verse from Songs, one that includes the key terms from the verse, "fragrance" and "oil." The three-part structure of the midrash begins with a declarative statement, continues with a brief parable, and concludes with a more specific elucidation of the message.

R. Yannai begins his comment in response to the first segment of Songs 1:3: "The fragrance of your oils is good." But he is also referring to the first verse of Songs: "The song of songs that are Solomon's." The sage describes these songs of the forefathers as scents. He then turns to the second segment of verse 1:3, declaring, "but ours are *oil poured forth, your name.*" As in the midrash on R. Akiba and his teachers, R. Yannai uses the dissimilarities between fragrance and oil to support his interpretation of the difference between the forefathers and later generations in terms of their songs. In the short parable that follows—"It is like a man who pours oil from one vessel to another"—R. Yannai indicates that he is interpreting the second segment of the verse, "oil poured forth, your name." In the explanation of the parable, R. Yannai not only repeats the comparison between the forefathers and the current generation, he also intimates what he means by "songs." He says, "All the commandments that the fathers did before You, they are scents, but ours are *oil poured forth, your name.*" Songs, that is, are commandments. Yet the commandments of the forefathers are only scents, whereas those of the current generation are oil. R. Yannai appears to value the substance of oil over the ephemerality of fragrance, a value reversal of the midrash on R. Akiba. But his interpretation should not be read as valuing his own generation over that of the forefathers. Rather, the sage distinguishes his own generation from earlier ones through access to "your name" (*shemekhah,* שמך); this is the new metaphor introduced in this segment of the original verse.

The forefathers may have sung songs, but they did not have the "song of songs"—that is, God's name—to sing to God. R. Yannai creates a metaphor of progression from fragrance to oil, in which fragrance is equated with the forefathers' songs, or commandments, before the giving of the law at Sinai, and oil is imagined as the covenant given at Sinai. The alliteration of the Hebrew words for "oil" (*shemen,* שמן) and "your name" (*shemekhah,* שמך) further aid the sage's interpretation of a deep connection between the commandments and God's name.[108] According to the sages, one comes to know God's name—that is, to experience God intimately—by following the commandments. In addition, R. Yannai makes a significant religious claim at the end of his comment by mentioning the 613 commandments. As these are the entirety of the scriptural commandments as reckoned by the rabbis, the focus becomes not just the generations after Sinai but specifically the rabbinic generations.

This midrash, like its "aromatic" counterparts, requires that the reader employ several latent understandings of the perception of scent in order to fully comprehend it. Although scent resides in substances, fragrance itself has no form and can waft in the air even if the substance that produces the scent is absent. Therefore, experience of fragrance can be uncanny, elusive, or transitory. On the one hand, fragrance can be evidence of the substance but lacking in source. The forefathers carry out commandments, but they do not have the actual law, or source, upon which to base their actions. After reception of the law at Sinai, the fragrance becomes oil. The oil, as God's name, pours from human to human, possibly even from teacher to student, through the rabbinic nomenclature of the 613 commandments. On the other hand, fragrance can also be evidence of the commandments the forefathers performed. The oil, as God's name and law, pours from one generation to the next in a continuous flow that emits fragrance along the way. With the mention of the 613 commandments at the end of the interpretation, the rabbis assert their authority over what the commandments entail.

R. Yannai's interpretation of Songs 1:3 incorporates the original verse from Songs but completely transforms the secular love scene it portrays. By focusing his interpretation on the second segment of the verse—"oil poured forth, your name"—R. Yannai takes the erotic intimacy of "the fragrance of your oils is pleasing," suspends this heightened sensation, and redeploys it toward a spiritual and esoteric knowledge of the divine name. The *eros* of the love of God is further transformed into the commandments. Through this atomization and reuse of the biblical verse, R. Yannai sets forth a thoroughly rabbinic theological concept: performance of the 613 commandments is the only path by which to know and to love God. In the course of his interpretation, R. Yannai incorporates oppositional ideas about fragrance and its ephemerality and oil and its substantiality. He focuses on the qualities of perfume—wafting, flowing, attraction—and a sense of proximity that leads to intimacy and intimate knowledge. The ways in which we draw perfume from outside our bodies into ourselves physically when we smell it, and the ways in which it, in turn, alters us emotionally and causes us to act differently, are also at work. R. Yannai uses all these characteristics of perfume to support his cultural assertions of rabbinic authority over the law, knowledge of the ineffable name of God, internal love of the Divine, and external manifestation of the commandments.

The next midrashic passage, which portrays the value of righteousness through righteous persons, also draws on a verse from Songs encountered earlier: "A lily among the thorns, so is my companion among the daughters" (Song 2:2). We have seen that the male lover compares the beauty of his beloved to the lily, and that in the midrash Israel is cast as the lily and God as the male speaker. Throughout the entire pericope (*Songs Rab.* 2:2), the comparison of Israel to the lily among the thorns is sustained, and the "thorns" variously represent Egypt during Israel's sojourn there and "the nations," or Rome, in her current situation.[109] The midrash below comes at the end of the cycle, and so ties together many of the preceding interpretations. In this portion of the unit, the lily is both Israel and the righteous:

> R. Abun[110] said, "Just as dry heat from the sun beats upon the lily and it withers, but when the dew falls, it blooms. So too as long as the shadow of Esau endures, as if it were possible, Israel appears withered in this world. But [when] the shadow of Esau passes, Israel goes on thriving, as it is written, *I will be as the dew to Israel; he shall blossom as the lily* (Hos 14:6)."
>
> Just as the lily ceases forever together with[111] its scent, so Israel perishes together with commandments and good deeds. Just as the lily is only for fragrance, so the righteous are created only for the redemption of

Israel. Just as the lily is placed on the table of kings at the beginning and at the end [of the meal], so [is] Israel whether in this world or in the next world. Just as the lily is recognized[112] among plants, so Israel is distinguished among the nations of the world. As it is said. *All who see them will know them [because they are a seed the Lord has blessed]* (Isa 61:9). Just as the lily is prepared for Sabbaths and festivals, so Israel are prepared for a redemption tomorrow.

R. Berekhiah said, "The Holy One, blessed be He, said to Moses, 'Go and say to Israel: My children, when you were in Egypt, you were like a lily among the thorns. Now that you are entering the land of Canaan, be [again] like a lily among the thorns. Be mindful that you follow the ways of neither the one nor the other.' Therefore it is written, *After the doings of the land of Egypt, in which you dwelt, you shall not do. And after the doings of the land of Canaan, where I will bring you, you shall not do [and their laws you shall not follow]*." (Lev 18:3). (*Songs Rab.* 2:2)

This midrash may be divided into three parts. First, R. Abun compares Israel's situation under Rome (Esau) to the withered lily that will thrive in the future.[113] In the second portion of the midrash, Israel and the righteous are compared on many levels to different aspects of the lily. The formulaic construction employed to accomplish this series of comparisons is "Just as . . . so." The third part of midrash acts as the prooftext and summary for the entire pericope.[114]

The supposition that Israel is the favored possession of God in comparison to the other nations is depicted in the parable we investigated earlier and in R. Abun's response to the verse "Like a lily among the thorns, so is my companion among the daughters." As the lily, Israel is in her withered state when Rome (the thorns, now overlaid with the metaphor of Esau) is in power. Her predicament though, is temporary, for in the future, when Rome no longer holds power over Israel, she will bloom. However, the metaphor becomes mixed. The initial image of Esau as the sun or dry wind that causes the flower, Israel, to wither is supplanted by the image of Esau's "shadow" (*tsel*, צל) passing—as if the tenebrous climate caused by Esau's shadow of power blocks Israel's sunlight and freedom, stunting her growth and preventing her from blossoming.[115]

The second segment of the midrash introduces a comparison of the lily and its aroma to Israel and its "commandments" (*mitzvot*, מצות) and "good deeds" (*ma'asim tovim*, מעשים טובים). The syntax of this version allows for several interpretive possibilities. The most obvious reading would be that when the lily dies, its fragrance also dies. Similarly, when Israel ceases to exist or is destroyed, so too her commandments and good deeds are gone forever. However, another assessment, in better accord with the rest of the piece,[116] is more probable: the lily dies "because of" or "by means of" (*'al gav*, על גב) its pleasant odor. In other words, because of its pleasant fragrance, the lily is picked and therefore dies. Likewise, Israel dies because she follows the commandments and performs good deeds. The formulation is highly suggestive of martyrdom: Israel and her adherents forfeit their lives because of their commitment to God.[117]

The reading that God plucks Israel, the fragrant flower, because of her aroma resonates with the sentences that follow. The lily's sole purpose is to create a pleasant scent. This becomes the metaphor for those of Israel who perform commandments and good deeds: the righteous. The only reason for their "creation" (*bara'*, ברא)[118] is to bring about redemption for Israel by means of their "death" (they "cease to exist"—*batal*, בטל). Here, in this stark contrast between death and creation, we begin to see the strange affinity fragrance has for images of the erotic and death.[119]

The ensuing lines strengthen these associations as they continue to build on the themes of election, death, and redemption. These lines also form bridges to the biblical text, as well as to everyday life. For example, the lily, placed on the table at the beginning and end of a meal, could represent a bouquet of flowers but more probably refers both to incense and to sacrifice. The reference to the "table of kings" alludes to the table of God (either the altar or God's table in heaven) and to the wealth of kings. The image of Israel placed on the table of the king in this world and the next is highly suggestive of sacrifice upon the altar, death and rebirth, and Israel's current situation and her future glory in the time of the messiah. In the line that follows, just as the lily stands out among the plants of the garden, Israel's unique features and position stand out among the nations. Like the lily and incense, she is exotic, different from all other nations. Similarly, the sense of Israel's exclusivity may be inferred, particularly with reference to her future redemption, which is explicitly stated, as she is "prepared for tomorrow's redemption," just as the lily or incense is prepared for Sabbath and festivals.

These images are highly reminiscent of the scent associations we have seen in the Bible for incense. They include atonement, wafting, a sense of travel upward (toward God), sacrifice, appeasement, exclusivity, and the exotic. Combined with the affinities of "the righteous," the scene suggests that the death of the righteous brings about atonement for Israel and the world, the appeasement of God's wrath, and redemption for Israel. Just as the plucking and smelling of the lily both kills the lily and creates a sense of pleasure and rest for the one who enjoys the aroma, so the death of the righteous wafts, like incense, up toward God, who inhales the scent, is appeased, and redeems Israel. But these biblical images that surround sacrifice are employed at the same moment in a new and highly erotic evocation of martyrdom in which the lover, or God, describes his beloved, the righteous of Israel, as the lily among the thorns, and her death—brought about through her commitment of love for the Divine—saves the world. The eroticism of the Songs is not only maintained but heightened by the exoticism of the king's table and the festive meal.

In these midrashim on rabbinic values, the biblical and cultural images work together—layering metaphor upon metaphor—until the message is wholly new and uniquely rabbinic. No longer situated in the garden or other natural setting, the images are applied to the intangible yet culturally real concepts with which the rabbis engage as their primary purpose. New metaphorical actors (forefathers, current generations of Israel, the righteous, the doers of good deeds) and actions (good deeds, acts of loving kindness, sacrifice of the body) are applied to the referent metaphors already present in the Songs (the lily, oil, fragrance, etc.). Yet, however striking the interpretation, the preservation of the original characteristics of those referents (wafting, flowing, attraction, *eros*)[120] as part of the interpretive process illustrates how everyday life enters into the process of interpretation and promotes the rabbinic agenda and theological claims.

Historical Moments and Aroma

One of the primary features of rabbinic interpretation is the "retelling" of Israel's history, and several of the midrashim presented so far have included within their interpretive frame what the rabbis consider historical events.[121] These include the giving of the law at Sinai, the period of wandering in the wilderness, and the future redemption of the Jewish people or the period of the messiah. Few of these biblical or cosmic events include aroma references in their original form, but by reading the verses from the Songs into them, the rabbis embellish and even radically change these narratives. One example of such a "retelling" is found in the midrash on the Israelite women who fumigate their garments using the spices they collect from manna (*Songs Rab.* 4:14). In this story the daily chore of feeding one's family, which had been linked with the miracle of the gift of food given personally by God, is joined to images of perfume and incense in the context of arousal and sexual repast. The tropes of scent are used in this case to structure place (the wilderness) and historical event (forty years of wandering). Naturally, not all scent-infused midrashim are as creative as this one about the "spices from manna." The images of frankincense and myrrh in the Songs inspire many midrashim on animal or incense sacrifice in the Temple. In other cases, a more subtle reference to scent gives rise to a biblical comparison. "Arise north wind and come south wind, blow on my garden that its spices will flow" (Song 4:16), for example, prompts a comparison between the sacrifices of the Tabernacle with those of the Temple.

This section evaluates three midrashim—all of which portray a historical event from the Bible and are drawn from the same familiar verse from the Songs: "While the king was in his enclosure, my spikenard gave forth its fragrance" (Song 1:12). Each interpretation employs scent images from the verse in different ways and reveals an underlying understanding of, and familiarity with, perfume and incense. Because of differences in the scope and nature of the midrashim, this section is divided into two parts. The first looks at a single midrash in which three rabbis successively interpret the same verse with reference to the same event: the giving of the law at Sinai. The second part examines two midrashim that are structurally similar but depict two different events. In each case, aroma and its multiple associations are employed as interpretive tools that restructure the places and events and even the interpretation itself.

The Sinai Event

No other moment in Israel's history is as important to the rabbinic interpreters as the covenant enacted at Sinai. There God gives the law, and Israel compliantly accepts it. Like the prophets before them, the rabbis envision the episode as a marriage in which the two parties come together freely and in love to enter into an eternal mutual commitment. That the event appears in several places in the biblical text does not stop the rabbis from giving it their own unique "spin." In the first example, the successive interpretations move the scene along in time and demonstrate an expanding creativity in the interpretive process:

R. Eliezer, R. Akiba, and R. Berekhiah [disagreed]. R. Eliezer says, *"While the king was in his enclosure.* While the king of kings, the Holy One, blessed be He, was in his enclosure, in the firmament, already Mount Sinai was sending up pillars of smoke. As it is said, . . . *And the mountain was burning with fire [until the heart of the heavens were darkness, clouds, and mist]* (Deut 4:11)." R. Akiba says, *"While the king,* the king of kings, the Holy One, blessed be He, was in his enclosure, in the firmament, already *the glory of the Lord abode on Mount Sinai . . .* (Exod 24:16)." R. Berekhiah says, "While Moses was in his enclosure in the firmament, [for] he may be called king. As it is said, *He was king in Jeshurun when the heads of the people gathered together . . .* (Deut 33:5), already *God spoke all these words . . .* (Exod 20:1)." (*Songs Rab.* 1:12)

This series of brief interpretations spans several generations and thus shows the hand of the redactor. As mentioned above, R. Eliezer, a second-generation Tanna, was one of R. Akiba's teachers. But R. Berekhiah is a fifth-generation Amora. The thrust of the comments appears as snippets on different parts of the chronological events at Sinai and less as an intergenerational disagreement. Each of the interpreters parses the verse from Songs into a scene at Sinai and provides a prooftext for his opinion.

The first interpretation, by R. Eliezer, depicts "spikenard" (*nerd,* נרד) and "gave forth fragrance" (*natan reḥo,* נתן ריחו) as the pillars of smoke that went up from Sinai. Mount Sinai thus becomes the spikenard that sends forth smoke or fragrance into God's chamber in the firmament. The interpretation calls forth an image of the sacrifices at the Temple. Like the aroma of the spikenard wafting horizontally toward the other room and drawing the lover toward his beloved, the smoke rises up to God and draws him down toward earth. However, unlike the male lover in Songs, who remains absent, God is present. The aroma has a positive effect on him, and he comes down to Mount Sinai and speaks from the midst of the fire (Deut 4:12).

Like R. Eliezer, R. Akiba uses "in his enclosure" (*bimesibo,* במסבו) to mean that God is in the firmament. But R. Akiba also uses *bimesibo* (במסבו) to mean "upon his couch," a reference to God's throne of glory. In this case, God sits on his throne on the mountain. Therefore, in addition to God's being in the firmament, a hypostasis of the Divine, his "glory," sits upon the throne: "*the glory of the Lord abode on Mount Sinai.*" Considered in its entirety, the biblical prooftext implies that the cloud that covers God's glory is the referent for "spikenard": "the cloud hid it for six days. On the seventh day, he called to Moses from the midst of the cloud" (Exod 24:16).

R. Berekhiah changes the referent of "the king" from God to Moses. He then interprets "gave forth fragrance" as the words of God, as in "God spoke all these words." Because "gave forth fragrance" applies to the words that God spoke, the term "spikenard" metaphorically represents God. In addition, "these words" are the most intimate and fundamental of God's enunciations, as they represent the Ten Commandments and are spoken directly to the Israelites. R. Berekhiah's interpretation, therefore, reaches a new metaphorical plane; in his view, the scent is the breath of the Divine.

Each of the interpretations demonstrates slight alliances and shifts in the scent associations employed. While the pillar of smoke (in R. Eliezer's midrash) and the cloud (in R. Akiba's midrash) are akin to animal or incense sacrifice that wafts upward and draws God downward, the commandments are spoken to the people once God has already come to rest on the mountain (Rabbis Akiba and Berekhiah). In this way, the association changes to a dialogical, horizontal orientation. The scent wafts to the Israelites and draws them toward God. Through an allusion to the intimacy of the relationship between God and Israel, R. Berekhiah's statement also conveys an erotic dimension of the scene at Sinai, as the Israelites are drawn to the spikenard that is the breath of God.

War and Redemption

While the next two midrashim also employ Songs 1:12 as their basis, the pertinent terms are "my spikenard" and "while" (*'ad she*, . . . עד ש). Unlike the passage above, which historicizes the Songs through scent imagery but leaves the foundation of the biblical narrative intact, the midrashim below adorn the biblical moments with so much new information that they seem more like creations than retellings. Although the two interpretations are similar in format, they are different in historical scene, message, and nuance.

In the first, R. Yudan interprets the verse from Songs to refer to the period of King Hezekiah's battle with Sennacharib of Assyria:

> [*While the king was in his enclosure, my spikenard gave forth its fragrance* (Song 1:12)]. R. Yudan said, "While Hezekiah and his forces[122] were still eating their paschal lambs in Jerusalem, God had already advanced [on the enemy][123] that night, as it is said, *And that night, the angel of*

the Lord went out and struck in the camp of the Assyrians (2 Kgs 19:35)."
(*Songs Rab.* 1:12)

The midrash employs the same structure as its counterparts above. Although the verse from Songs is not repeated in the midrash, R. Yudan draws his comments from specific terms in the verse and then cites a prooftext in conclusion.[124] The rabbi uses the term "while" to set the historical scene of Sennacharib's attack against King Hezekiah. More specifically, the time period is the night before the assault. God sends out the "angel of the Lord," who may also be understood as the angel of death, to strike the Assyrian camp. The scene presents three possibilities for the referents to "spikenard" and "fragrance." The first is that King Hezekiah's observance of the law, for which he is well known in the Bible, acts like perfume or sacrifice upon God and encourages God to attack the enemy. In this case, the aroma suggests attraction, appeasement, and an upward spatial orientation of the scent that brings God down toward earth.[125] The second referent for "spikenard" may be God, who sends the angel out like fragrance. A third possibility is that the angel is the spikenard and his fragrance is his strength in attacking the camp. The affinities of the last two "aromatic" images include strength, victory, and death (of the enemy). In addition, the angel of death and fragrance are similar in that neither can be seen and both often go undetected. They are both ethereal and insubstantial. Similarly, Sennacharib's men perceive the angel of death only after it has come and gone and the men are dead.

More significantly, there is no scent reference or Passover sacrifice or meal in the biblical text. R. Yudan has created a subplot by pairing the verse from Songs with the verse from 2 Kings and inserting a strong religious marker (the eating of the paschal lamb) into the story. This subplot also contains deep cultural markers (specific to the rabbis) and serves as a paradigm for the complex rabbinic reading of the biblical narrative. In the biblical account, when King Hezekiah discovers Sennacharib's plans, he is frightened (2 Kgs 19:1–4) and turns to the prophet Isaiah for guidance. Sennacharib's forces are much larger and more powerful than King Hezekiah's, and it is likely that Sennacharib will rout Hezekiah's army and capture Jerusalem handily. In the midrash, R. Yudan reverses the images. The king is portrayed as feasting the night before the battle, while the enemy is killed by the angel of death. Metaphorically, it is the enemy who smells of fear, not Hezekiah. The Israelite king experiences victory, while the enemy is defeated before the battle can take place. The aroma of victory and the stench of death, decay, and defeat are identical in terms of smell but represent opposite values here. The single aroma is multivalent—both positive and negative at the same time but connoting two different meanings to two different audiences. The juxtaposition of King Hezekiah's celebration of Passover eve and the stress of impending battle allows the reader to infer that it is Hezekiah's piety and observance that bring about the death of his enemy by means of God's agent. The midrash also deftly communicates a message of hope and future power for the Jews, which will be brought about by their faithful observance of the law.

The next and final midrash in this category employs the same structure in its opening sentences as the interpretation by R. Yudan. However, the creative subplot articulated by R. Abbahu takes a different turn. The scene takes place during the days of the final plague in Egypt:

> R. Abbahu said, "While Moses and Israel were still reclining and eating their paschal lambs in Egypt, God had already advanced [on the Egyptians]. As it is said, *And it came to pass at midnight, that the Lord struck every firstborn in the land of Egypt* (Exod 12:29)." (*Songs Rab.* 1:12)[126]

The structure of R. Abbahu's comment parallels that of R. Yudan's.[127] The new referents are inserted into the literary structure of the verse from Songs and followed by a prooftext. Therefore, "while" becomes the moment of the tenth plague and the first celebration of the Passover, and "his enclosure," or "on his couch," places Moses and Israel at the festive table. R. Abbahu clarifies and strengthens the reading of "my spikenard" by clearly articulating God as the referent. In this narrative, God is the agent of destruction in Egypt, as he personally redeems Israel.[128] The next portion of this midrash differs from the Hezekiah midrash in structure but reintroduces some of the same thematic concerns:

> It is the opinion of R. Abbahu to say, "My stench[129] gave forth its odor," in order to teach that the odor of the blood was bad and so the Holy One, blessed be He, brought forth for them a pleasant fragrance from the spices of the garden of Eden, and they were dying[130] to eat. They said to him, "Our master Moses, give us something to eat." Moses said to them, "Thus the Holy One, Blessed be He, said to me, '*No stranger shall eat of it* (Exod 12:43).'" They arose and separated all the strangers from among them, and they were still dying to eat. They

said to him, "Our master Moses, give us something to eat." And he said to them, "Thus the Holy One, Blessed be He, said to me, '*Every male slave that is bought with money, when you have circumcised him, then he may eat of it* (Exod 12:44).'" They arose and circumcised their slaves, and they were still dying to eat. They said to him, "Give us something to eat." And he said to them, "Thus the Holy One, Blessed be He, said to me concisely,[131] '*Anyone who is uncircumcised may not eat of it* (Exod 12:48).'" Immediately, every single one put his sword to his thigh and circumcised himself. (*Songs Rab.* 1:12)[132]

Structured as a dialogue between the Israelites and Moses, the passage defines all who must be circumcised in order to participate in the Passover rite. At first glance, the midrash appears similar to the argument, analyzed in the beginning of this chapter, between Rabbis Meir and Judah on the same verse from Songs. However, whereas R. Meir's position is that the "odor" (*reaḥ*, ריח), in the phrase "gave forth its odor," was pleasant and evil, R. Abbahu claims that the "odor" stinks.[133] Further, R. Abbahu interprets "spikenard" positively, as the aroma of the spices God wafts from the Garden of Eden. This pleasant fragrance arouses hunger in the Israelites.

As in the midrash on the golden calf, the subplot of this episode is triggered by a confusion in chronology. In Exodus 11:4–8, God tells Moses that the plague of the firstborn is imminent, but what follows in Exodus 12:21–28 is an outline of the laws governing the paschal lamb and observance of the Passover feast days. Thus it appears that the Israelites eat the paschal lamb while they are still in Egypt, while the firstborn are being killed. In the biblical text this is problematic for a number of reasons. First, God states in verse 48 that every male who participates in this ritual must be circumcised. The Israelite male slaves are not in the habit of circumcision, as proved by the need for Joshua to perform a mass circumcision forty years later, just before the Israelites enter Canaan (Josh 5:2–3). Because the verse in Joshua may be construed to mean that Joshua circumcises the males "again" (ושוב), however, the rabbis are free to understand the occasion of the first paschal feast as evidence for the first group circumcision.[134] Another, more obvious problem with the chronology is that the ordinances for Passover say that "slaves" must be circumcised in order to participate in the festivity. This passage is irrelevant to the Israelites, who are slaves themselves!

R. Abbahu alters significantly the narrative of the final plague and Israelite redemption from Egypt. In so doing, he includes several of perfume's characteristics, such as wafting, attraction, seduction, and the aroma of the garden, which in turn awaken the hunger of the Israelites. In R. Abbahu's interpretation, it is God who wafts the pleasant scent (rather than the beloved, the Israelites). The erotic nature of the Songs is maintained in the midrash through God's demonstrated love for the Israelites and his arousal of their hunger, which is both real and a metaphor for the lovers. The sexually charged eating imagery already present in the Songs also remains, but it is now transformed into the religious rite of eating the lamb.

By using his special perfume—the spices of the Garden of Eden—God stimulates his beloved, Israel. And as her hunger is aroused, God is able to entice her to ritual piety. More precisely, he takes on the typically female role of seductress to get Israel to do his bidding.[135] Two primary rabbinic concerns are rearticulated here: the importance of redemption from Egypt and observance of the commandment of circumcision. In each of the midrashim covered here, God's intervention in history and his immanence in the world are depicted by the rabbis through the embellishment of historical moments as well as the articulation of ritual observance. The Songs, with its multilayered scent images already encoded with their own affinities and associations, provides the means by which the rabbis vigorously and creatively reinterpret these events. God acts personally on behalf of the Israelites; he actively cares for them and lures them as a lover might his beloved; he is concerned for them above all others and interacts with them intimately. The selection process the rabbis employ in deciding which events to narrate and which to expunge through their interpretive choices represents yet another cultural assertion. Rarely do we see midrashim on the peaceful reunion between Esau and Jacob or the installation of the Aaronide priesthood. In addition, the highly embellished narratives are examples of an active *poesis*—a literary creative force that is not otherwise present in the biblical text and that is both culturally constructed and reflective of the concerns of the rabbis themselves.

Conclusion

As the rabbinic interpreters analyze the Songs and other passages in the biblical corpus, they interpret the aroma imagery as well. As a result, these images are reframed and often transformed dramatically. This chapter evaluated midrashim in terms of four basic categories: those that pertain to geography; references to the "other"; those that display the values and people the rabbis hold in high esteem; and depictions of significant "historical" moments. Each midrash was subjected to contextual reading in order to tease out its significance and relation to the biblical verse as well as its message, structure, and other particularities. As part of this exercise, the associations and characteristics of the scent images were highlighted—particularly with respect to which images might be textually and which might be culturally derived. In many instances the rabbis begin with the biblical references to aroma and then "massage" and reemploy these images or alter them dramatically to signify new symbols and referents. We have seen that as the rabbinic interpreters layer new metaphors on top of those already present in the Songs, they entwine the old associations with the new.

In many instances, older terms resurfaced with new meaning. For example, "soothing odor," referring in the biblical text to a properly performed sacrifice, was employed to connote the role of Israel in the world, the commandments, or righteousness. The significance of incense in the priestly writings—its connotations of exclusivity, chosenness, and acceptance—are associated in the midrashim with Israel, Jacob, and scholars. Inversions also occur. So, for example, the absence of perfume on the Abtinas women is depicted positively. Likewise, the bad breath of R. Eliezer, interpreted as perfume, signifies an even stronger inversion. Metonymic images of items that produce fragrance, such as the lily, spice, and spikenard, which are linked in the biblical text to "the female," "attraction," and "seduction," are applied in the midrashim to the righteous, scholars, and even God. In the midrashim pertaining to scholarship, the human sense of olfaction is engaged to describe the highest form of Torah study. In addition, we have seen that many of the associations of incense and perfume in the biblical text are carried into the rabbinic literature with significant changes in nuance and new forms of layering of ideas and metaphors. The righteous, who are first identified with perfume, love, and images from the garden of the Songs, are then identified with incense. Their sacrifice, as depicted in acts of both love and death, atones for Israel or the world and appeases God by generating a soothing odor. The geographic or directional valences are also realigned in these midrashim, as the horizontal wafting of perfume in the Songs is reinterpreted as an incense sacrifice that floats upward to God and, in turn, brings him downward toward earth.

The midrashim also reflect the rabbis' everyday experience with perfume and incense. One rabbi draws a comparison using his personal opinion about the fragrances he most enjoys. Another demonstrates his awareness that fumigated scents enter into the weave of clothing and hair. Other voices draw on a deep understanding of how perfume operates emotionally—calming anger, encouraging emotional impulsiveness, creating a sense of well-being, and arousing sexual desire. Personal knowledge of and experience with perfume, oil, and incense inform each of these interpretations, providing not only some interesting artifact or anecdote but supplying the spark behind what is creative and new in these interpretations.

As with the biblical material, the four categories used in this analysis are really a subjective classification that serves as an organizing principle in the evaluation of the streams of tradition and ideas. In fact, almost every midrash could be seen through one or more of these lenses, because each of them employs metaphors and symbols that are in flux. That said, the divisions allow us to determine the extent to which the themes, metaphors, and associations set forth in the Bible are continued in the rabbinic interpretations with slight and significant alterations, and in which areas complete transformation occurs. In many of the midrashim on "historical moments," aroma is deployed as an interpretive tool—bringing scent into discussions where it had not been before—in order to render new frames, scenes, events, and meanings. This chapter has reviewed the scent associations that are sustained or arise through the interpretive process and has determined that in almost every instance, those that originally appear in the Songs, and some that appear in other places, remain and are reemployed. Moreover, in the discussion of the role of Israel and the righteous, in particular, the priestly valences (such as atonement, appeasement, and exclusivity) are combined with the erotic elements of the poetry of the Songs and are highly suggestive of emotional and physical sacrifice, suffering, and death. The next chapter takes up these issues and locates them within the fragrant garden, the life of Abraham, and as the ultimate result of Jewish observance. Here, the strange triangulation that Rindisbacher draws among scent, death, and the erotic is fully laid out, even as it confounds explanation or justification.[136]

Soothing Odors: Death, Suffering, and Sacrifice

When people die, rather than sigh the exhalation of soothing, calm sleep, they gulp and gasp, suck and swallow air as their bodies begin to shut down. Without sedatives or painkillers, death can be a painful, writhing agony—a face contorted, red and splotchy, crying out until it growls or moans for release. At best, death has no smell; at worst, it stinks of a fetid and rotted body unable to care for itself. And sometimes death is messy. It is an ugly business; little of it, save maybe its victim, is beautiful or tranquil, and nothing about it is desirable except that its finality surely ends the suffering of dying. There is nothing here that makes one think of perfume, of the erotic, of beauty. Naught that might draw us to it, to embrace it or yearn for it. Yet in the hands of the rabbis, death is utterly transformed. With its ample capacity for creative, imaginative force, interpretation is able to harness enough metaphor, simile, and allusion to change all that death and dying truly are. By recombining poetry, forming new associations, and layering their elucidations, the rabbinic voices redeem death by the most sublime imagery and sensual comparisons. That is to say, these exegetes delicately translate their deepest theological conceptions about suffering, death, and martyrdom onto the frames of erotic pleasure and biblical sacrifice.

Like the righteous who act as the blossom among the bramble and atone for the sins of the world, the midrashim examined in this chapter employ the images of the flower, the beloved, the garden, and all the attendant imagery of perfume—its wafting, attraction, and enticement—to describe the reciprocal love of man and God as evidenced in the suffering and death of the upright. But not only this; these interpretations also draw on the images of incense found in the priestly writings of the Hebrew Bible—sacrifice, atonement, and exclusivity—and thus hint at both the intimacy and desolateness that these rabbis feel in their love of the Divine. Throughout, images of perfume float horizontally to draw people in, and those of incense rise upward to be inhaled by God. In the most dramatic of these cases, the sacrifice and death of the righteous person both draw in the convert and produce a "soothing odor" for God's benefit, triggering God's immanence and immediate human atonement and redemption. This chapter, therefore, seeks out the righteous—whether rabbis, students, Abraham, or martyrs. It groups the midrashim in order to explore the layered and interlocking *topoi* of death, suffering, sacrifice, and martyrdom, and it highlights the awareness of perfume, incense, and the flow of scent that is an integral part of the interpretive process and message.

Flowers, Perfume, and the Angel of Death

As they did with almost all the events of daily life, the rabbis imbued the practices and rituals surrounding death with multiple meanings and significance. And while few of these connotations surface in the legal writings, midrash is replete with them. But even as the legal notations depict preparation of the body in the home, the making and carrying of the bier through town, and burial in caves, there is little attestation in these legal notes to the wide-reaching association of death with the garden that is so apparent in the many midrashim on the subject. Similarly, just as the specific rationale for burial with perfume is elusive because it is nowhere discussed in the rabbinic legal texts, the sustained comparison of the scholar to perfumed oil is linked to death in the midrashim and may point toward some of the underlying motivations for the ritual practice.

Plucking the Righteous

Although it lacks a direct reference to scent, the opening of R. Shimon's eulogy for R. Ḥiyya is indicative of many midrashim that draw on the garden from the Songs in reference to death: "R. Shimon entered and eulogized him, '*My lover has gone down to his garden, to the beds of spice, to graze in the gardens and to gather lilies* (Song 6:2).[1] The Holy One, Blessed be He, knows the deeds of R. Ḥiyya ben Aviyah and has removed him from the world.'"[2] R. Shimon begins his eulogy for R. Ḥiyya by quoting Songs 6:2. In the poetry of the Songs, the female speaker variously compares her body to the garden, to beds of spice, and to lilies. She imagines the male as coming down to her body the garden, grazing in it, and gathering flowers. Each of the verbs—going down, grazing, and gathering—suggests a sexual encounter. The movement in the verse travels along two spatial axes. The horizontal moves through or across the garden, and this axis also extends from broad to narrow. The garden is the large place in which the beds of spice are located. Even more specific are the lilies, a particular plant among the rows of various flora. As for the vertical axis, the male lover travels downward, and the flowers travel upward as he plucks them.

R. Shimon's interpretation is not triggered by the verse but by the fact of R. Ḥiyya ben Aviyah's death; thus R. Shimon's desire and need to eulogize his colleague. The metaphor that R. Shimon employs already assumes the male lover from the Songs as representing the Divine. However, instead of the female lover representing Israel, R. Shimon assumes the role of the speaker, and his comment focuses on an interpretation of the garden as the world. Like the structure of the verse, in which articulation of the geography begins with the broad and ends with the specific object, R. Shimon narrows the area of the world to a single person. He also maintains the vertical imagery as he depicts the Divine traveling down to the earth and gathering up the rabbi.

This gathering is personal, even intimate, and demonstrates that the structure of the comparison also corresponds to its subject. The flower in the poem stands for one small part of the garden and is singled out for special attention by the male grazer; so too R. Ḥiyya is singled out from all the other people of the world by God.[3] As the flower is considered special because it is both visually beautiful and wonderfully fragrant, so too R. Ḥiyya is considered exceptional because of his good deeds. Although scent is suggested only at a very deep level of embedded imagery (the flower: the rabbi), the pleasant scent of the righteous is a prevalent theme that R. Shimon likely intends, even though he does not openly articulate it. The strong eroticism present within the Songs verse is transformed in the midrash into a subtext of mutual sensual ardor and intimacy. The rabbi loves God and displays his love through a lifetime of devotion dedicated to study and observance of the commandments. Likewise, God responds intimately to the rabbi by gathering up his soul as one gathers lilies.

A recitation similar to R. Shimon's personal reflection occurs with reference to the righteous more generally: "*My beloved,* this is the Holy One, blessed be He; *to his garden,* this is the world; *to the beds of spice,* this is Israel; *to browse in the gardens,* these are the synagogues and houses of study. *And to gather lilies* [means] to remove the righteous who are in Israel."[4] The message and theme of the midrash are essentially the same as those of the eulogy. God gathers the righteous and personally removes them from the world at death. However, through atomization of the *lemma,* the interpretation takes on a four-part structure. The garden represents the world, the beds of spice are Israel, the gardens are synagogues and houses of study, and the lilies are the righteous. As in the eulogy, the geographic spaces in both the poem and the midrash proceed from large to small and from the general to the particular. The description of the garden moves from the entire garden, to the terraces of spices (or rows of plantings), to the specified lilies. The midrash mirrors this continuum by moving its focus from the world, to Israel, to the synagogues and schools, and finally to the righteous individual. Notably, God does not remove the righteous from the world but from the synagogues and houses of study. And although the righteous individuals may or may not be rabbis, the suggestion remains self-referential, as the house of study is synonymous with the rabbinic community.[5]

As in the eulogy, a sense of the erotic remains in the transition from the poetry to the midrash through the intimate bond between God and the righteous. This eroticism is also suggested by the articulation of the garden scene alone—the garden is a place imbued with erotic overtones of potency and sensual arousal. That the garden is a metaphor for this world rather than for heaven or the afterlife seems at once to awaken a receptivity to sentience and sensuality in the reader as well as to heighten the mood of pathos and loss. At the same moment, though, both midrashim transform the natural world into the cultural world of rabbinic values. This is apparent in the chosen referents: rabbis, synagogues and houses of study, the righteous. The rabbis accomplish this transformation by blurring the identity of geography with people. As the areas move from large to small and general to particular, the world becomes a subset of the people in it. That is, the world is not a place; it is the people who live there. Likewise, the synagogues and schools are not buildings; they are the righteous who pray and study there. The associations of the encoded scent messages are similar to those of the priestly literature of the Bible. God is drawn downward toward earth in order to take the rabbi and the righteous upward. In accordance with the lily's special position within the garden, those taken up may be considered chosen; they are the elect of God. Finally, they are as far inside as one may go: they are inside the world, inside the Jewish community, and inside the rabbinic community specifically.

Enticing the Angel of Death

In the midrashim quoted above, the role of aroma is veiled; it is embedded and assumed within the interpretation but remains subtle, subdued. In other interpretations, though, particularly those involving the rabbis or their students, perfume plays a much more dramatic part. For example, in *Genesis Rabbah*, the righteous are shown their reward by God just before they die, but for R. Abbahu this is specified as rivers of balsam (*Gen. Rab.* 62:2). In this way, perfume is called upon to express both a constellation of fundamental rabbinic values (as seen in chapter 4) and to articulate the images of love and death. And, as it does so, a strand of the ambivalent and suspicious feelings that the rabbis exhibit toward perfume, as seen in the legal texts, also emerges in the more lyrical literature. Concurrently, such midrashim reveal a profound understanding of how perfume operates and demonstrate the valences of attraction, desire, and irrationality.

A late Babylonian midrash triggered by the now familiar verse "The fragrance of your oils is good; oil poured forth, your name. Therefore the maidens love you" (Song 1:3) illustrates these points. In the biblical verse, the female beloved speaks to the male lover, and this becomes the point of contention between two rabbis. The midrash, based on *m. 'Abod. Zar.* 2:5, opens with Rabbis Joshua and Ishmael walking down a road.[6] Along the way, R. Ishmael asks his teacher, R. Joshua, several questions. In order to deflect these questions, R. Joshua asks Ishmael whether he thinks Songs 1:2—"Thy love is better than wine"—is directed toward a male or a female. As recounted in the Mishnah, Ishmael replies incorrectly that it is to the female, and R. Joshua quotes Songs 1:3 as his proof ("The fragrance of your oils is good").[7] The Amoraic discussion of this passage and the reasons for R. Joshua's deflection are given extensive treatment in the Talmud Bavli and *Songs Rabbah*. This midrash appears at the very end of the Talmud's discussion:[8]

> Rab Naḥman[9] the son of Rab Ḥisda interpreted: What is the meaning of the verse, *The fragrance of your oils is good [oil poured forth, your name]* (Song 1:3)? To what may a scholar be compared? To a flask of foliatum.[10] When opened, its scent wafts. Covered up, its scent does not spread. And not only this, but also things that are hidden (from him) become revealed to him, as it is said, *Therefore the maidens love you* (Song 1:3), which is read as, "the hidden [love you]." And not only this, but also the angel of death loves him, as it is said, *Therefore the*

maidens love you, which is read as, "The one [appointed] over death [loves you]." And not only this, but also, he inherits both worlds. One is this world and the other is the world to come. As it is said, *maidens,* which is read as, "worlds [love you]." (*b. 'Abod. Zar.* 35b)[11]

The midrash is structured around a parable that compares the scholar to an open and closed bottle of perfume. The *nimshal* of the parable provides several different interpretations of the term *'alamot* (עלמות, maidens),[12] each of which relates to the scholar and builds upon the interpretation before it. One of the difficulties of the piece is that in relation to the midrashic stimulus (the discussion between Rabbis Joshua and Ishmael), the scholar should align with the image of the closed vial of perfume rather than with the open bottle. That is, the scholar who remains quiet rather than incessantly asking questions should be the preferred model, but the images for the term "maidens" (*'alamot,* עלמות) all appear to align with the metaphor of the open flask. This disjunction indicates that the passage may have been appended to the Talmudic discussion. It is possibly a late addition or, more likely, has been imported from another source because of its relevant subject matter. Nevertheless, it reveals deeply held beliefs—some positive, others negative—about the allure and representational force of perfume.

In the first association, Rab Naḥman employs the term "maidens" to describe the scholar, who, motivated by his love of God, pursues knowledge. That which is "hidden" (*'alumot,* עלומות) from the scholar becomes manifest. In this case, the portion of the verse "oil poured forth, your name" recollects R. Yannai's comments on the same verse, wherein he emphasized the importance of the *mitzvot,* access to God's name, and the pouring of commandments from one generation to the next as the primary purpose of the rabbinic enterprise. Moreover, the affinities for pleasing scent and scholarship depicted in the hierarchy of the men of Israel and articulated by R. Akiba's rank are also strongly present here. The scholar, scholarship, and perfume are conjoined with an already agreed upon understanding of the type of scholarship at stake: that of the commandments and the rabbinic interpretations of Scripture. Particular scholars (e.g., R. Akiba, R. Ḥiyya ben Aviyah, etc.) are not named; rather, the midrash includes all scholars as an assumed ideal type.

In the next comparison, the angel of death, the one who is appointed "over death" (*'al mavet,* על מות), is attracted to the scholar who exudes the pleasant scent. The metaphor of the flask of uncorked oil imagines that as the scholar studies, and oil both is poured into him and pours out of him, he emits a pleasant fragrance.[13] The portion of the verse "the fragrance of your oils is pleasing" is stressed. However, as a result of his studies and his love for God, the scholar dies. Like the lily (the righteous person) that God plucks from the world because of its beauty and aroma, the angel of death is attracted to the scholar's fragrance and so kills him. The representation of the angel of death as the male lover and the scholar as the beloved demonstrates the contradictory physical and cultural connotations of perfume. Here, the perfume of knowledge attracts the angel of death and arouses his desire for the scholar. Likewise, the death of the scholar is brought about by perfume, for this same desire works on both the lover and beloved; it turns off rational thought and awakens and arouses an inherent eroticism, the uncontrollable nature of which causes both supreme pleasure and also death.[14] The final comparison of "the maidens" is to the "two worlds" (*'olamot*, עולמות) that the scholar inherits: this world and the next. His reward in this world is both his scholarship (knowledge of the things hidden) and his assurance of a position in the world to come. As for the scholar's reward in the next world, this is probably more personal than eternity or an eternal place of redemption in which all Israel takes part; no doubt, the next world extends to a postmortem heavenly realm in close proximity to God.[15]

The figurative structure of the scholar as a vial resembles that of the righteous person as a lily, as we saw in the previous chapter. And this collocation entails not only the primary images but many of the terms and characteristics attached to them as well. As such, the metaphors and valences that describe the righteous are transferred and applied to the scholar and vice versa. Likewise, the rabbinic values of scholarship, righteousness, and even the *mitzvot* themselves are intricately tied together through reapplication and layering of the fragrance metaphors and their affinities (wafting, attraction, desire, etc.). But the lily and perfume exemplify only half of this equation. The other half is the role of incense and its accrued imagery of sacrifice, atonement, and exclusivity drawn from the priestly literature of the Bible. In the hands of the rabbis, these images are reanimated and reformulated—using methods similar to those of the prophets—in order to frame suffering and death as rabbinic virtues.

Abraham, the Suffering Servant

In rabbinic depictions of Abraham, images of the flower, perfume, and incense come together to create new stories and perpetuate new ideologies because, according to the rabbis, Abraham combines all the elements of righteousness, scholarship, and suffering. And although he does not have access to the commandments of the covenant, the patriarch is accorded special status because of his legacy in being the first to believe in God as a unique and inimitable force in the world. In fact, it is this belief in God that causes much of Abraham's suffering and marks him as a potential martyr.

God Saves Abraham

Although unarticulated in the Bible, the fact of Abraham's suffering can be readily discerned from the events of his life: God asks Abraham to sacrifice his son, Isaac. But Abraham's suffering also derives from a rabbinic legend in which King Nimrod throws Abraham into the fire for his belief in one God and his efforts to proselytize.[16] In these interpretations, Abraham's experience in the fire is compared and contrasted with that of Daniel's three friends, who, the Bible recounts, were thrown into the fiery furnace of King Nebuchadnezzar for their refusal to bow down to his statue. Although the midrash is stimulated by many different verses, it is commonly triggered by reference to the wafting of fragrance, particularly Songs 1:12, "While the king was in his enclosure, my spikenard gave forth its fragrance":

> R. Eliezer ben Jacob and the rabbis [disagreed]. R. Eliezer says, "*While the king*, [this refers to] the king of kings, the Holy One, blessed be He; *was in his enclosure*[17] [this refers to] the firmament [of heaven], the great prince, Michael had already gone down from heaven to rescue Abraham, our father, from the fiery furnace." But the rabbis say, "The Holy One, blessed be He, went down to save him, as it is said, *I am the Lord who took you out of Ur of the Chaldees* (Gen 15:7)." And when did Michael go down? In the days of Ḥananiah, Mishael, and Azariah. (*Songs Rab.* 1:12)

The three-part structure of the midrash is based on a difference of opinion between R. Eliezer and some anonymous rabbis.[18] R. Eliezer's position is presented first, without a prooftext. The opinion of the rabbis is then established and bolstered by a prooftext. The additional line at the end of the midrash furthers the point of the rabbis, as it directly contradicts R. Eliezer's assertion.

As in other midrashim on this verse from Songs, the term "while" (*'ad she,* עד ש) refers to a period of time. In this case, both sides agree that this period of time marks Abraham's unfortunate incident with King Nimrod and confirms that God was in heaven. R. Eliezer asserts that because God was in the firmament of heaven (i.e., in a remote place), he sent the archangel Michael down to save Abraham.[19] It thus appears that R. Eliezer interprets "my spikenard" as God and "gave forth its fragrance" as the archangel Michael. The anonymous rabbis disagree with R. Eliezer's assertion and insist that God personally saves Abraham.[20] At first glance, the rabbis appear to interpret the verse much as R. Eliezer does but assign the phrase "gave forth its fragrance" to God's strength or will in removing Abraham. There is, however, another possibility. The rabbis may understand "spikenard" as Abraham and "gave forth fragrance" as the burning of Abraham's flesh. They may also draw on the understanding of the term "while" to mean that Abraham's flesh burns "until" God comes down from the firmament to rescue him.[21] This interpretation is based on both parts of the verse: "While the king was in his enclosure, my spikenard gave forth its fragrance." It is the scent of Abraham burning that notifies God that he must go down to earth to save Abraham. The prooftext "I took you out of Ur of the Chaldees" (Gen 15:7) bolsters the claim that God personally saves Abraham through reference to God's own words and by employment of a pun. The city of Ur has the same spelling in Hebrew as the word for "light" or "fire" ('*or,* אור). Therefore, the verse is understood as "I took you out of the fire."

This midrash and others like it are found in several sources throughout rabbinic literature, and many of them are quite ancient.[22] As in this one, a comparison is often drawn between the legend of Abraham and the three friends of Daniel (Dan 3).[23] Invariably, both Abraham and Daniel's friends are presented in the midrashic texts as potential martyrs; that is, these characters choose to die public deaths rather than recant their belief in God. So, for example, in *Genesis Rabbah* 39:8, God declares, "I was with you when you willingly offered for my name to go down to the fiery furnace."[24] However, unlike the later martyrologies of the rabbis themselves or other early Christian martyrdom accounts, these vignettes are much less narratival in form and one must read almost every reference in order to grasp and reconstruct the entire narrative that lies behind any single midrash. Each midrash, therefore, is missing some of the key elements that academics employ in order to define the genre of martyrdom.[25] Nevertheless, the rabbis depict both Abraham and Daniel's friends as martyrs. Daniel's friends, even without the help of the rabbinic imagination, declare their love and faith in God. And in almost every midrashic example, God's love for Abraham impels

God to rescue the patriarch. And this love is in no way one-sided; on the contrary, the reciprocity depends completely on Abraham's virtues with respect to his love of God.[26] In addition, in several midrashim, Abraham is closely tied to the conversion of gentiles—a motif common to some of the Christian martyrdoms and apologies.[27] Sedition against the government, another important theme in Christian and Jewish martyrdom accounts, also plays a role in the depictions of Abraham and Daniel's cohort. In the case of Ḥananiah, Mishael, and Azariah, their declaration of faith is coupled with their refusal to bow down to the image erected by the king of himself. In the case of Abraham, his active conversion of the gentiles means that they will no longer view King Nimrod or other gods as divine.

The martyrdom motif is most evident, though, as the connecting tie between aroma and sacrifice. Like Ignatius, who desires to be the sacrifice on the altar, or Polycarp, whose body, though refusing to burn in the oven-shaped fire, gives off the scent of incense, the characteristics of the *spikenard*, or perfume, in the verse from Songs, which entailed horizontal wafting, spreading, and attraction, are now structured with reference to the burning of Abraham.[28] Abraham and God are separated from each other (like the female and male lovers in the Songs). And, like the priestly conception of the aroma of sacrifices depicting a spatial verticality, the fragrance of Abraham's burning flesh travels upward to God and motivates movement of the Divine downward toward earth to save the human. God responds to Abraham through immanence; that is, God makes himself manifest not only in the world but in that spot, as seen in the theological constructions of the priestly literature. God also plays the role of the lover, though, as he is awakened and aroused by the perfume of the beloved—by Abraham's burning flesh.

Abraham, Myrrh, and Incense

The identification of Abraham's near martyrdom with spices, perfume, and attraction, on the one hand, and the characteristics of incense, sacrifice, and suffering, on the other, are even stronger in other midrashim. These two spheres come together most notably around the term "myrrh," which could be used in both perfume and incense. As a result, almost every reference to myrrh in the Songs triggers a midrashic reference, whether explicit or implicit, to Abraham's virtue, his close relationship with God, and his episode in the fire.[29] And these tropes are expressed in terms of the relevant cultural valences that attach to perfume and incense. A midrash on Songs 1:13—"A bundle of myrrh is my beloved to me, he lodges between my breasts"—demonstrates this association:[30]

> *A bundle of myrrh is my beloved to me* (Song 1:13). What is a *bundle of myrrh*? R. Azariah in the name of R. Yehudah expounded the verse with [respect to] Abraham, our father. Just as myrrh is the chief of all spices, so Abraham is the chief of all the righteous. Just as myrrh has no scent until it is in the fire, so Abraham did not make known his deeds until he was sent into the fiery furnace. And, just as anyone who gathers myrrh feels his hands smart, so Abraham afflicted himself and plagued himself with sufferings. *He lodges between my breasts,* [this is Abraham] who was placed between the Divine Presence and the angel, as it is said, *He looked up and he ran to meet them* (Gen 18:2); [that is,] he saw the Divine Presence and he ran to the angel. (*Songs Rab.* 1:13)

The midrash consists of two parts. The first segment is arranged as a series or list of similes that compare the characteristics of myrrh to those of Abraham. The second section interprets the second half of the verse as a metaphor for Abraham's encounter with God and the angels in Mamre (Gen 18:1–5), which in turn becomes an allegorical allusion to Abraham's martyrdom.

Each proof of the midrash describes a different aspect of Abraham's righteousness. Abraham's deeds, his belief in one God, and his efforts to convert gentiles to this belief are not touted by the ancestor himself; they are not known until he is cast into the fire. Abraham's self-inflicted suffering also demonstrates his virtue, as the reference is assuredly connected to his willingness to sacrifice his son.[31] The reference to breasts seeks to define Abraham's righteousness further, as the breasts are said to refer both to the divine presence and to the angel. Just as other martyrs and saints metaphorically serve God on earth through death and come to sit in heaven with God and the angels, so Abraham literally rushes to serve God and the angels on earth (Gen 18:1–5), thereby being "placed between" them on earth and in heaven.

R. Yehudah chooses to compare Abraham to the properties of myrrh by means of wordplay rather than as real associations with the spice. The first assertion, that myrrh was considered the "chief of all spices," is inaccurate, since balsam held this position in the rabbinic community. Further, in the

Hebrew Bible, myrrh is more widely associated with perfumed oil than with incense. It is thus incorrect for R. Yehudah to declare that the spice gives off an odor only when brought near fire or burned. The point is that Abraham is the most righteous of all ancestors, and he is brought near fire and burned. Similarly, "myrrh," or *mor* (מר) in Hebrew, when pronounced *mar*, means "bitter." Abraham's life is not only bitter, the righteous ancestor also "embitters" (*memarer*, ממרר) himself through suffering. However, bitterness is not naturally associated with the spice, and there is no evidence that myrrh was used in food; therefore, this pun is also indicative of a desire to make the word conform to the interpretation rather than to describe any real characteristic of the spice. Finally, the root can be reconfigured into a verb that means "to smart" or "to burn" (*hithmarmer*, התמרמר). Again, there is no evidence outside the rabbinic literature itself to substantiate the claim that myrrh burned the hands of those who worked with it. Because myrrh was used extensively in embalming practices and is obliquely referred to in rabbinic literature as a depilatory,[32] it is possible that it caused "burning." But this quality is not discussed by the ancients who studied flora and fauna, and so it is much more likely that rabbinic references such as this one are derived from the desire for wordplay rather than from some intrinsic quality in the spice.

At the same time, it is no accident that Abraham is compared to myrrh. The motive of these midrashim is to align Abraham with concepts of love and sacrifice, perfume and incense, and their associated signifiers. Because myrrh can be used in perfume and was also widely used as an incense ingredient, the spice may be employed both in erotic metaphors from the Songs and in images of incense sacrifice. The midrash attempts to retain the mood of ardent love of the Songs as it reformulates this love into a description of the relationship between the burning sufferer and the Divine. Thus the associations with the myrrh perfume images (attraction, passion, intimacy) in the Songs are taken up in the relationship between Abraham and God and Abraham's near martyrdom. And this near martyrdom is further associated with myrrh incense images (suffering, sacrifice, and death).

But how do the rabbis make this connection between myrrh and incense sacrifice? They cannot draw on the biblical text because no mention of myrrh appears there. Rather, they establish this connection by reconfiguring the Temple incense recipe and then assuming that myrrh is in the recipe. The following interpretation depicts this process. It is based on the same verse—"My lover is a bundle of myrrh" (Song 1:13)—and it focuses on "bundle of myrrh" as the means of describing the Temple incense:

R. Yoḥanan interpreted [the verse with reference] to the incense of the House of Abtinas. *Bundle of myrrh* (Song 1:13), this is one of the eleven spices that they placed in it. R. Huna said of it: *And the Lord said to Moses: take spices* (Exod 30:34), this is two; *stacte, onycha, and galbanum,* this makes five; *spices*—if you say of the matter that this is two, then didn't it already say "*spices?*" *Let there be an equal part of each,* these are five against the five; that is ten. *And pure frankincense,* that is eleven ingredients. From there the sages investigated and found that nothing is more beautiful for the incense than these eleven ingredients that are in it. (*Songs Rab.* 1:14)[33]

While the midrash is triggered by Songs 1:13, it is structured around a parsing of Exodus 30:34, the description of the incense recipe. Here, R. Huna turns an elaborate, although vague and incalculable, incense recipe from the Hebrew Bible into an even more elaborate and equally vague and incalculable accounting of eleven spices. This is a pure rabbinic creation that is no doubt based on personal experience—either with incense lit after meals or perhaps in the synagogue or even encountered in idolatry or in other "unapproved" settings. R. Yoḥanan inserts myrrh into the recipe by reading the verse from Songs together with the verse from Exodus.[34] Once this connection between myrrh and incense is established, the rabbis are free to associate Abraham with images of incense sacrifice.

Martyrdom and Conversion of the Maidens

Aggadic representations of Abraham's martyrdom event, as well as those of other characters, address more than just the circumstances of impending death. The midrashim also assert theologically significant and complex ideologies as part of their narrative structure. In this way they are similar to other martyrdom accounts, both Christian and Jewish, that often incorporate other motifs and religious messages into the structure of their narratives. Two motifs common to these other martyrdom narratives are "otherness" and conversion. Often the martyr is the "other," or outsider, with respect to the hegemon. As a result, the willing victim stands in stark contrast to the authority figure, who identifies the victim as a threat because of his or her beliefs, or sees the martyr as a solitary figure or iconoclast whose intransigence is a sign of hubris and who therefore deserves death. But because the martyr's "otherness" is driven by steadfast love of God, it is always presented positively—thereby undermining the power of the government or ruling elite and drawing attention to the folly and futility of the perpetrator's actions rather than the victim's. The second motif, that of conversion, is related to the first. Because of the strength and spiritual fortitude of the victim, he or she serves as a model and may inspire witnesses to convert.

Some of the rabbinic midrashim not only demonstrate these thematic elements but also employ metaphors of aroma to express them. One such series or cycle of midrashim links Abraham's "otherness" to his work in converting the gentiles and pairs these images with Daniel's friends and other martyrs. Throughout, fragrance is employed both to convey these thematized points and to link images of love with those of death. The cycle is drawn from the verse "The fragrance of your oils is good; oil poured forth, your name. Therefore the maidens love you" (Song 1:3). In the midrashic sequence, each part of the verse is taken up and reemployed in the interpretation. The first segment of the midrash appears as a homiletic interpretation of Genesis 12:1:

> R. Yoḥanan applied the verse to Abraham our father. When the Holy One, blessed be He, said to him, "*Go forth from your land and from your birthplace* (Gen 12:1)," to what can this be compared? To a flask of scented oil[35] that was resting in one corner and whose scent wasn't spreading. One came and moved it from its place, and its scent spread. Just so the Holy One, blessed be He, said to Abraham, "Abraham, you have many good deeds; you have [done] many commandments; move yourself over the world and your name will grow great in my world." (*Songs Rab.* 1:3)

Although the *lemma* does not appear in the printed edition, the placement of the verse from Genesis 12:1 at the beginning of this section gives the appearance of enjambment, so that Songs 1:3 is synthesized with Genesis 12:1.[36] This is followed by a parable that compares Abraham's impending journey from his homeland to a flask of perfume as yet unopened, the scent of which is therefore not spreading.[37]

The trope of Abraham's pleasant scent, which derives from his continual affinity with myrrh, is so ubiquitous that R. Yoḥanan is able to interpret "the fragrance of your oils" as Abraham without requiring the word "myrrh" for a foundation. Through his observance of the commandments and performance of good deeds, Abraham takes on the metaphorical characteristics of myrrh oil. Like a corked bottle of perfume, the patriarch emits no scent when he stays in the land of his birthplace. To release odor, he must travel the world. At this point in the midrash, "Go forth" (Gen 12:1) is repeated and the narrative thread of Abraham's journey continues:

> *Go forth* (Gen 12:1). What is written after it? *And I will make you a great nation* (Gen 12:2). *Therefore the maidens love you* (Song 1:3). The Holy One, blessed be He, said to him, "Here are many worlds for you." As it is written, *And Abram took his wife, Sarai, and Lot, his brother's son, and all the property they had acquired, and the souls*[38] *that they had made*[39] *in Haran* (Gen 12:5). If the entire world comes together in order to create one gnat, they are not able to create it. Rather, these are the foreign men and women that Abraham and Sarah were converting. Therefore it says, *the persons they made in Haran*.

The midrash extends the scene of Genesis 12:1 by quoting the succeeding verses from Genesis with interspersed portions of the verse from Songs. The final lines of commentary in this segment explain the meaning of the strange term from Genesis 12:5, "they made." Another enjambment occurs in this segment, but the placement of the verses is reversed. The second half of Songs 1:3 follows Genesis 12:5. As a result, the midrash interprets "maidens" (*'alamot*, עלמות) as "worlds" (*'olamot*, עולמות) and describes Abraham's efforts at conversion as "creating souls."[40]

Although this segment of the midrash quotes only the "maidens" portion of the *lemma*, the metaphorical images in the first half of Songs 1:3—"The fragrance of your oils is good, oil poured forth, your name"—are deftly employed in the commentary. Abraham's message is compared to fragrance that spreads; the righteous ancestor travels the world and spreads the message of belief in the one God. As the message spreads, people convert—the creation of "worlds." Consequently, two associated interpretations are encoded with respect to the phrase "oil poured forth, your name." Abraham is the oil that is poured; as the oil flows, God's name spreads to the gentiles. Similarly, as Abraham's scent spreads throughout the world, he becomes famous and the founder of a great nation (i.e., Abraham's name is also like oil poured forth).

The passage continues with details of Abraham's efforts:

> R. Hunya' said, "Abraham was converting the men and Sarah, the women." And why does Scripture teach: *that they made in Haran?* It teaches that Abraham, our father, was bringing them into his house,

and feeding them and giving them drink and making them beloved, and bringing them near, and converting them, and bringing them under the wings of the Shekhinah.

The structure of this segment is an elucidation of two terms from Genesis 12.5, "the persons" by R. Hunya' and "they made." Once again, the text highlights Abraham's role as proselytizer and his metaphorical role as perfume. The narrative inverts the situation depicted in the Genesis account. As the person traveling to distant lands, Abraham is the "foreigner" (*ger*, גר) and therefore should be treated as the guest. But the Bible also presents Abraham as a hospitable host who rushes to welcome his guests and serve them by washing their feet and feeding them good food (Gen 18:1–5). In the midrash, Abraham "converts" (*megayer*, מגייר) the gentiles or "foreigners" (*gerim*, גרים) to belief in God by treating them as special guests. Abraham is not the stranger; the converts are. Twice the word for "bringing" (*makhnisan*, מכניסן) is used. First, Abraham brings these people into his house, and then he brings them under the wings of the Shekhinah. The foreigners do not actively "enter" but are passively "brought." Through the use of this term, location also becomes part of the metaphor. The converts move spatially from the outside to the inside of Abraham's home and figuratively from outside Israel to inside the covenant.[41]

Repetition of the root "to like" or "to love" (*a-h-v*, אהב) forges a direct link between the midrash and the original verse from Songs. This root is found in the *lemma* "Therefore the maidens love you" and in the midrash in Abraham's making the foreigners "beloved." Through Abraham's perfumed scent ("the fragrance of your oils"), already determined as his message of belief in one God, the "foreigners," now in the role of the maidens, are drawn to God and come to love him. As the maidens in the verse from Songs are drawn to the male lover by the fragrance of his perfume, so the foreigners are drawn to God through the perfume that is Abraham and his message. The feeling of being drawn in by perfume is alluded to in the passivity of the converts and in the employment of the term "to bring near," "to invite," "to attract" (*meqarban*, מקרבן).[42] Just as perfume attracts the lovers to each other, lures one to the other, so Abraham acts as an agent of attraction between his guests and the Divine.

These three expressions—"bringing in," "loving," and "bringing near"— are all associated with the operation of perfume through its strongest characteristic, attraction. But as soon as perfume is invoked, all the other associations of perfume also acquire a subtle presence. These include desire, arousal, and irrationality, or, at the very least, the idea that the maidens turn off their rational thought in favor of their erotic impulses. The act of imposing this metaphor on the metanarrative, that of Abraham's efforts at conversion, which result in his near martyrdom in Nimrod's furnace, demonstrates the impulsivity of the converts, for they too may end up in the fire. Although this potential result is strictly implicit in the text, the layering of images and valences from the Songs, combined with the verse and account from Genesis as well as all the other midrashim on Abraham, is extremely suggestive. Each time Abraham, here identified with perfumed oil, is mentioned, his association with myrrh and incense will also be recalled—and with these images the faint lines of suffering, embitterment, and martyrdom may also be perceived in the text. Therefore, not only does the constant layering of images ensure this light tracing of affliction, but the scene itself, in which the patriarch has left his homeland and all that is familiar for travel to unknown places, where he will live among unpredictable people, also implies a hardship of sorts.

In the next section of the midrash, this outline begins to be filled in, as the discussion moves to the topic of redemption:

> R. Berekhiah said, "Israel said before the Holy One, blessed be He, 'Ruler of the universe: Because You bring light to the world, Your name is magnified in the world.' And what is that light? Redemption. In the moment when You bring light to us, many converts come and convert and are added to us."

This portion of the midrash is constructed as a dialogue between Israel and God, in which the reader is privy only to Israel's statement. R. Berekhiah[43] follows the quotation with an explanation of "light." The surface reading of the text draws a parallel between "light" and knowledge of the covenant. As people learn of the one God, they convert and glorify God's name. Similarly, when the covenant comes into the world and people follow it, redemption becomes possible. But throughout this literature redemption is continually identified with the righteous, whose suffering and demise bring about this salvation. So, for example, as depicted in the midrash on Songs 2:2—"a lily among the brambles"—the purpose of the creation of righteous people is to effectuate deliverance for the world by means of their martyrdom.[44] Granted, R. Berekhiah's allusion to suffering and death is much less explicit, at least at this point in the midrash. Here, the reference is merely a hint that rises to the surface through the combination of trigger words and ideas: Abraham, the converts, and redemption.

In the next section, however, R. Ḥaninah's[45] comments extend the interpretation intimated by R. Berekhiah by openly introducing the martyrdom of Daniel's three friends:

> R. Ḥaninah said, "In the moment that the Holy One, blessed be He, did [the] miracle for Ḥananiah, Mishael, and Azariah, many converts were converted. As it is written, *For when he [rather][46] his children see the deed[s] of my hands in his midst, they will make my name holy and they will make holy the holy-one of Jacob, and they will be in awe of the God of Israel* (Isa 29:23). And what is written after that? *The confused[47] will come to know understanding and the murmurers will learn instruction* (Isa 29:24)."

The midrash is formulated as an opinion and a prooftext, and the conversion legend is now applied to Daniel's three friends at the moment at which King Nebuchadnezzar places them in the fiery furnace. Although Abraham's experience is not mentioned (probably because this event would have occurred prior to his "going forth" from his homeland), the articulation of the near martyrdom of Daniel's friends recalls Abraham's experience and is no doubt motivated by the earlier reference to him.[48] This midrash is much more explicit in its reference to martyrdom than R. Berekhiah's allusion, and whereas R. Berekhiah's midrash focused on redemption, this one mentions deliverance only in the prooftext. The comments of both rabbis must be read together if the reader is to get the full sense of martyrdom and its salvific efficacy. The passage from Isaiah 29:23—"they will make my name holy" (*yaqdishu shemi,* יקדישו שמי)—serves as a direct reference to martyrdom, for it incorporates a Hebrew form of "sanctification of the divine name" (*kiddush hashem,* קדוש השם).[49] The next portion of the verse—"they will make holy"—refers to those who commit the martyrs or saints (God's elect) to fire; the "holy-one of Jacob" are those righteous Jews who, like Abraham and the three friends, are willing to die for God's name and thereby bring about the redemption of all Jews. As extended to the descendants of Jacob, martyrdom makes these Jews like holy sacrifices and ensures for them a place in heaven. The final part of this verse—"they will be in awe of the God of Israel"—refers to those who convert, that is, the gentiles, who are represented as the "confused" and the "murmurers" in Isaiah 29:24.

The passage suggests that the perfume of Abraham, the friends, and other righteous Jews is the scent of their burning flesh ("the fragrance of your oils"). As myrrh releases its scent when brought near fire, so too

Abraham's scent—and that of the righteous sufferers—spreads when they are sacrificed or martyred. However, the conception of Abraham's fragrance as his message is also sustained, as glorification of the divine name occurs through both the act of martyrdom ("oil poured forth, your name") and the conversion of the foreigners ("therefore the maidens love you").[50]

The midrash incorporates many of the associations of incense and perfume found in the Bible, and most remarkably it melds two categories of antinomic characteristics together. In the "secular" poetry of the Songs, the wafting of fragrance, which is associated with seductive perfume and the arousal of the lover, has a horizontal valence. But the aroma of the sacred incense sacrifice in the priestly literature wafts vertically, upward toward God, and has a calming and soothing effect on the deity's wrath. In this case, the scent of the burning flesh of the potential martyr travels up toward God and causes God to come down toward the earth for redemption. God may be said to be both soothed and aroused. At the same moment, the fragrance of Abraham's message as well as his burning flesh—both represent his belief in one God—wafts horizontally like perfume toward the foreigners, who are motivated to convert. They are drawn toward Judaism and attracted to conversion at the moment of martyrdom. R. Ḥaninah amends the legend of the fiery furnace by asserting that gentiles become Jews when they witness martyrdom. He also indicates that it is the "miracle" that the people witness that compels them to convert. This is an indication that Daniel's three friends, and Abraham by association, are delivered safely from the fire (in agreement with the biblical text).

But the potential for martyrdom no longer belongs only to Abraham and Daniel's three friends. It now extends to the "holy ones of Jacob," that is, to all Israelites or Jews. The suffering and potential martyrdom of Jews constitute a transformative religious experience for the witnesses and motivate God's deliverance of the martyr. This near martyrdom is thus a sacrificial rite the performance of which affects God and influences his response. These righteous martyrs perform a function similar to that of the lighting of sacred incense in the priestly literature of the Bible. God's immanence is desired as the sign of arousal, acceptance, and response. In this case, the response is prevention of death. And, as with the prophetic voice, the rabbinic focus on perfume and incense together produces its own radically new construction: that of a Jewish sufferer whose affliction redeems himself and others.[51] This aspect of suffering, while seen in the Christ figure, does not appear in other accounts of Christian martyrdom. In those narratives new adherents may be drawn to conversion as they witness the event, but the martyr's dying body does not encourage God to save the victim's life; rather, the victim is saved by means of his or her death. Ultimately, this midrash is a self-referential and fundamentally direct theological statement by and about the rabbis and their perceived position in the world. After all, Abraham and Daniel's friends are a metaphor for the rabbis themselves. These men are the conduits who "pour" the oil of covenant into and out of themselves. It is really they who are perfume and incense, they who are at once teachers, proselytizers, and potential martyrs.

The Scent of Sacrifice

In the midrash just discussed, the willingness to die effectuates divine clemency for the martyrs. But most commonly in the priestly literature, properly performed sacrifice removes collective guilt and sin. Incense in particular assuages divine anger and serves as a concrete form of repentance—not only on the Day of Atonement, when it accompanies the high priest into the innermost sanctum of the Temple, but also in situations of crisis, when death has become an active, destructive force. In the course of rabbinic interpretation, a similar nexus emerges among incense, sacrifice, and penitence, as midrash too inscribes the victim with biblical sacrificial imagery. This person is often young, pure, and innocent and is put to death by burning. And, as in the priestly literature, where burning on the altar both calms divine anger and stimulates God's reaction, the sacrifice of the victim soothes God and brings about divine deliverance. However, unlike the priests, who retain total control over the process of sacrifice, especially that of incense, the rabbinic voices are not exclusive in this respect. They are more than happy to ascribe images of sacrifice and incense to their fellow adherents so that the group may be forgiven, albeit not usually in terms of martyrdom. In the rabbinic estimation, atonement is brought about through observance of the covenant. Therefore, whether one is a special sufferer—the righteous, Abraham, or the rabbis themselves—or an ordinary believer, collective atonement is commonly depicted as sacrifice of the body, observance of the commandments, or both.

Circumcision as Sacrifice

In the Bible, the legal term that describes an accepted sacrifice is "soothing odor." But this term rarely appears in midrash in connection with the sacrifice of humans. One notable exception is found in *Genesis Rabbah* 34:9, in which soothing odor appears in the *lemma* as a reference to Noah's sacrifice after the flood, and the midrash explains that this term refers to the burning of Abraham, Ḥananiah, Mishael, and Azariah.[52] But these characters, as noted above, are special sufferers: they are particularly connected to perfume and incense imagery; they are usually saved at the last moment; and, while they cause others to convert, they ensure deliverance only for themselves. Midrashim that address repentance for collective guilt are driven by other terms from the biblical corpus, such as direct mention of the term "incense" or, even more common, "frankincense." In addition, sacrifice as atonement for sin is bound up with suffering and therefore often recollects Abraham. An example of such a midrash is based on Songs 4:6: "Until the day breathes and the shadows flee, I will go myself to the mountain of myrrh and the hill of frankincense."

> R. Abbahu and R. Levi [disagreed]. One said in the hour that Abraham our father circumcised himself and his sons and the sons of his house, he made their foreskins into a hill. And the sun shone upon them, and they became worm-eaten. The smell of them went up before the Holy One, blessed be He, and it was like the smell of the ingredients of the incense offering and like the smell of the fistful of frankincense that is on the fire offerings. And the Holy One, blessed be He, said, "And when the sons of this man come [to do] transgressions and evil deeds, I will remember for them this smell and I will be filled with mercy for them. And I will convert for them the Attribute of Justice to the Attribute of Mercy." On what grounds? *I will go myself to the mountain of myrrh and the hill of frankincense.*[53]
>
> R. Levi said that in the hour that Joshua circumcised the children of Israel, he erected for them their foreskins into a hill . . . (*Songs Rab.* 4:6)

The overall structure of this midrash is a disagreement between Rabbis Abbahu and Levi[54] about whether the protagonist of the midrash should be Abraham or Joshua. R. Abbahu derives his comments on Abraham from Genesis 17:23–27, in which Abraham circumcises himself and all the males of his house, while R. Levi bases his interpretation on Joshua 5:3, in which Joshua circumcises all the males of Israel before settling in the land of Israel. The narrative structures of the two interpretations are parallel: circumcision as sacrifice, smell as soothing odor, atonement, mercy.

In relation to the *lemma*, the midrash sustains the reading of Israel as the female and God as the male lover by indicating that the mountain and hill, typically identified as the beloved's breasts, are piles of foreskins shed by the Israelites. And yet the scene is cross-gendered, as those hills are made from pieces of male genitalia. The midrash also creates a directional reversal, as the Songs verse depicts the male lover traveling to the female ("I will go myself to the mountain"), while the midrash asserts that the odor of the foreskins drifts up to God. The image of decomposing, rotting foreskins is highly unusual in comparison with the texts engaged so far. In almost every instance of scent, the connotation of a pleasant aroma is either positive or negative depending on its characteristics, but "stench" is almost always perceived negatively. The case of R. Eliezer's bad breath, discussed in chapter 1, could almost be considered unique if it were not for this one.[55] Here, a horrible odor is not only associated with positive images and results but the smell is actually pleasant to God. Further, in the story about R. Eliezer, his bad breath is a metaphor for his hard work and study. The foreskins, however, are not a metaphor for the covenant, since circumcision is *part* of the covenant.

God's response to the heaps of foreskins stems from their significance as sacrifices. The scent of the foreskins travels up toward God and, like other sacrifices, gets his attention focused downward on earth. The piling and decay of the foreskins are compared to the "ingredients of the incense offering" and are akin to the "fistful of frankincense that is on the fire offerings." As a result, the foreskins also have an affinity with myrrh, frankincense, pleasant fragrance, and death. Because of the association with incense sacrifice in particular, the foreskins are also linked to images of atonement, appeasement, and election or exclusivity. The act of circumcision has its own set of associations, including covenant, election, conversion, and observance of the commandments. Although not articulated directly in the midrash, aspects of perfume are also subtly deployed throughout by means of the *lemma* (i.e., evocation of memory, attraction, and impulsive reaction, etc.). To encourage ardor in her lover, Israel adorns herself with myrrh and frankincense—the stench of the foreskins. When he smells them, God is both enticed and encouraged to turn off his rational thought—read as his "Attribute of Justice"—and to follow his more passionate, spontaneous, and emotive side—read as his "Attribute of Mercy."

The initial act of sacrifice has a continuing efficacy in the future, when the Jews, who bear the marks of circumcision, sin. At that time, this initial sacrifice is reactualized and becomes a means of atonement for the people.

More significantly, the sacrifice of the body brings about a change in God, and this response is twofold. As a sacrifice, the hill of foreskins calms divine wrath and produces a soothing odor.[56] In addition, God's inhalation of the aroma of the foreskins is comparable to the male lover's smelling the myrrh and frankincense of the woman. Judgment is turned off and love and compassion activated. The activating agent in this change is the scent itself. The sacrifice works as a soothing odor in order to transform the "mood" of the deity. He is encouraged to be pacified and then to approach the world and the people. The simulated death engenders love.

Reminiscent of other midrashim, this midrash assumes several characteristics of olfaction, the most intriguing of which is the evocation of memory. Scent is closely tied to memory and emotions because of the location in which scents are stored (the limbic system). It is common to smell a particular scent and remember precisely where or when it was first experienced. Specific scents may prompt very strong emotional responses. In this midrash aroma operates on God in many of the same ways it operates in humans. God first smells the foreskins when Abraham or Joshua circumcises the men and boys. God then declares that he will recall this odor in the future. The strength of the initial memory is so profound that it reignites God's initial experience and feeling of well-being. In other words, the soothing odor is reexperienced when the Israelites and Jews sin. However, God's recollection is dramatically different from that which takes place with human olfaction, because God must also recall the scent itself: "I will remember for them this smell."[57] It is as if God remembers smelling the scent and thereby reexperiences it again in order to evoke memory and emotion.

As yet unaddressed is the issue of disagreement between the two rabbis, that is, whether the verse in question relates to Abraham or Joshua. R. Levi's interpretation, although missing its prooftext, is clearly drawn from Joshua 5:3: "And Joshua made knives of flint and circumcised the Israelites at Gibeath-haaraloth" (the hill of foreskins). The hill of foreskins parallels the hill of frankincense, and this is the obvious motive for linking the two texts.[58] The identification of Abraham with Songs 4:6 is less obvious. Although Abraham's link with circumcision occurs as the result of his role in the first episode of circumcision in the biblical narrative, the bridge between this event and the verse from Songs is unclear. R. Abbahu neither establishes any direct tie between Abraham and Songs 4:6 nor employs any wordplay, atomization, enjambment, or prooftext. Rather, the rabbi bases his commentary on object association—the representation of myrrh for the incense sacrifice, frankincense for the other sacrifices, and the creation of a new referent—namely, the hill of frankincense (as proved by Josh 5:3) for the hill of foreskins. But the association between the *topoi* of Abraham, myrrh, incense, and sacrifice is already so well established that no other bridge is necessary. The progenitor is linked to these images as well as those of conversion, covenant, suffering, love, and death.[59] Therefore, the interpretation of Joshua's hill may be strong because of its prooftext, but the interpretation of Abraham's hill is stronger still. Abraham's excessive merit and virtue can be stored up to be called upon and used by his progeny in future generations.

The Martyr Who Atones

Clearly, *Songs Rabbah* and *Genesis Rabbah* are filled with images of martyrdom, potential martyrdom, and sacrifice of the body as a form of ritual simulation and substitution for martyrdom.[60] In many cases, atonement not only makes an appearance but becomes both the motivation for and the hoped-for result of the sacrifice. Woven into these scenes is a thicket of perfume and incense metaphors, with all their encoded imagery. Every permutation can be found of the willing martyr, who in choosing such a fate, is able to accrue enough righteousness and suffering to bring about repentance and redemption for all Jews. The most commonly invoked and therefore best known of these martyrs, or "near martyrs," is Isaac. In *Genesis Rabbah*, the sacrifice of Isaac is reformulated again and again with slight nuances to produce diverse messages and results.[61] In the example below from *Songs Rabbah*, the primary purpose of Isaac's sacrifice is to atone for Israel, and this message is articulated through a scent reference. The midrash is based on Songs 1:14: "A cluster of henna is my beloved to me in the vineyards of Ein Gedi."[62] This verse follows Songs 1:13: "A bundle of myrrh is my beloved to me. He lies between my breasts." As in the midrash on Songs 1:13, in which Abraham is identified with the bundle of myrrh (*Songs Rab.* 1:13), in this midrash Isaac is associated with the cluster of henna:

> *A cluster of henna is my beloved to me* (Song 1:14). *A cluster*, this is Isaac who was tied on the altar like a cluster. *Henna*, that he atones for the iniquities of Israel. *In the vineyards of Ein Gedi*, this is our father Jacob who went to his father . . . (*Songs Rab.* 1:14)

The verse is atomized in order to teach that Isaac is considered a cluster because he lay bound like a cluster on the altar. His near sacrifice, which is described as atoning for the iniquities of Israel, is achieved through a pun. The words for "henna" (*kofer,* כפר) and "atone" (*kipper,* כיפר) contain the same letters but use different vowels. In combination with the midrash, discussed earlier, on Abraham as the bundle of myrrh (Song 1:13), the midrashim as a unit list all three patriarchs in order: Abraham, Isaac, and Jacob. However, only Isaac and Abraham are associated with images of sacrifice and scent.[63]

Isaac's role as the sacrifice that atones for the sins of Israel and Abraham's role as the suffering servant are undeniably similar to descriptions of Jesus. And these theological constructions are not built upon the Hebrew Scriptures; they either evolve within the Jewish tradition itself or develop as shared traditions between Christians and Jews.[64] That is, while much of the imagery employed in these descriptions is biblical, the message, and even how the imagery is used, is a cultural construction of the Amoraic period, probably during the early Byzantine period. A dramatic example of this is built on the two verses "A bundle of myrrh is my beloved to me, he lodges between my breasts. A cluster of henna is my beloved to me in the vineyards of Ein Gedi" (Song 1:13–14).

> R. Berekhiah said, "The congregation of Israel said before the Holy One, blessed be He: 'In the hour that you afflict me, when you embitter me, even then you are *my beloved.* You act as my beloved and you see if there is a great man in me who is able to say to the Attribute of Justice, "Enough!" And you take him as a levy for me.' And so it is written, *A cluster of henna.* What is meant by *cluster*? A man in whom there is everything: Scripture, Mishnah, Talmud, Toseftas, and Aggadot. [What is meant by] *of henna*? He atones for the transgressions of Israel." (*Songs Rab.* 1:14)

As in his earlier midrash on converts and redemption (*Songs Rab.* 1:3), R. Berekhiah structures his comments as a dialogue between Israel and God. Once again, only the enunciations of Israel are depicted. As part of Israel's statement, several words from the verses are reworked and employed as part of the interpretation. The midrash incorporates the categories and many of the associations addressed so far. The bundle of myrrh is the righteous and knowledgeable Jew who lives within the community. He is beloved both of the community and of God. He is "chosen"—even among the chosen—and serves as God's elect when God seeks him out. At the same time, God is the bundle of myrrh that lies between the breasts of Israel, for God is also represented as the male lover.

God plays a role in bringing about martyrdom, for he "afflicts" (*metser,* מצר) his beloved Israel and "embitters" (*memer,* ממר) her—employing a pun on the word *myrrh* (*mor,* מר) and incorporating a phonic wordplay on *bundle* (*tseror,* צרור). As a result, myrrh and henna acquire two valences. They represent love or *eros* as well as suffering, for God's people are afflicted and suffer on behalf of the Divine. Although Israel, the beloved, is tempted to reject her lover in her hour of affliction, he nevertheless remains her beloved. She says that God seeks a martyr, akin to the representation of Jesus on the cross, a "ransom for the many," a tax or penalty payment for her transgressions. By means of a pun on the word "cluster" (*'eshkol,* אשכל), in due course God finds such a person, the "everything man" (*'ish shehakkol,* איש שהכל). And who is this man? He is the one who knows all things Jewish and, more specifically, all things rabbinic (the Mishnah, Talmud, Toseftas, etc.). In the most obviously self-referential and messianic expression yet, R. Berekhiah elucidates the deep connection between the righteous martyr and the rabbis. Like the incense sacrifice he represents, this chosen man, the elect of God, serves as a compensatory atonement for Israel. No longer does the metaphorical understanding of incense, and its special role as an atoning sacrifice, symbolize the election of the priesthood. Scholarship supersedes birthright in the hierarchy of rabbinic interpretation, and this scholarship points directly to the rabbinic community itself as the divinely elected leadership.

Unlike other midrashim, this one presents an outright indictment of God—even as it expresses extreme sentiments of pathos and love. By aligning Israel with the beloved of Songs, the rabbi describes her as the distressed woman, abused by her husband, her lover, for no apparent reason. We are not told of any sins she has actually committed, yet her lover afflicts her. It is noteworthy that it is the "Attribute of Justice"—the violent, impatient, and stern aspect of God—to which the martyr must address himself. The martyr serves as an appeasement to the wrathful attribute of God's justice. This righteous Christlike figure stops the affliction by becoming a "soothing odor." His burning stays the wrath even as it says to justice, "Enough, no more."

The love relationship between God and Israel depicted in the midrash is one of holy and yet passionate suffering. The sensual evocations of the lovers in the Songs are transformed in order to introduce an ideology of pain and suffering for love of the Divine. *Eros* and *thanatos* are completely intertwined in the event of the sacrifice of the human. Similarly, the characteristics attributed to the secular scent poetry of the Songs are intermingled with those of the priestly literature on sacred sacrifice. The deity is described in the most alluring and loving of terms, as a bundle of myrrh that lies between the breasts of Israel, but her arousal of his desire comes through her own destruction and burning death. As a result of this intermingling, the valences that attach to the secular conceptions of the spices, such as love, attraction, and wafting, are brought together with those of incense sacrifice, such as atonement, appeasement, and exclusivity. In addition, the layering of metaphorical images that produces this multiplicity of characteristics also echoes other scent associations specific to the midrashic formulations, such as righteousness, scholarship, and suffering.[65]

Conclusion

As the rabbis interpret the poetry of the Songs, the many scent metaphors for love, passion, and intimacy are reemployed as new metaphors for dying, bodily sacrifice, and martyrdom. What James Fernandez describes as "organizing and subordinate metaphors" are actualized within the texts, as the rabbinic voices articulate these new and transformative perceptions of the Songs.[66] The images and scenes of the lovers are converted into overarching metaphors of the love relationship between humans and the Divine—really to be read as the rabbis and the Divine—and the result of that love is often depicted as suffering and death as well as hope for God's immanence and redemption of the world.

The rabbinic use of spices in perfume and incense lends itself to complex interpretations in which the valences of perfume (embedded within the Songs) and incense sacrifice may be expressed within the same interpretation. Images of wafting, attraction, and the evocation of memory are combined with the characteristics of atonement, appeasement, and exclusivity. Ultimately, these associations and characteristics are intermingled and become part of the single category of *eros* and *thanatos* as expressed in martyrdom and sacrifice of the body.

As demonstrated in the first part of this chapter, the life of the rabbi is plucked like a flower in the field, and scholars lure the angel of death with the precious perfume that is their knowledge. Although aspects of suffering are left unarticulated in these midrashim, when they are read in conjunction with the array of self-referential interpretations on aroma and death, it becomes clear that to be a scholar—to pour covenant into and out of oneself—means that one will suffer and die. Likewise, Abraham is thoroughly associated with spices in general and myrrh in particular in order to draw out his role as the righteous and suffering martyr who is willing to die for his love and belief in one God. His near martyrdom becomes the paradigm for all martyrs. He is both perfume and incense, as he attracts the converts and is brought near fire to release his scent in the "fiery furnace." Isaac as well is the "soothing odor" of sacrifice, identified with henna and frankincense. The burning of these types—the righteous suffering ancestor and the pure sacrificial victim—effect atonement for the Israelites. Even the events of mass circumcision performed by Abraham and Joshua have efficacy in this regard. But none of these examples is as direct and powerful as that of the "everything man." He surely represents the pinnacle of rabbinic learning. Expert in Scripture and rabbinic law and legend, his suffering on behalf of all Jews speaks directly to God's attribute of justice, and his martyrdom secures redemption for all Jews.

Although several of the examples presented in this chapter involve characters from the biblical text, the characteristics with which they are imbued are entirely fixed within the rabbinic hierarchy of values and perceptions. The mention of Abraham's name is not only symbolic of martyrdom but illustrative of the values of righteousness, suffering, and commandment observance. Similarly, Isaac is identified with atonement.

The chapter also presents what may be considered literary or historical developments in the martyrdom narrative. Those martyrdoms that depict Abraham or Daniel's three friends appear in older texts, such as *Genesis Rabbah*, while those that depict "Israel" in dialogue with God or include all the descendants of Jacob as potential martyrs most often transmit the name of R. Berekhiah, a fifth-generation Amora, within their structure. It would seem, therefore, that perceptions of martyrdom have less to do with actual violence or death, since the motif extends well beyond the time period of the worst violence and persecution (the Bar Kokhba revolt). Rather, as we see by R. Berekhiah's interpretations in particular, the motif is expanded, spiritualized, and intensified to reflect the rabbinic understanding of a newly Christian world and the position of the rabbis and Israel within it.[67] Even more striking, however, are the deep and complex theological messages encoded within this literature, which express at once the mutual love experienced by God and Israel and the suffering that Israel endures in that relationship—tied together by aroma.[68]

6

Ephemerality and Fragrance: Desire for Divine Immanence

By its very nature, fragrance is fleeting and elusive. When we smell a pleasant scent and it brings about in us feelings of well-being, the scent itself may be almost imperceptible. It seems to enter us at the fringe of our awareness. Once inhaled and inside us, aroma can either calm or excite, arouse or soothe. Too much of a pleasant odor may repel us, while a mere whiff may unaccountably draw us toward its source. Aroma's ephemerality and liminality mirror love, with its expectant possibilities, its lonely yearning, and its sometimes obsessive infatuation. And fragrance is also intimately tied to death—perhaps as a representation of what we desire in that finality—that death too will be fleeting, temporary, of no consequence. Or it may be that fragrance and death unite with the bonds of love and longing we feel in mourning those whom we have lost. Curiously, the psyche bundles fragrance with its constituent images of love and memory and death and buries them so deeply within human consciousness that it becomes an unreflective part of who we are. Each of these characteristics, and in some cases all of them at once, were experienced by the rabbis, reflected upon by them, and deployed as a generative force in their interpretation.

Conclusions

This book has examined the "aromatic" midrashim and how rabbinic personal experience with pleasing fragrance was put to use in the interpretive effort. The discussion began with a review of the history and material remains, and then drew upon the references to perfume and incense that are referred to in passing in the rabbinic legal texts. The history, wider cultural context, and evaluation of material culture set the scene for both the possibility and the fact of rabbinic encounters with aroma in the second through fifth centuries C.E.—the most reasonable period for the rise of the interpretations and tropes that appear in the midrashim. Reading the material culture with the references to perfume, incense, and spices in the rabbinic literature demonstrated that the rabbis not only were exposed to pleasant fragrances through the Roman and Byzantine culture in which they lived; they also employed aromatics in much the same way as their non-Jewish counterparts.

Aromatics were part of rabbinic everyday life in the Galilee, and by accounting for the context of these ordinary settings—the home, the bathhouse, the marketplace, the grave—we could begin to color in the feelings and cultural associations attached to these settings and their odors. The smell of incense lit after a dinner with invited guests produced an air of festivity, relaxation, and camaraderie. The scents used to fumigate garments might stir the imagination with thoughts of exotic lands, sensual awakenings, or evenings of warm embrace. Or maybe the residual aroma of fumigated clothing simply filled one with pleasurable feelings of tidiness, fresh attire, a clean and well-kept home, or perhaps it reminded one of the drudgery of household chores. Perfumed oil rubbed on the hands might merely have indicated cleanliness, while buried in the hair of one's wife it might remind a husband of the desire he felt for her on their wedding day. But those same smells found in the marketplace could be dangerous: an instantaneous arousal of inappropriate ardor felt for the casual female passerby or, even worse, a male. Perfume used to massage the body at the bathhouse gave rise to both feelings of calm and tranquility and latent anxiety about the dangers of the market. And in death it seems that perfume and incense did much more than simply cover some unwanted odor. Anointment symbolically prepared the person in death as it did in life for the next step in the cycle; like a bride for a wedding, the corpse was bathed, anointed, and dressed, and then carried to its final dwelling place. Similarly, incense wafting through the streets in attendance of the burial reminded residents of the fact of death and of their responsibility toward the mourners. Burial with perfume bottles might do for the entombed what their loved ones could do no longer: care for them and surround them with memories of comfort, ease, and well-being. By focusing on these contexts for perfume and incense, we see not only the evidence of rabbinic experience but more deeply how scent would permeate rabbinic interpretation—where anxieties might be carried from one literary genre to the next, where analogies would give rise to further correspondences, and where expression of the sublime could be layered and thickened.

Before studying the interpretations, we scrutinized the scent terms of the Hebrew Bible and discovered that clusters of images seem to be drawn to, and form around, such terms as perfume, incense, frankincense, and myrrh. In placing the terms and their associations back into their contextual settings, it became apparent that these terms held different associations depending on their frameworks. In the priestly writings, clusters of scent images include the formal structures of the priesthood, outlining the exclusive purview of the priests to offer incense sacrifice. Incense also has a close affinity with the Day of Atonement and was employed as a protective shield for the priest as well as a tool to draw the Divine earthward. In some cases, clusters moved from one context to another. Anointment with perfumed oil is associated with power and preferred selection by God, as it was used to consecrate priest and king. However, perfumed oil is also deeply connected to images of women and sensuality. In the biblical book Song of Songs, the aromatic garden is a description of the woman's body, and her aroma flows out to the male lover and draws him toward her. He too is described as flowing oil, the fragrance of which reminds the beloved of her time with him. In some cases, the valences attached to perfume—seduction, wafting, arousal, and impulsivity—could be depicted negatively, as in the case of the woman in Proverbs 7. The prophetic writings take hold of both "aromatic" spheres, priestly and sensual, and apply the images of women and perfume to incense sacrifice and vice versa. This interpretive process seems to foreshadow the interpretative layering the rabbis employed in the creation of the midrashim.

But what of the interpretations themselves? Here, the rabbinic voices took hold of the biblical literature, shook it, and sprinkled it upon their own bodies, minds, and hearts. They inhaled the biblical images and were forever changed by them. Infringing on the priestly perception of incense and its valences of exclusivity, sacrifice, and atonement, the rabbis created midrashim that were as self-referential as the priestly code itself. Likewise, from the sensual garden of the Songs, they captured the lovers and tenderly brought them into the midrash to express the mutual affection and devotion of the righteous and the Divine—now read as the blossom in the king's thorny and overgrown orchard. These voices sought to turn the female "other" first this way and then that, sometimes pointing toward real women who, in the rabbis' opinion, either needed to perfume their bodies or, once perfumed, might bring about the ruin of men. At other times, the interpretation traces the mere outline of some woman or biblical women whose aromatic practices define them as honorable because they comply with the wishes of men. Drawing on the aroma valences of the Songs, the rabbis describe the propagation of rabbinic tradition as scented oil poured from one vessel into the next. Abraham's wandering is rendered as an unstoppered perfume vial whose contents attract converts to belief in the one God. But more than drawing on and interpreting the fragrance images of the Songs, the rabbinic voices also allowed these images to migrate into other narratives. Perfume, with its horizontal wafting, arousal, and seduction, becomes an interpretive device, a tool used to rewrite the most important events of Scripture, such as the Passover and the Sinai covenant.

Most arresting are those midrashim in which the lovers of the Songs, with their perfume and incense, become articulations of righteousness, suffering, and ritual death. In these, the valences of perfume (wafting, seduction, and arousal) are joined to those of priestly incense (sacrifice, death, chosenness, and "soothing odor") to utterly transform the garden into a sacrificial altar. Here, Deuteronomy's mandate to "choose life" by clinging to the covenant is inverted; instead of life, adherence to God and commandment inexorably leads to potential or realized death. At the moment of human sacrifice, the smoke from the burning flesh of the victim drifts horizontally toward the gentile to promote conversion and upward toward heaven to persuade the deity to act. In some cases, God delivers the victim. In others, the sacrifice has a theurgic effect that causes God to engage his "attribute of mercy." In still others, the death of the human is a salvific force in the world. Although thematic aspects of martyrdom (desire for death, the eventual reward in the world to come, sedition against the hegemon, power through victimhood, love of God) arise time and again in these interpretations, the death is not always completed. In fact, actual death seems not to be the point. Rather, the victim's power, or "merit," to vindicate Israel and save her adherents can be called upon long after he (and they are all "he") is gone. Isaac's near-death experience, Abraham's suffering, and even the circles of men who circumcise themselves at the time of Abraham and Joshua, all provide enough merit for future generations to be looked upon with mercy, to be forgiven, to be redeemed.

Trajectories of Interpretation

While the main objective of this book was to study pleasing odor in all its many facets in rabbinic life and literature, and that has been accomplished, scholarship is always ready with other questions once any single inquiry is undertaken. During the course of this study, two themes seemed to arise in the midrashim—neither ever coming into full focus through the study of the scent imagery but rather floating in and out of view. The first is an apparent indictment of God that begins to emerge in the fourth century C.E., and the second is a late strand of interpretation that desperately cries out for divine immanence. Together, these two subsurface themes form a trajectory that, by innuendo, blames God for the predicament of Jews under Christendom and calls on divine pathos and mercy to be present within the world and thereby rectify the plight of the Jews.

Indictment

Throughout the literature, midrashim that employ scent images in relation to death, and in particular the thematic strands of martyrdom, almost always focus on Abraham, Isaac, the unnamed "righteous," or named rabbis from the period of the Bar Kokhba revolt (e.g., R. Akiba).[1] However, none of these actually indicts God for his role in those martyrdoms. In the fourth century, this begins to change. For example, we saw that in one midrash R. Berekhiah describes the righteous martyr as "the everything man," the man in whom all forms of rabbinic discourse may be found (*Songs Rab.* 1:14). The man remains unnamed, but the description of him opens up the topic of martyrdom to the prospect of R. Berekhiah's current day as it also narrows the definition of who may be considered righteous. The most dramatic and disturbing element of this midrash is the accusation of God for his role in the persecution of Israel. Israel assumes the personality of the battered wife who calls out to her husband, whom she loves, to stop abusing her. R. Berekhiah deftly executes his allegation through the speech act of Israel: "The congregation of Israel said before the Holy One, blessed be He: 'In the hour that you afflict me . . .'" The power of this martyr lies in his ability to stay the hand of God's attribute of justice by means of his own death; and the invocation of justice sets up a structural dichotomy that entails the death of the martyr, bringing about a "soothing odor" that in turn activates God's attribute of mercy.

R. Berekhiah was a fourth- or fifth-generation Amora, which means that he was active sometime in the middle of the fourth century C.E. (ca. 320–75 C.E.). This period coincides not only with the rise of a Christian hegemony in the person and rule of Constantine (306–37 C.E.) but is also witness to new sanctions against Jews (the laws of Constantius in 339 C.E.) as well as the Jewish revolt against Gallus in the Galilee (350–51 C.E.). It appears that R. Berekhiah and his cohort perceived a similarity between their predicament and that of the rabbis during the Bar Kokhba revolt approximately two hundred years earlier.

Similarly, in another midrash that evokes images of martyrdom, R. Berekhiah again employs the device of the speech act, but this time, rather than accuse, he affirms: "Israel said before the Holy One, blessed be He, 'Ruler of the universe: Because You bring light to the world, Your name is magnified in the world.' And what is that light? Redemption" (*Songs Rab.* 1:3). However, the affirmation quickly turns to focus on death with the comment that follows in R. Ḥaninah's name. He makes clear that "redemption" is brought about through "sanctification of the name." Although not a direct accusation, the arrangement of the remarks gives rise to some ambiguity in R. Berekhiah's interpretation. If God's light is redemption that he brings into the world, and redemption occurs by means of the death of the martyrs, then it stands to reason that God is in some respect instrumental in persecution and martyrdom. As for dating R. Ḥaninah's remarks, it is difficult to ascertain with certainty that R. Ḥaninah is a fifth-generation Amora.

But these accusatory midrashim also appear in reference to verses other than those in the Songs that refer to scent, and these too can be dated to the fourth century, although a bit earlier than R. Berekhiah (who is by far the most explicit in this respect). On a verse from Songs that has no scent image—"I adjure[2] you daughters of Jerusalem by the gazelles or does of the field" (Song 2:7a)—indictment seems to evolve within the cycle itself (*Songs Rab.* 2:7). First, R. Eliezer says that God adjures Israel by the "hosts" of heaven and earth.[3] Next, R. Ḥaninah bar Pappa argues that God adjures Israel by the patriarchs and the matriarchs (tribes).[4] R. Yehudah bar Simon states that God adjures by the circumcision.[5] He goes on to state that the Israelites pour out "their blood" like the gazelles and does. It is possible that this reference is to Leviticus 17:13–14, wherein God stipulates that one must pour out and not eat the blood of an animal. However, "their blood" could also refer to the Israelites' own blood, and no prooftext is cited to clarify to whom the blood belongs. In the current arrangement of interpreters, it appears that R. Yehudah bar Simon speaks of the Israelites' own blood, since the next elucidation seems to understand the reference this way. The assertion is from an anonymous group of rabbis who stipulate that God adjures Israel by the generation of the persecution (Bar Kokhba revolt) because "they carried out my (God's) will in the world, and I did my will with them. . . . They poured out their blood for sanctification of my name." It would seem that the editor has arranged the quotations of the rabbis so far, from R. Eliezer to the anonymous group, in historical order. R. Eliezer is a Tanna, R. Ḥaninah bar Pappa and R. Yehudah bar Simon are third- and fourth-generation Amoraim, respectively, and "the rabbis" usually indicates a later generation.

However, the editor does not allow this cycle to end with this accusation. Rather, he pulls back from the precipice of irreverence through the words of R. Ḥiyya bar Abba, a third-generation Amora: *"For your sake, we are killed all day long* (Ps 44:23). R. Ḥiyya bar Abba said, 'If a man said to me, "Give your life for the sanctification of the name of the Holy One, blessed be He," I would give it if they killed me immediately. But I am not able to endure [that which] the generation of the persecution [endured].'"

This interpretation serves as the pivot for the cycle. By beginning his comment with one of the most oft cited verses from Psalms, the indictment is clearly laid bare for any to see. He has done no less than bring a prooftext for God's role in martyrdom: "We are slain for you all day." But from here, the comments move toward a reconciliation. First, R. Ḥiyya quiets the tone of accusation by referring to his own cowardice. Then R. Oshaiyah, a first-generation Amora, says the verse means that God will make Israel like the hosts of heaven. She need only wait patiently for it. The rest of the comments instruct Israel not to seek redemption by means of force (i.e., rebellion) or to hasten it (e.g., by moving back to the land) in any way. Comments from no less than five tradents are brought to bear on the topic of Israel's acceding to the rule of the other nations and the disastrous consequences that resulted when she did not. It is almost as if, once the blame is articulated, the voices fear their own emotion and set about realigning their attitudes as quickly and thoroughly as possible. The historical order of the rabbinic statements is abandoned in favor of theological capitulation and acceptance. It almost appears that the historically earlier positions, closer in time to actual persecution, are resigned to God's judgment of Israel and Israel's role in her persecution. Her revolt makes her culpable in the fact of her historical position. The later midrashim, however, seem to indicate, at least on the part of some rabbis, an ideology of divine indictment—the message that God too is responsible for the persecution of Jews—and that while redemption can only take place according to the word and action of the Divine, fealty and devotion to God and covenant will not necessarily rectify the situation. This God remains the lover but is unknowable and transcendent.

Redemption and Divine Immanence

If redemption is what the rabbis seek, then, we must ask, what is it? What do they really mean by deliverance? Is their distress political? Do they simply desire an end to perceived discrimination, or do they want to *be* the hegemony? Is their concern of a spiritual nature—a freedom from religious persecution, the dream of a unified Jewish praxis, or a resurrection of sorts, a rebirth, a time when the righteous will live and others will not? Or is their vision a combination of these: a renewal of the people in the land, when the dead will live again and all Jews will be together? While the specifics are vague, the instrument by which this future is actualized is clear. It is divine immanence. Among the shifting layers and valences of scent interpretation, those that involve the triangulation of scent, love, and death and in which the suffering faithful are willing to die for their love of God, the desire to overcome divine transcendence and the need for God's presence on earth arise as part of the layering of metaphors. In fact, no less than every rabbinic prescription for practice—every prayer and blessing—is in some measure an articulation of this desire for God to inhabit the world he has created.

In the later midrashim, Israel's exile is also bound up with this yearning; and beseeching God, the rabbinic voices commingle images of heaven, Eden, and exile with the lovers of the garden and their spices. On Songs 8:14—"Flee my beloved, and be like a gazelle or a young stag on the mountains of spices"—the rabbis pull at the beloved's speech, which belies her true intent. She calls to her lover to flee, but she is really asking him to turn about, to return.[6] Incorporated into the midrash, the beloved once again becomes Israel, who says to God, "'Flee my beloved, and be like a gazelle': like the host of above who are like your glory with one voice, with one chant. 'Upon the mountains of spices': in the very highest heavens."[7]

The interpretation echoes the mood and motivation of the original biblical verse; Israel declares, "Flee my beloved," but what she means is, "Return, please stay." After the destruction of the Temple and Israel's initial and succeeding exiles, God has ascended back into heaven, to the mountains of spices. Israel asks to be like the host[8] of angels in heaven, who in turn resemble God's glory both in their beauty and in their unified chant.[9] The mountains of spices are taken to mean the highest heavens; that is, the place of pleasant fragrance is heaven—God's abode. The orientation in this midrash is entirely upward: toward the "highest heavens" and the mountains of spices.

In the other midrashim that employ images of God's abode (see chapter 4), we have seen a fusion of Eden, heaven, and the garden of the Songs. In many of these interpretations, the fragrance of the spices from the garden floats up to God in heaven like the "soothing odor" of sacrifice. But the geographical representations in this midrash present a distinct category. Here, the spices are already located above, in heaven; that is, they do not float to that position, and they cannot be construed as being on earth (as Eden can). The geography itself indicates God's transcendence, and the next interpretation continues in that vein:

> Another interpretation: *Flee my beloved:* from the exile in which we are at present living and in which we are soiled[10] with inequities. *And be like a gazelle:* purify us like a gazelle, *or a young stag:* that you will receive our prayer like an offering of kids and rams. *Upon the mountains of spices:* It comes to you like the good odor on account of the merit of our forefathers whose scent went up to you like the spices. This is the garden of Eden, which is full of spices. Therefore it is said, *Upon the mountains of spices.* (*Songs Rab.* 8:14)[11]

The anonymous interpreter asks God to accept prayer in lieu of sacrifice as a means by which the people will be redeemed. The signified representation of "mountains" shifts between heaven and Eden and includes an allusion to the Temple as well. While structured, like its predecessor, around a series of itemizations, the organization of this midrash moves from statement of condition, to request, to hoped-for result.

Israel, in the role of the beloved, describes herself to God as dirty and soiled in her state of exile.[12] As such, her Diaspora is both geographic and spiritual. Her sins have exiled her from God and sullied her appearance. But though she is dirty and impure in her current predicament, in her future redemption she will be beautiful and purified.[13] In the next phase of the midrash, Israel asks to be cleansed and purified of her sins so that her sacrifice, now interpreted as prayer, may be accepted by God. The plain sense of this portion of the midrash, "accept our prayer like a sacrifice," echoes Psalm 141:2: "Let my prayer be established like incense before You." In the psalm, prayer and sacrifice are two different but contemporaneous methods of addressing God. However, now Israel's prayers serve as a replacement for the sacrifices she can no longer offer.

Comparison of Israel to animals and sacrifice adds yet another layer that recalls other midrashic images of human sacrifice. Israel's sullied condition in exile not only implies that she may not sacrifice; it also indicates that she may not serve as sacrificial victim. She is both the sacrificer and the sacrificed. She offers up prayer and becomes like the purified rams that were offered in the Temple. The "good odor" symbolizes the scent of her own burning as well as that of her sacrificial offering. The reference to "our forefathers, whose scent went up to you like the spices," no doubt refers to the sacrifices offered by Israel's ancestors before and during the time of the Temple, but also serves as an allusion to the burning bodies of Abraham and Isaac.

An alternative translation of the sentence—"It comes (*'ata,'* אתא) to you like the good odor . . ."—in which the subject of the sentence is "the scent" facilitates another significant interpretive move. Michael Sokoloff understands this form of the verb "to come" (*'ata'*, אתא, or *'aty* אתי) as an unusual formulation of the imperative. Sokoloff's translation thus interprets Israel as directing God to come toward the scent: "Approach the pleasant odor."[14] This rendering maintains a parallelism with the Songs verse, since it provides a directive in the midrash comparable to the imperatives "flee" and "be like" in the verse. While this translation reverses the recurrent biblical and midrashic image of the scent of sacrifice wafting up toward God, it strengthens the feeling of desire and need for God's immanence. Israel asks God to come down from the mountains of spices to earth, to approach her, and to allow the good odor to draw him toward her.[15]

Here, fragrance is the connective tissue in a new landscape that intermittently shifts heaven, the Temple, and Eden as the referents for mountains of spices, now the symbolic place of God's abode. However, like the female lover in the Songs, who wishes to meet her lover wherever he might be, Israel desires and attempts to meet God through prayer—the new sacrifice—in any of the geographic or spiritual places of her exile. Geographical scent, therefore, involves the melding not only of geographical images but also of spiritual identity and circumstance. In this interpretation, geography and spices express the spiritual condition of exile, of separation, and the desire for divine immanence. At the same time, the images of aroma recollect the forefathers, whose fragrant suffering accrued merit for just this moment of hoped-for intercession. The soothing odor emitted by the forefathers through self-sacrifice and suffering is compared to that emitted by exiled Israel's prayer.

The rabbinic voices pull the images of sacrifice from the biblical material (communication with the Divine, atonement, and upward direction), but they also combine these with valences of their own creation: suffering, the efficacy of human death, cessation of harsh justice in favor of mercy, and ultimately redemption, manifested first through divine immanence. Therein they produce their own clusters of images and meanings surrounding aroma, and these are significantly different from the Bible's, theologically new and poignant.

What lies behind this revolution is the unique combination of the associations of perfume and incense in the Scripture and the experience of perfume and incense in everyday life—at the bath, after dinner, in the home, and at the market. The feelings that perfume and incense engender in the rabbis are those they wish to arouse in God when he thinks of Israel, his beloved. The imagined sacrifice of the martyr should bring about in the Divine feelings of impulsivity, enjoyment, attraction, and arousal, so that he will approach the beloved lovingly, with his attribute of mercy engaged. In this way the everyday is infused into the theological—not just in the sense of thinking about how olfaction works, how scent spreads, its ephemerality, its liminality, or that it brings about a sense of well-being, but in understanding God as both the same as and utterly different from humans. The rabbis understand aroma as having the same effect on the Divine that it has on us—it inspires arousal, forgiveness, patience, tranquility—but they also perceive God as radically dissimilar in that God can reexperience the scent of the original circumcision or be soothed by the burning flesh of martyrs. But most of all, in the parlance of the Songs, the rabbis hope for their lover's quick return—that he will come down from the mountains of spices—and they will be together in the garden once again.

NOTES

Chapter 1

1. Adapted from *Genesis Rabbah* 42:1. J. Theodor and Ch. Albeck, eds., *Midrash Bereshit Rabba* (Jerusalem: Shalem Books, 1996). Another version of this narrative is found in Avot d'Rabbi Natan, Recension A, chapter 6, and Recension B, chapter 13, in Menahem Kister, *Avoth De-Rabbi Nathan: Solomon Schechter Edition, with References to Parallels in the Two Versions and to the Addenda in the Schechter Edition* (New York: Jewish Theological Seminary of America, 1997).

2. Either through comparison (the plain to the mountain) or explication (R. Eliezer fled from his brothers).

3. Midrash (the singular of the word "midrashim") derives from the root *d-r-sh* (דרש), "to seek." Midrash is the biblical commentary, interpretation, or exegesis created by the rabbis from approximately the first century C.E. onward. Although midrash usually centers on the narrative and poetic sections of the Hebrew Scriptures (i.e., the Torah and Writings), it can also focus on other sources (e.g., the Jewish celebratory calendar, legal literature). A midrash can be *lemmatic* (exegetical), based on a specific line of Scripture, or it can be part of a sermon, homily, or teaching. Midrashim can be found both in *aggadic* (nonlegal) material and in *halakhic* (legal) material.

4. By "valence" I mean not only the apparent characteristics of an aroma but all the subsurface images and connotations, as well as cultural constructions, that may also adhere to it and to related terms or images. Similarly, certain scent terms attract other terms, with all of their latent meanings intact.

5. For example, *Genesis Rabbah,* a work edited in the fifth century C.E. and thus representative of earlier strands of tradition, ties the patriarch Abraham to a verse in Song of Songs simply by stating the verse and affirming, "This refers to Abraham." In some instances the text includes an ambiguous reference to an event in the patriarch's life, or to a character trait, but these rabbinic formulations are nearly impenetrable without comparison to a fuller description. Fortunately, elaborations can often be found in the much later collection of *Song of Songs Rabbah,* which may clarify the earlier vague remark while at the same time include new images.

6. Scientists argue about whether it is possible to recall and thereby reexperience an odor from memory alone. There is anecdotal evidence that a few people can do this; I have yet to meet any.

7. Diane Ackerman, *A Natural History of the Senses* (New York: Vintage Books, 1990), 10.

8. See also D. Michael Stoddart, *The Scented Ape: The Biology and Culture of Human Odour* (Cambridge: Cambridge University Press, 1990), 12.

9. For instance, people "born before 1930 in less urbanized and industrialized times . . . mentioned such natural odors as pine, hay, horses, sea air, and meadows as reminiscent of childhood. But those born after 1930 were more apt to mention food and artificial odors such as plastic, scented markers, airplane fuel, Vaporub®, and Play Doh®

as reminiscent of their childhood." Alan R. Hirsch, "Nostalgia, the Odors of Childhood, and Society," *Psychiatric Times* 9, no. 8 (1992): 29.

10. Ackerman, *Natural History of the Senses*, 11.

11. On long-term memory and olfaction, particularly in comparison to vision, see Donald A. Wilson and Richard J. Stevenson, *Learning to Smell: Olfactory Perception from Neurobiology to Behavior* (Baltimore: Johns Hopkins University Press, 2006), 196.

12. Trygg Engen, *The Perception of Odors* (New York: Academic Press, 1982).

13. This fact is not to be confused with synesthesia, "a sensory blending, where stimulation of a single sense arouses a mélange of sensory images. Stimulation evokes not just those sensations that are normally considered proper to that modality, but also evokes sensations or images that are normally considered proper to other modalities." Lawrence Marks, *The Unity of the Senses: Interrelations Among the Modalities* (New York: Academic Press, 1978), 83.

14. For an interesting explanation of instances that contradict this assertion, including pungent cheeses and strong fish, see William Ian Miller, *The Anatomy of Disgust* (Cambridge: Harvard University Press, 1997).

15. Ibid., 67.

16. Dan Sperber, *Rethinking Symbolism*, trans. Alice Morton (Cambridge: Cambridge University Press, 1975), 115–16.

17. Ackerman, *Natural History of the Senses*, 6.

18. Martha McClintock, a psychologist at the University of Chicago, is one of the names most commonly associated with pheromone research.

19. In 2004, Linda Buck, of the Fred Hutchinson Cancer Research Center, and Richard Axel, of Columbia University, won the Nobel Prize for Physiology or Medicine for their work on odorant receptors and how the olfactory system is organized. Their work together began when Buck won a postdoctoral fellowship in Axel's lab at the Howard Hughes Medical Institute. There they identified a family of genes that control the process of olfaction. There are more than a thousand genes in this family, making it the largest family in the human genome. http://nobelprize.org/Nobel_Prizes/Medicine/Laureates/2004/Press.html (accessed 4 October 2004).

20. For more on scholarly reaction to research in olfaction, see the introduction to Constance Classen, David Howes, and Anthony Synnott, *Aroma: The Cultural History of Smell*, 2d ed. (London: Routledge, 1997).

21. Hans J. Rindisbacher, *The Smell of Books: A Cultural-Historical Study of Olfactory Perception in Literature* (Ann Arbor: University of Michigan Press, 1992), 5–6.

22. Classen, Howes, and Synnott attribute the higher status of sight, and therefore the greater number of studies on sight, to our contemporary need to "distance ourselves from the emotions, that societal structures and divisions be seen to be objective or rational and not emotional, that personal boundaries be respected. Thus . . . sight, as the most detached sense (by Western standards), provides the model for bureaucratic society." *Aroma*, 5.

23. Rindisbacher notes that Kant includes "touch" as one of the "higher senses." *Smell of Books*, 34n17.

24. From G. W. F. Hegel, *Ästhetik*, ed. Friedrich Bassenge, 2 vols. (Berlin: Das Europäische Buch, 1985), 1:48–49, quoted in Rindisbacher, *Smell of Books*, 18.

25. Alain Corbin has written extensively on the control of odors in Paris in the late eighteenth and nineteenth centuries in *The Foul and the Fragrant: Odor and the French Social Imagination* (Cambridge: Harvard University Press, 1986). See also Rindisbacher, *Smell of Books*, 21.

26. Sigmund Freud, *Civilization and Its Discontents*, trans. James Strachey (New York: W. W. Norton, 1962), 46–47n1. See also Miller, *Anatomy of Disgust*, 70–71.

27. Classen, Howes, and Synnott cite both Darwin and Freud as proponents of the theory that "the sense of smell had been left behind and that of sight had taken priority." *Aroma*, 4.

28. In fact, if one considers the evidence that the subtleties of taste are strongly connected to smell, then how does this theory account for the large number of men who are sommeliers, chefs, and food and wine critics?

29. It is true that in comparison to humans, some animals have more olfactory genes, while others have significantly larger olfactory epithelium areas.

30. Most humans recognize approximately two thousand odors (odor patterns); those highly trained in odor detection (e.g., sommeliers, perfumers, etc.) may detect upward of ten thousand scents.

31. One of Rindisbacher's goals is to devise such a lexicon.

32. Cathy Newman, "Perfume: The Essence of Illusion," *National Geographic*, October 1998, 102.

33. Hegel, *Ästhetik*, 1:48–49.

34. See, for example, the essays by Georgia Frank, Susan Harvey, and Steve Weitzman in *Religion and the Self in Antiquity*, ed. David Brakke, Michael Satlow, and Steven Weitzman (Bloomington: Indiana University Press, 2005). Yael Avrahami has also written recently on the senses in the Hebrew Bible, in "The Sensorium and Its Operation in Biblical Epistemology: With Particular Attention to the Senses of Sight and Smell" [in Hebrew] (PhD diss., University of Haifa, 2008). On food and eating, see the SBL journal *Semeia* 86, no. 2 (1999), "Food and Drink in the Biblical Worlds," edited by Athalya Brenner and Jan Willem van Henten. Andrea Lieber also focuses on eating in "God Incorporated: Feasting on the Divine Presence in Ancient Judaism" (PhD diss., Columbia University, 1998).

35. See Marcel Detienne, *The Gardens of Adonis: Spices in Greek Mythology* (1977), trans. Janet Lloyd (Princeton: Princeton University Press, 1994).

36. This literature is far too vast to list here, but some of the pioneers in this field include Samuel Krauss, *Talmudische Archäologie*, vols. 1–3 (Leipzig: Buchhandlung Gustav Fock, 1910; reprint, New York: Arno Press, 1979); Erwin R. Goodenough, *Jewish Symbols in the Greco-Roman Period*, vols. 1–13 (New York: Pantheon Books, 1953–68); and Yehoshua Brand, *Ceramics in Talmudic Literature* [in Hebrew] (Jerusalem: Mossad Harav Kook, 1953). More recent scholarship includes Steven Fine, "Archaeology and the Interpretation of Rabbinic Literature: Some Thoughts," in *How Should Rabbinic Literature Be Read in the Modern World?* ed. Matthew Kraus (Piscataway, N.J.: Gorgias Press, 2006); Eric Meyers, "The Use of Archaeology in Understanding Rabbinic Materials," in *Texts and Responses: Studies Presented to Nahum N. Glatzer on the Occasion of His Seventieth Birthday by His Students*, ed. Michael Fishbane and Paul Flohr (Leiden: Brill, 1975), 28–42; Daniel Sperber, *Roman Palestine, 200–400: Money and Prices* (Ramat Gan, Israel: Bar-Ilan University Press, 1974); Yehuda Feliks, *Trees: Aromatic, Ornamental, and of the Forest* [in Hebrew] (Jerusalem: Rubin Mass Press, 1997); Lee I. Levine, "Bet Šeʿarim in Its Patriarchal Context," in *"The Words of a Wise Man's Mouth Are Gracious" (Qoh 10, 12): Festschrift for Günter Stemberger on the Occasion of His Sixty-Fifth Birthday*, ed. Mauro Perani (Berlin: Walter de Gruyter, 2005).

37. For more information on the debate about the history of the rabbinic community from the second through the fourth centuries C.E. and its political power relative to the Jewish patriarchate and the wider Roman culture, see, among others, Lee I.

Levine, *The Rabbinic Class of Roman Palestine* (Jerusalem: Yad Izhak Ben-Zvi, 1989); Seth Schwartz, *Imperialism and Jewish Society, 200 B.C.E. to 640 C.E.* (Princeton: Princeton University Press, 2001), 101–76; Jacob Neusner, *Judaism in Society: The Evidence of the Yerushalmi; Toward a Natural History of a Religion* (Chicago: University of Chicago Press, 1983); and for discussion of the power (or lack thereof) of the rabbis within the larger Jewish community and their "disdain" for "the masses" during the period of the Tannaim (20–200 C.E.), see Shaye J. D. Cohen, "The Place of the Rabbi in Jewish Society of the Second Century," in *The Galilee in Late Antiquity*, ed. Lee I. Levine (New York: Jewish Theological Seminary of America, 1992). For discussion of the role, status, and power of the patriarch (*nasi*), see Martin Goodman, "The Roman State and the Jewish Patriarch in the Third Century," in Levine, *Galilee in Late Antiquity*, 127–39. On issues of titles, roles, institutions, and power within and outside the communities in Palestine as perceived in the literature, see Alexei Sivertsev, *Private Households and Public Politics in Third-Fifth-Century Jewish Palestine* (Tübingen: Mohr Siebeck, 2002).

38. For example, on rabbinic social construction as loose formations of personal networks or clusters, see Catherine Hezser, *The Social Structure of the Rabbinic Movement in Roman Palestine* (Tübingen: Mohr Siebeck, 1997). For aspects surrounding urbanization of the rabbis in the third through fifth centuries, see Hayim Lapin, "Rabbis and Cities in Later Roman Palestine," *Journal of Jewish Studies* 50, no. 2 (1999): 187–207. For the relationship between village and city and rabbinic representations of them and in them, see Lapin, *Economy, Geography, and Provincial History in Later Roman Palestine* (Tübingen: Mohr Siebeck, 2001).

39. A *baraita* is considered by the rabbis an authoritative Tannaitic ruling that does not appear in the Mishnah. It is commonly introduced by the phrase "the rabbis taught" (תנו רבנן).

40. H. L. Strack and G. Stemberger, *Introduction to the Talmud and Midrash*, trans. Markus Bockmuehl (London: T & T Clark, 1991), 342–43. On the new material, innovations, and creative force of the redactor (sixth or seventh century C.E.), see Tamar Kadari, "On the Redaction of Midrash Shir Hashirim Rabbah" [in Hebrew] (PhD diss., Hebrew University, 2004).

41. Tradents are those rabbis who quote a verse under someone else's name. They usually appear in the form of "Rabbi X said in the name of Rabbi Y" and may extend backward several generations.

42. To be sure, there is some slippage in the dates, and many scholars would view the fourth century C.E. as the *terminus post quem* for such a study. This is particularly true for discussion of the Talmud Yerushalmi, in which the last Babylonian scholar cited is Raba, who died in 350 C.E., and in which the last historical event is either the unrest under Gallus in 351 C.E. or the emperor Julian's mobilization for his Persian campaign in 363. For more on redaction of the Talmud Yerushalmi, see Strack and Stemberger, *Introduction to the Talmud and Midrash*, 188–89.

43. Susan Ashbrook Harvey, *Scenting Salvation: Ancient Christianity and the Olfactory Imagination* (Berkeley and Los Angeles: University of California Press, 2006).

Chapter 2

1. See *b. Šabb.* 62b. On this passage and the topic of women as seductresses, see also Michael Satlow, *Tasting the Dish: Rabbinic Rhetorics of Sexuality* (Atlanta: Scholars Press, 1995), 158ff.

2. Strack and Stemberger, *Introduction to the Talmud and Midrash*, 98.

3. E.g., *Lev. Rab.* 16:1. All references to *Leviticus Rabbah* are from Mordecai Margulies, ed., *Midrash Wayyikra Rabbah: A Critical Edition Based on Manuscripts and Genizah Fragments with Variants and Notes* (Jerusalem: Jewish Theological Seminary of America, 1958).

4. Recent evidence suggests that the Cypriots may have mastered a technique for extracting scented oils and begun mass-producing perfumes as early as 1900 B.C.E. See Esther Wolff, "Notes on the Act of Perfuming Clothes and on the Cypriot Origin of Minoan and Greek Perfumery," in *From Aphrodite to Melusine: Reflections on the Archaeology and History of Cyprus*, ed. Matteo Campagnolo and Marielle Martiniani-Reber (Geneva: La Pomme d'Or, 2007), 45–46.

5. Amihai Mazar, *Archaeology of the Land of the Bible: 10,000–586 B.C.E.* (New York: Doubleday, 1990; new ed., 1992), 492–502. See also Seymour Gitin, "Incense Altars from Ekron, Israel, and Judah: Context and Typology," *Eretz-Israel* 20 (1989): 52–67.

6. Gabriel Barkay, "The Iron Age II–III," in *The Archaeology of Ancient Israel*, ed. Amnon Ben-Tor, trans. R. Greenberg (New Haven: Yale University Press; Tel Aviv: Open University of Israel, 1992), 326. On incense burners and altars, see Wolfgang Zwickel, *Räucherkult und Räuchergeräte: Exegetische und archäologische Studien zum Räucheropfer im Alten Testament* (Freiburg, Switzerland: Universitätsverlag, 1990), 74–90, 110–28. During the First Temple period, there is evidence that the Philistines imitated the horned incense altars of the Israelites and their "secular" use of incense. Gitin, "Incense Altars."

7. That is, YHWH, according to William G. Dever's "Asherah, Consort of Yahweh? New Evidence from Kuntillet 'Ajrûd," *Bulletin of the American Schools of Oriental Research* 255 (1984): 21–37.

8. Elizabeth Bloch-Smith, *Judahite Burial Practices and Beliefs About the Dead* (Sheffield, U.K.: Sheffield Academic Press, 1992), 75.

9. Mazar, *Archaeology of the Land of the Bible*, 131, 82, 214–16, 62.

10. Michal Dayagi-Mendels, *Perfumes and Cosmetics in the Ancient World* (Jerusalem: Keter, 1991), 8.

11. Ibid., 19. Dayagi-Mendels notes that the strigil eventually became a personal accessory for men and women.

12. Ibid. And also from *kilekes* (drinking cups).

13. J. Innes Miller, *The Spice Trade of the Roman Empire: 29 BC to AD 641* (Oxford: Clarendon Press, 1969), 134.

14. Andrew Dalby, *Empire of Pleasures: Luxury and Indulgence in the Roman World* (London: Routledge, 2002), 183.

15. Miller, *Spice Trade of the Roman Empire*, 193.

16. E. Marianne Stern and Birgit Schlick-Nolte, *Early Glass of the Ancient World: 1600 B.C.–A.D. 50* (Osfildern: Verlag Gerd Hatje, 1994), 81.

17. The earliest evidence of glassblowing comes from the first century B.C.E. in Jerusalem (ca. 50 B.C.E.). Nahman Avigad, "Excavations in the Jewish Quarter, Jerusalem," *Israel Exploration Journal* 22 (1972): 195–200.

18. Jodi Magness, "Qumran Pottery," in *Methods of Investigation of the Dead Sea Scrolls and the Khirbet Qumran Site: Present Realities and Future Prospects*, ed. Michael O. Wise et al. (New York: New York Academy of Sciences, 1994), 44.

19. Yael Israeli, "Glass in the Roman-Byzantine Period" [in Hebrew], in *Ancient Glass in the Israel Museum: The Eliyahu Dobkin Collection and Other Gifts*, ed. Yael Israeli (Jerusalem: Israel Museum, 2003), 219. See also Rachel Hachlili, *Jewish Funerary Customs, Practices, and Rites in the Second Temple Period* (Leiden: Brill, 2005), 383–85.

20. If these even differed dramatically from Etruscan practices.

21. Fikret Yegül notes, "The terminology and formal designations given to these special rooms should be taken only as a general guide since the meanings of some of the terms are not entirely consistent in ancient sources and inscriptions over the centuries of usage and coming from vast geographical spans." Yegül, *Baths and Bathing in Classical Antiquity* (New York: Architectural History Foundation, 1992), 39n59.

22. This form of exercise should not be confused with the exercise of the Greek athlete; it was intended only to produce a light sweat. Heavy exercise was considered deleterious to health.

23. Strabo and Pliny, quoted in Dalby, *Empire of Pleasures*, 198.

24. Paul Faure, *Parfums et aromates de l'antiquite* (Paris: Fayard, 1987), 264–65.

25. On Plutarch, compare ibid. and Dalby, *Empire of Pleasures*, 244.

26. The medicinal use of oils began with Galen and continued through the Byzantine period. Miller, *Spice Trade of the Roman Empire*, 25–26.

27. Joseph Patrich and Benny Arubas, "A Juglet Containing Balsam Oil (?) from a Cave Near Qumran," *Israel Exploration Journal* 39 (1989): 43–59.

28. Yizhar Hirschfeld, "Early Roman Manor Houses in Judea and the Site of Khirbet Qumran," *Journal of Near Eastern Studies* 57, no. 3 (1998): 185. Most scholars disagree with Hirschfeld on this claim regarding Qumran as a manor house. See Jodi Magness, *The Archaeology of Qumran and the Dead Sea Scrolls* (Grand Rapids, Mich.: William B. Eerdmans, 2002), 69–70.

29. Among others, see Joseph Patrich, "Agricultural Development in Antiquity: Improvements in Cultivation and Production of Balsam," in *Qumran: The Site of the Dead Sea Scrolls; Archaeological Interpretations and Debates,* ed. Katharina Galor, Jean-Baptiste Humbert, and Jürgen Zangenberg (Leiden: Brill, 2006), 241–48.

30. These too are lacking at the Qumran site. In addition, if one considers that the Essene community served as "cheap labor" for the family that owned the manor house (as Hirschfeld asserts), then one must account for this remark of Josephus: "Oil they consider defiling, and anyone who accidentally comes in contact with it scours his person; for they make a point of keeping a dry skin and of always being dressed in white." Josephus, *The Jewish War*, trans. H. St. J. Thackeray, 7 books in 3 vols. (Cambridge: Harvard University Press, 1927–97), book 2:123. It is possible that Josephus got it wrong and that Essenes refrained from anointing because they worked with balsam (perhaps extracting oil) and therefore wanted to keep their sense of smell as attuned as possible to the subtle nuances of the oil, but this seems unlikely. In light of the cultural attitudes surrounding perfume use, eschewing oil seems appropriate for this ascetic sect.

31. On the increased urbanization of the rabbis during the third through fifth centuries C.E., see Lapin, "Rabbis and Cities in Later Roman Palestine."

32. E.g., at Meiron, where small glass bottles and cosmetic implements dating to 250–365 C.E. appear in abundance. Eric M. Meyers, James Strange, and Carol Meyers, *Excavations at Ancient Meiron* (Cambridge, Mass.: American Schools of Oriental Research, 1981).

33. Kenneth G. Holum et al., *King Herod's Dream: Caesarea on the Sea* (New York: W. W. Norton, 1988), 11.

34. See Pliny, *Naturalis historia*, trans. H. Rackham, 4 vols. (Cambridge: Harvard University Press, 1945–2000), 5.14.69.

35. Lee I. Levine, *Caesarea Under Roman Rule* (Leiden: Brill, 1975), 41; Lee I. Levine, "The Archaeological Finds and Their Relationship to the History of the City," in

Excavations at Caesarea Maritima: 1975, 1976, 1979—Final Report, ed. Lee I. Levine and Ehud Netzer (Jerusalem: Institute of Archaeology, Hebrew University of Jerusalem, 1986), 178.

36. Levine, "Archaeological Finds," 178–79, 84; Kenneth G. Holum, "Identity and the Late Antique City," in *Religious and Ethnic Communities in Later Roman Palestine,* ed. H. Lapin (Potomac: University Press of Maryland, 1998), 155–77.

37. Eric Meyers, "Roman Sepphoris in Light of New Archaeological Evidence," in Levine, *Galilee in Late Antiquity,* 321.

38. Of note, unguentaria and incense shovels were found in the caves in which it is thought that Bar Kokhba and his supporters hid (near the site of Qumran and the Dead Sea). Yigal Yadin, *Bar-Kokhba: The Rediscovery of the Legendary Hero of the Last Jewish Revolt Against Imperial Rome* (New York: Random House, 1971), 108–9, 14–17.

39. Meyers, "Roman Sepphoris," 327.

40. Lapin, "Rabbis and Cities in Later Roman Palestine."

41. On rabbinic schools and circles of disciples, see Hezser, *Social Structure of the Rabbinic Movement.*

42. Charlotte Elisheva Fonrobert and Martin S. Jaffee, *The Cambridge Companion to the Talmud and Rabbinic Literature* (Cambridge: Cambridge University Press, 2007), xv, xix.

43. Mordechai Aviam, *Jews, Pagans, and Christians in the Galilee: Twenty-Five Years of Archaeological Excavations and Surveys; Hellenistic to Byzantine Periods* (Rochester: University of Rochester Press, 2004), 12. I was present at the excavation of the temple to Augustus in Caesarea in 2000 and catalogued unguentaria.

44. See, e.g., *m. Ber.* 8:6 and its related discussion in *b. Ber.* 53a, or any reference in *b. 'Abod. Zar.* Note also that some editions of the Mishnah insert "Samaritans" for "worshippers of the stars," which, in turn, can be a medieval substitute for "gentiles."

45. On the relationship among Esau, Edom, and Rome and how this changes over time in Jewish literature, see Gerson Cohen, "Esau as Symbol in Early Medieval Thought," in *Jewish Medieval and Renaissance Studies,* ed. Alexander Altmann (Cambridge: Harvard University Press, 1967), 19–48.

46. For example, on daily life in Tiberias, as discussed by the rabbis themselves, see Yaron Z. Eliav, "Sites, Institutions, and Daily Life in Tiberias During the Talmudic Period," [In Hebrew.] *Mi'tuv T'veria* 10 (1995): 1–106.

47. E.g., *y. 'Erub.* 9:4 (25d).

48. Theophrastus, *Historia plantarum,* trans. A. F. Hort (Cambridge: Harvard University Press, 1926), 9.6.2. "Balsam of Mecca" is another common name for opalbalsam, since Mecca was its region of origin.

49. Pliny, *Naturalis historia,* 12.111–12. It should be noted that balsam is a shrub; Pliny describes it as being the size of a myrtle tree (12.111–23).

50. Also found in 1 Kgs 10:10.

51. Josephus, *Jewish Antiquities,* trans. H. St. J. Thackeray et al., 10 vols. (Cambridge: Harvard University Press, 1926–65), book 8:174, book 9:7; Josephus, *Jewish War,* book 1:136–41, book 1:358–62, book 4:467–72.

52. Josephus, *Jewish War,* book 4:402–5.

53. Ze'ev Safrai, *The Economy of Roman Palestine* (London: Routledge, 1994), 147–55. Safrai cites Galen (end of the second century C.E.), a curious inscription of the sixth century C.E. on the Ein Gedi synagogue, and *b. Šabb.* 26a for his assessment. It is doubtful that Galen knew much about balsam production in Palestine, particularly

considering that other authors relied heavily on Theophrastus and Pliny. The synagogue inscription, while intriguing, is based entirely on the reading by Yehuda Feliks that the "secret" that those of Ein Gedi might reveal to the non-Jews (and therefore have their names blotted out of the world forever) concerns the production of balsam. See Feliks, *Trees*, 54–57. For the complete inscription, which only speaks of those who "reveal the secret," not what the secret is, see Joseph Naveh, *On Stone and Mosaic: The Aramaic and Hebrew Inscriptions from Ancient Synagogues* [in Hebrew] (Jerusalem: Ha-Ḥeverah le-Hakirat Erets Yisrael ve-'Atikoteiha, 1978), 106. The last piece of evidence, *b. Šabb.*, assumes that Rav Joseph is speaking about his own time (third century C.E.) even though he is referencing the Persian period.

54. E.g., *y. Ber.* 6:6 (10d).

55. E.g., *y. Ber.* 8:5 (12b); and *'Abot R. Nat.*, Recension A, 18.5.

56. This is the *pu'al* form; see *b. Ber.* 43b.

57. E.g., *m. B. Bat.* 6:3; *y. B. Bat.* 6:1 (15b). Fragrant wine seems to be different from wine that has frankincense mixed into it. The frankincense mixture appears to have narcotic effects (see 3 Macc 5:2, 45, and *b. Sem.* 2:9).

58. But almost all the terms are more prevalent in the Talmud Bavli—no doubt owing to its size and breadth.

59. For an in-depth discussion of these two resins and their relationship to other spices, such as *nataph*, see Kjeld Nielsen, *Incense in Ancient Israel* (Leiden: Brill, 1986), 61–62, 65–66; Miller, *Spice Trade of the Roman Empire*, 101–2; and Feliks, *Trees*, 38–43. Feliks notes a *baraita* (*y. Yoma* 4:5, 41d) in which Rabban Simeon b. Gamaliel states that "*tsori* is none other than the resin that seeps (נטף) from the trees of *qetaf*," demonstrating how enmeshed the terms are in rabbinic literature. Although Miller draws an association of *qetaf* with balsam because of its botanical relationship (*Commiphora kataf*), Feliks seems to argue that *qetaf* was a particular shrub, grown in the land of Israel, that produced resin. He notes that the resin was produced near the Dead Sea. As we have seen, this is one of the places where balsam was thought to have grown. Feliks also argues against the association of *tsori* with storax; Nielsen, however, disagrees.

60. Also מרחץ.

61. It is quite possible that as the primary caretakers of children and other household members, women may have been apothecaries and formed close networks in order to share information and recipes. For more on women and networks in the biblical period, see Carol Meyers, "Guilds and Gatherings: Women's Groups in Ancient Israel," in *Realia Dei: Essays in Honor of Edward F. Campbell, Jr., at His Retirement*, ed. Prescott H. Williams and Theodore Hiebert (Atlanta: Scholars Press, 1999).

62. Although I have not found references to very small oil presses for perfume, Brun believes he has found evidence for these many centuries before in Greece. Jean-Pierre Brun, "The Production of Perfumes in Antiquity: The Cases of Delos and Paestum," *American Journal of Archaeology* 104 (2000): 277–308.

63. See *t. Šeb.* 5:12. The appellation could also be translated as "spice dealer"; literally, the term is "the balsam" or "the spice" (הבשם). Regarding *qetaf*, Lieberman notes that it means "spice wood, and in the Talmuds its meaning is *tsori*." Saul Lieberman, *Tosefta Ki-Fshuṭah: A Comprehensive Commentary on the Tosefta* (New York: Jewish Theological Seminary of America, 1992), 188. R. Akiba is considered a second-generation Tanna (90–130 C.E.). It is thought that he died during the Bar Kokhba revolt. Strack and Stemberger, *Introduction to the Talmud and Midrash*, 79.

64. See *y. Yoma* 4:5 (41d). The term used here is "the pounders" or "the mixers" (הפטמין).

65. On "spice peddler" (apart from the context), Jastrow defines *rokhel* (רוכל) as "peddler, esp. seller of spices, perfumes." Marcus Jastrow, *Dictionary of the Targumim, Talmud Babli, Yerushalmi, and Midrashic Literatures* (New York: Judaica Press, 1903), 1459.

66. *'Abot R. Nat.*, Recension A, 18.5. Although *'Abot* is redacted somewhat late, the material is from the third and fourth centuries C.E. Strack and Stemberger, *Introduction to the Talmud and Midrash*, 247.

67. Others: "idolaters."

68. See *m. Ber.* 8:6. All quotations of the Mishnah are from Chanokh Albeck, *Shishah Sidre Mishnah*, 6 vols. (Jerusalem: Bialik Institute and Dvir Co., 1959; reprint, 1973). On the phrase "use it for light," literally "enjoy," in the sense of "deriving benefit" from it, see p. 30.

69. See *y. Ber.* 8:6 (12b). Reading "burning" or "causing a fumigation," במעשין (Vatican MS), or במעשן (Constantinople MS), rather than "does" or "places," במעשיו (Venice and Leiden). See Guggenheimer, who renumbers this passage *y. Ber.* 8:7 and maintains that R. Jacob does not formulate this law but "quotes the Tannaitic formulation." Heinrich Guggenheimer, *The Jerusalem Talmud: First Order; Zeraim (Tractate Berakhot)* (Berlin: Walter de Gruyter, 2000), 584.

70. This can be inferred with reference to *t. Ber.* 5:32: "The one who stands in the spice store all day blesses only once. The one who enters and goes out, enters and goes out, blesses each time." Lieberman, *Tosefta Ki-Fshutah*, 32. This also appears in *b. Ber* 53a.

71. On the issue of idolatry and the heretical use of spices, the passage states further on, "Not over the lamp and spices of idolatry. Isn't it that of the gentiles [the same] as that of idolatry? You explain it with the idolatry of Israel." In the *b.*, the discussion from *y.* is reorganized to include several other fragrances and to focus attention on women and idolatry. See chapter 4.

72. Rather than *mugmar* (מוגמר), the Tosefta uses *shemen arev* (sweet oil, שמן ערב). Lieberman notes that this oil is for washing the hands after the meal (see also Rashi). However, cleansing oils do not receive blessing, while the oil used for lighting does. In addition, the Bavli clearly understands this oil as being lit after meals, since Rabbi Ze'ira comments that the blessing is not said until the smoke column rises (*b. Ber.* 43a).

73. See *t. Ber.* 5:29 and *y. Ber.* 8:5 (12b). The Yerushalmi has מבושם.

74. See *b. Ber.* 43b. A range of meanings for גנאי would include "insulting" at one end of the spectrum and "obscene" at the other.

75. See *b. Ber.* 43b.

76. Fumigation of clothing is the one area that is considered the sole domain of women in rabbinic literature.

77. Note that in the midrash on the women of Jerusalem, they required a means (albeit a strange one) of splashing the perfume onto the young men because otherwise the scent would have gone undetected.

78. Zeev Weiss and Ehud Netzer, "Zippori—1994–1995," *Excavations and Surveys in Israel* 18 (1998): 22–27, 31–38.

79. Katharina Galor has restated the case for *miqva'ot* at Sepphoris. Assessing the material evidence separately from the literary data and employing the term "stepped pool," Galor interprets the pools to be for ritual immersion but leaves aside the issue of "priests." Galor, "The Stepped Water Installations of the Sepphoris Acropolis," in *The Archaeology of Difference: Gender, Ethnicity, Class, and the "Other" in Antiquity: Studies in*

Honor of Eric M. Meyers, ed. Douglas R. Edwards and C. Thomas McCollough (Boston: American Schools of Oriental Research, 2007), 201–13. Hanan Eshel refutes claims that these pools were used for ritual immersion; see Eshel, "A Note on 'Miqvaot' At Sepphoris," in *Archaeology and the Galilee: Texts and Contexts in the Graeco-Roman and Byzantine Periods,* ed. Douglas R. Edwards and C. Thomas McCollough (Atlanta: Scholars Press, 1997), 131–33.

80. Stuart Miller employs a close reading of rabbinic texts to explore the shifting valences of *miqveh* and the possibilities of the *miqveh*'s other uses. Miller, "Stepped Pools and the Non-Existent Monolithic 'Miqveh,'" in Edwards and McCollough, *Archaeology of Difference,* 215–34.

81. The hot springs of Ḥammat Gader, located southeast of the Sea of Galilee, should also be mentioned. Its large bathing complex was built during the second century C.E. and was well known throughout the empire for the healing effects of its waters. Yizhar Hirschfeld, *Hammat Gader Excavations: 1979–1982* (Jerusalem: Israel Exploration Society, 1997). For a thorough assessment of Ḥammat Gader and Ḥammat Tiberias and spas throughout the Roman empire, see Estēe Dvorjetski, *Leisure, Pleasure, and Healing: Spa Culture and Medicine in the Ancient Eastern Mediterranean* (Leiden: Brill, 2007).

82. Although the Mishnah is sparse in its discussions of bathing, the famous passage concerning Rabban Gamaliel and the Aphrodite of the bathhouse can be found in m. *'Abod. Zar.* 3:4.

83. See *y. Ber.* 2:8 (5c).

84. See *y. Šabb.* 1:2 (3a).

85. Yaron Eliav has collected several stories that refer to the baths at Tiberias. Eliav, "Sites, Institutions, and Daily Life," [In Hebrew.] 22–32.

86. See *y. Ber.* 9:5 (14d).

87. See *y. Ketub.* 12:3 (35a), and *y. Kil.* 9:3 (32b).The language of the text is problematic. The term for *unctorium* should be סכותה rather than סכנתא, which means "danger" or "dangerous place." While the problem is one of orthography or transcription, the merging of these concepts (i.e., the place where oil is applied and one is massaged with its being a dangerous place) is intriguing. See Michael Sokoloff, ed. *A Dictionary of Jewish Palestinian Aramaic of the Byzantine Period* (Ramat Gan, Israel: Bar-Ilan University Press, 1992), 376. He also cites Saul Lieberman's introduction to *Hayerushalmi Kiphshuto* (Jerusalem: Hotsa'at Darom, 1934), 11.

88. On the issue of whether the rabbis (and other Jews) bathed nude, see Yaron Z. Eliav, "The Roman Bath as a Jewish Institution: Another Look at the Encounter Between Judaism and the Greco-Roman Culture," *Journal for the Study of Judaism* 31, no. 4 (2000): 416–54.

89. See *t. Ber.* 5:32. This sentence is followed by the examples of the person who sits in the spice shop all day and says the blessing (for experiencing a pleasant scent) only once, and the person who goes in and out and so says the blessing each time.

90. See *t. Šabb.* 16:16.

91. See *t. Ter.* 10:10; *t. Dem.* 1:23; *t. Šeb.* 6:9; *t. Šabb.* 16:14. Although it is not clear that this marble table is in the bathhouse, I cannot imagine where else it would be. The only situation in which it was likely that a gentile would lie down on a marble table to oil himself, and then be followed by a Jew (*t. Dem.* 1:23) is in the bathhouse. Furthermore, the bathhouse (מרחץ) or sweet oil (שמן ערב) is mentioned near these passages several times; cf. *t. Ter.* 10:10; *t. Dem.* 1:22 (with reference to the oil for a wound, which was likely to have been scented), *t. Šeb.* 6:8; *t. Šabb.* 16:16.

92. See *m. Šabb.* 22:6. See Saul Lieberman, *Greek in Jewish Palestine* (New York: Jewish Theological Seminary of America, 1942; reprint, 1994), 93–97.

93. See *b. B. Bat.* 53b.

94. Exercise at the *kordimah* is an example.

95. On the question of whether the rabbis considered bathing and its related activities "Roman," the example of the slave seems to argue in the negative. On its surface, the case of a slave carrying jars of unguents and other oils may seem more suitable to Roman literature than rabbinic; nevertheless, the Talmud employs this example in a simple and straightforward style. As such, the rabbis appear to be just like others of the wider society—employing images of slaves at the bathhouse. In none of the accounts in the Yerushalmi or the Talmud Bavli does there seem to be any indication that the rabbis consider the act of bathing or anointing, the bathhouse, or the oil to be in some way "Roman" or foreign. For more on this issue, see Eliav, "Roman Bath as a Jewish Institution."

96. In fact, lighting incense after a meal may have been considered entirely an act of festivity and as having nothing to do with covering up an odor. In most cases, a blessing was said when one "enjoyed" or "derived benefit" from the aroma. If the scent was produced for utilitarian reasons such as fumigation, then no blessing was said.

97. See *m. Ber.* 6:6.

98. Guggenheimer notes that the text should say Rav Ze'ira throughout since he was the student of Rav Jeremiah in Babylonia and the teacher of Rabbi Jeremiah in Galilee. Guggenheimer, *Jerusalem Talmud*, 501. This discussion and what follows also appears in *b. Ber.* 43.

99. "Filth" in the sense of something that smells bad and that requires using oil to remove the odor.

100. Guggenheimer, *Jerusalem Talmud*, 501.

101. See *b. Ber.* 53a. This reference in the Talmud seems to counter Rashi's comment on *b. Ber.* 43b that with reference to the disagreement between the houses of Hillel and Shammai on which blessing is said first—that of oil or that of myrtle—the purpose of the oil is to clean the hands after eating. If the Talmud claims that no blessing is said over the oil for cleaning, then this oil must not be for cleaning; rather, it is for anointing and lighting, and the oil of the myrtle is for smelling (either lit or unlit).

102. See *y. Ber.* 6:6 (10d), where a substance referred to as *'olentith* (אלינתית) is discussed. Some consider this ointment *'aluntith* (אלונטית), related to *œnanthe* or *oenanthinus*, while others believe it to be *olens, olentis*, or "sweet smelling" in the Latin. Cf. Jastrow, *Dictionary of the Targumim*, 68; Guggenheimer, *Jerusalem Talmud*, 501.

103. See *b. Ber.* 43a.

104. "Helmeted" refers to an animal roasted whole, with its legs over its head. See Jastrow, *Dictionary of the Targumim*, 1379.

105. See *m. Beṣah* 2:7. See also *m. 'Edu.* 3:11.

106. A *megufah* (מגופה) is commonly a "stopper," or the clay that is used to seal wine. Jastrow cites this reference and describes it as "an air-tight vessel." However, it is also possible that the term simply means "burner," as the point of the narrative is to recall that Rabban Gamaliel's house used a special type of burner for the incense employed on a festival day. Jastrow, *Dictionary of the Targumim*, 726–27.

107. Many different forms of this word are found: MS Vienna: ערדסקאות; MS London: אפרטקסאות; Yerushalmi: פרדיסקיס. On the basis of the similarity of the Yerushalmi's word to the Latin *pyrdiscos*, Lieberman defines this as boxes or drawers.

It also may have a relationship to the Greek πυργισκος, box, crate, or chest. Lieberman, *Tosefta Ki-Fshuṭah*, 956–57. However, Lieberman's ערדסקאות may also have a relationship to the Latin verb *ardescōs*, to catch fire, become ignited, or become lit. See P. G. W. Glare, ed. *Oxford Latin Dictionary*, combined ed. (Oxford: Clarendon Press, 1982), 165. Jastrow identifies ערדסקאות as Damascene plums or plum-shaped. Jastrow, *Dictionary of the Targumim*, 1114.

108. See *t. Beṣah* 2:14. See M. S. Zuckermandel, *Tosephta: Based on Erfurt and Vienna Codices* (Jerusalem: Wahrmann Books, 1970).

109. See *b. Beṣah* 22b.

110. Reading the somewhat obtuse construction of the infinitive "to perfume" (*legamer*, לגמר) with no direct object, according to Rashi.

111. See *y. Ber.* 8:7 (12b) and *b. Ber.* 53a. On *y. Ber.* 8:7, cf. Guggenheimer, *Jerusalem Talmud* (*y. Ber.* 8:6), and Schäfer (*y. Ber.* 8:7). Peter Schäfer and Hans-Jürgen Becker, eds., *Synopse zum Talmud Yerushalmi*, vol. 1 (Tübingen: J. C. B. Mohr [Paul Siebeck], 1991).

112. See *b. Šabb.* 18a.

113. See *m. Ber.* 8:5 This passage is followed by the passage regarding the spices and lights of the gentiles. See also *t. Ber.* 5:30; *y. Ber.* 8:1 (12a); and *b. Ber.* 51b.

114. These would be European Jews, who were actually smelling myrtle leaves rather than spices, according to Mordechai Narkiss, "Origins of the Spice Box," *Journal of Jewish Art* 8 (1981): 35.

115. See *t. Ber.* 5:30 (6:6 in the Erfurt edition).

116. See *y. Ber.* 8:5 (12b).

117. Notably, *b. Ber.* 52b presents another version in which it is Hillel who advocates that the blessing for the spices comes before that of lights, and R. Yoḥanan asserts that Hillel is followed.

118. In fact, almost all of the references in the rabbinic legal literature to spices as part of ritual acts concern idolatry or witchcraft and explain how to avoid blessing fragrances used in those contexts.

119. Ismar Elbogen, *Jewish Liturgy: A Comprehensive History*, trans. Raymond Scheindlin (Philadelphia: Jewish Publication Society, 1993), 101. Although highly speculative, see also Jacob Lauterbach, "The Origin and Development of Two Sabbath Ceremonies," *Hebrew Union College Annual* 15 (1940): 367–424.

120. Narkiss, "Origins of the Spice Box," 31.

121. This may be said of synagogues as well. Destruction of the glass at the synagogue at Gush Ḥalav was so extensive that the team was unable to record it. Eric M. Meyers, Carol Meyers, and James Strange, *Excavations at the Ancient Synagogue of Gush Halav* (Winona Lake, Ind.: Eisenbrauns, 1990), 123. Another issue raised by Meyers et al. is the placement of glass finds (at Khirbet Shemaʻ it is difficult to ascertain whether the glass belongs to the synagogue or to the house next door). Eric M. Meyers, A. Thomas Kraabel, and James Strange, *Ancient Synagogue Excavations at Khirbet Shemaʻ, Upper Galilee, Israel, 1970–1972* (Durham: Duke University Press, 1976), 245–47.

122. Personal communication with Ken Holum and Eric Meyers.

123. See, e.g., Yadin, *Bar-Kokhba*, 93ff.

124. Marva Balouka, "Ceramic Vessels and Objects," in *Sepphoris in Galilee: Crosscurrents of Culture*, ed. Rebecca Martin Nagy et al. (Winona Lake, Ind.: North Carolina Museum of Art, 1996), 206.

125. As quoted in Leonard Victor Rutgers, "Incense Shovels at Sepphoris?" in *Galilee Through the Centuries: Confluence of Cultures*, ed. Eric M Meyers (Winona Lake, Ind.:

Eisenbrauns, 1999), 194n102. My personal communication with Eric Meyers also confirms this assessment.

126. Ibid. Note that Eric Meyers considers in detail the issues in this disagreement. Eric M. Meyers, "The Ceramic Incense Shovels from Sepphoris: Another View," in *"I Will Speak the Riddles of Ancient Times": Archaeological and Historical Studies in Honor of Amihai Mazar on the Occasion of His Sixtieth Birthday,* ed. Aren M. Maeir and Pierre de Miroschedji (Winona Lake, Ind.: Eisenbrauns, 2006), 874–76.

127. See Rutgers, "Incense Shovels at Sepphoris?"; Meyers, "Ceramic Incense Shovels," 869. Although the findings of the shovel fragments were not yet published when Rutgers and Meyers reviewed the evidence, see now James F. Strange, Thomas R. W. Longstaff, and Dennis E. Groh, *Excavations at Sepphoris,* vol. 1, *University of South Florida Probes in the Citadel and Villa* (Leiden: Brill, 2006), 61.

128. On the evidence in rabbinic sources for priests at Sepphoris, see Stuart S. Miller, *Studies in the History and Traditions of Sepphoris* (Leiden: Brill, 1984), particularly chapter 3.

129. Meyers, "Ceramic Incense Shovels," 877. The idea of potpourri was first suggested to Eric Meyers by Carol Meyers in reference to "cup-and-bowl" vessels that date to the late Bronze and Iron Ages. Carol L. Meyers, "Fumes, Flames, or Fluids? Reframing the Cup-and-Bowl Question," in *Boundaries of the Ancient Near Eastern World: A Tribute to Cyrus H. Gordon,* ed. Meir Lubetski, Clare Gottlieb, and Sharon Keller (Sheffield, U.K.: Sheffield Academic Press, 1998), 30–39. Although Meyers suggests that the vessels could have been used for potpourri, she is more inclined to believe that they were used to burn incense or other aromatics (e.g., leaves). These vessels are fairly common in Carthage and other areas of Tunisia. From private conversation with Abdelmajid Ennabli, the former director of the National Museum of Carthage and conservator of the site of Carthage, I learned that he and his colleagues also believe that these vessels are incense burners.

130. It should also be noted that the incense shovels as depicted on synagogue floors are most often square (e.g., Beit Alpha), but those found at Sepphoris are both round and square. Censers, which are a completely different shape, are also depicted. Dan Bahat, "A Synagogue at Beth-Shean," in *Ancient Synagogues Revealed,* ed. Lee I. Levine (Jerusalem: Israel Exploration Society, 1981), 82–85. We might further surmise that the depiction of shovels and burners on the synagogue floors suggests fumigation in the synagogue. See Steven Fine, *This Holy Place: On the Sanctity of the Synagogue During the Greco-Roman Period* (Notre Dame: University of Notre Dame Press, 1997), 85.

131. See *m. Šabb.* 8:1 and *y. Šabb.* 8:1 (11b).

132. See *y. Šabb.* 8:6 (11c).

133. See *m. Šabb.* 6:3 and *b. Šabb.* 62a. In addition, *m. Šabb.* 9:6 holds that anyone who carries spices on the Sabbath is culpable. The term for perfume in the Mishnah is פליטון, which is usually considered to be "ointment," and therefore we expect some form of the word for "jar." However, because it is preceded by the term for "bottle" (צלוחית), "perfume" seems to be the better translation. Albeck describes the women's jewelry as something like a "crown worn around the head," and a "bundle." Albeck, *Shishah Sidre Mishnah,* 31. Saul Lieberman identifies this piece of jewelry as a bead probably made from some kind of peeled (or thin) shell, such as tortoise shell, that may have been worn between the eyes. Lieberman, *Tosefta Ki-Fshuṭah* (*t. Šabb.* 9:11), 19n35, 67n59 (34–35).

134. See *b. Šabb.* 62a–b.

135. See *t. Šabb.* 5:9.

136. See Nissan Rubin, *The End of Life: Rites of Burial and Mourning in the Talmud and Midrash* [in Hebrew] (Jerusalem: Hakkibutz Hameuchad, 1997). For a full discussion of the relationship between unguentaria found in burials and the rabbinic literature, see Deborah Green, "Sweet Spices in the Tomb: An Initial Study on the Use of Perfume in Jewish Burials," in *Commemorating the Dead: Texts and Artifacts in Context; Studies of Roman, Jewish, and Christian Burials,* ed. Laurie Brink and Deborah Green (Berlin: Walter de Gruyter, 2008).

137. See *m. Kil.* 9:4; *m. Šabb.* 23:4, 5; *m. Ma'aś. Š.* 5:12.

138. See *m. Šabb.* 23:5 and *t. Šabb.* 17:18.

139. See *m. Meg.* 4:3; *m. Ber.* 3:1; *m. B. Bat.* 6:7; *m. Sanh.* 2:1 (2:3).

140. See *m. B. Meṣi'a* 6:1; *m. Meg.* 3:3, 4:3; *m. Mo'ed Qaṭ.* 3:8; *m. Ket.* 4:4 (which also discusses the playing of flutes); *t. Šabb.* 17 (which also discusses the playing of instruments); *m. Menaḥ.* 10:9. For a more detailed description of these activities and their significance, see David Kraemer, *The Meanings of Death in Rabbinic Judaism* (London: Routledge, 2000).

141. Zeev Weiss, "The Location of Jewish Cemeteries in Galilee in the Mishnaic and Talmudic Periods" [in Hebrew], in *Graves and Burial Practices in Israel in the Ancient Period,* ed. I. Singer (Jerusalem: Yad Izhak Ben-Zvi, 1994), 230–40. I have been unable to obtain Zeev Weiss's master's thesis, which is considered a standard in the field. I am grateful to him, however, for sharing his thoughts with me in conversation in 2004, for subsequent communication via e-mail, and for pointing me in the direction of his article "Hellenistic Influences on Jewish Burial Customs in the Galilee During the Mishnaic and Talmudic Period" [in Hebrew], *Eretz Israel* 25 (1996): 356–64.

142. See *m. Mo'ed Qaṭ.* 1:6; *m. B. Bat.* 6:8.

143. See *m. Sanh.* 6:6; *m. Mo'ed Qaṭ.* 1:5.

144. Rachel Hachlili, *Ancient Jewish Art and Archaeology in the Land of Israel* (Leiden: Brill, 1988), 97; L. Y. Rahmani, *A Catalogue of Jewish Ossuaries in the Collections of the State of Israel* (Jerusalem: Israel Antiquities Authority, Israel Academy of Sciences and Humanities, 1994), 16, 21; Gideon Avni and Zvi Greenhut, *The Akeldama Tombs: Three Burial Caves in the Kidron Valley, Jerusalem* (Jerusalem: Israel Antiquities Authority, 1996), 118–20; Baruch Arensburg and Patricia Smith, "Appendix: Anthropological Tables," in *Jericho: The Jewish Cemetery in the Second Temple Period,* ed. Rachel Hachlili and Ann E. Killebrew (Jerusalem: Israel Antiquities Authority, 1999), 192–95; Jodi Magness, "The Burials of Jesus and James," *Journal of Biblical Literature* 124, no. 1 (2005): 132; Hachlili, *Jewish Funerary Customs,* 94, 322–24, 483.

145. See Rahmani, *Catalogue of Jewish Ossuaries,* 21.

146. This has not deterred scholars from trying. For a recent discussion and review of opinions, see Magness, "Burials of Jesus and James," 129.

147. These phases should not be confused with the three-stage pattern of funerals first outlined by Arnold van Gennup, *The Rites of Passage* (1909), trans. Monika B. Vizedom and Gabrielle L. Caffe (Chicago: University of Chicago Press, 1960); and Robert Hertz, *Death and the Right Hand* (1907), trans. Rodney Needham and Claudia Needham (reprint, Glencoe, Ill.: Free Press, 1960).

148. This passage raises a fascinating question: why is "anointing" mentioned before "rinsing" (or washing)? With reference to bathing, "washing" usually occurs prior to "anointing." See, for example, *m. Ta'an.* 1:6, where one is not allowed to "wash or anoint" (ברחיצה ובסיכה) during a fast.

149. Although "limb" could also refer to the genitals or penis, it is unlikely in this passage.

150. See *m. Šabb.* 23:5.

151. For the "stopping up" of the orifices, see *t. Šabb.* 17:18.

152. E-mail communication from Arpad Vass, research chemist and forensic anthropologist, Life Sciences Division of the Oak Ridge National Laboratory, Oak Ridge, Tennessee.

153. See *m. Ber.* 3:1; *m. Meg.* 3:3, 4:3; *m. Mo'ed Qaṭ.* 3:8; *m. B. Bat.* 6:7, 8; *m. Sanh.* 2:3; and *m. Menaḥ* 10:9.

154. זלח, that is, "sprinkled fluid" or "perfume." However, this is not the usual word for perfume or spices (בשׂמים).

155. Zuckermandel has בפני ("in front of") (*Tosephta*, 651). Lieberman has לפני ("before" or "in front of") (*Tosefta Ki-Fshuṭah*, 204).

156. See *t. Šeqal.* 1:12. Lieberman also cites the *y. Šeqal.* 2:7 (47a) and *Sem.* 12:9 (*Tosefta Ki-Fshuṭah*, 673). However, the issue in *b. Sem.* 12:9 is whether one should sprinkle wine and oil on the bodies at the time of burial (or on the bones at the time of secondary burial, as Kloner reads—see below), as instructed by Rabbi Akiba. R. Simeon ben Nanos disagrees and states that oil but not wine should be sprinkled, and the later sages affirm that neither wine nor oil should be sprinkled.

157. Or "intestines."

158. See also Jacob Mann, who discusses the employment of spices in the burial of Jesus according to the Gospels. Mann, "Rabbinic Studies in the Synoptic Gospels," *Hebrew Union College Annual* 1 (1924): 350–51.

159. This terminology is very similar to the term "before his bier" (בפני מיטתו or לפני מיטתו) in *t. Šeqal.* 1:12.

160. See *y. Ber.* 8:6 (12b).

161. That is, they are not there for "enjoyment" and so do not receive a blessing. This rabbi's rationale may be based on two different possibilities. The first is that one should "not have any use from things given to the dead." Thus Guggenheimer, *Jerusalem Talmud*, 587. The other is that the function of the spices is to cover up the odor. This is the reason given in *b. Ber.* 53a.

162. This language of "honor" appeared in the *t. Niddah* passage as well but with respect to the dead. In that reference, we saw that the purpose of those spices was to "honor the dead." In both cases, "honor" can be construed as "use" or "employment." In other words, if the spices are used by the dead (i.e., belong to the dead) or are used to honor the dead, then no blessing is said. However, if the spices belong to the living (i.e., are experienced by the living for no other purpose than smelling), then one should say a blessing. The trajectory of this logic appears in the Talmud Bavli, where recitation of the Mishnaic passage triggers a reorganization of the Yerushalmi's version (see *b. Ber.* 53a).

163. Ironically, *semaḥot* means "happy occasions." Strack and Stemberger date the tractate, also known as *'Ebel Rabbati*, to the eighth century C.E., noting that Zlotnick and Meyers date it to the third century C.E. Strack and Stemberger, *Introduction to the Talmud and Midrash*, 249. David Kraemer dates *Semaḥot* to the Geonic period (ninth century C.E.). Kraemer, *Meanings of Death*, 9.

164. This phrase appears in *m. Šabb.* 6:10 and *m. Ḥul.* 4.7.

165. The use of bride and groom as a paradigm of the deceased is significant, for weddings and funerals (marriage and death) are deeply connected. Both events entail the

movement of the participants from one "home" to another, from one family to another. The participants are in a liminal, transitory period, which can cause its own anxiety or fear. They cannot be easily defined as single or married, alive or dead. They are in a sense between communities and alone. At the same time, they will soon be a part of a new community and partake in a sort of rebirth as they enter that community.

166. *Sem.* 8:2. However, "sweet oil" (צלוחית של שמן מתוק) is forbidden. Another reference that appears in this same list of "nonsuperstitious" customs is to tubes through which wine and oil are poured for the honor of the bride and groom (*Sem.* 8:4). The custom of pouring libations of oils and wine through tubes for the dead is strongly associated with earlier Roman practices.

167. Kraemer, *Meanings of Death*, 39.

168. Ibid., 103–5, 108–9; Saul Lieberman, "Some Aspects of After Life in Early Rabbinic Literature," in *Harry Austryn Wolfson Jubilee Volume* (Jerusalem: American Academy for Jewish Research, 1965), 495–532.

169. Moshe Schwabe and Baruch Lifshitz, *Beth She'arim: The Greek Inscriptions*, vol. 2 (New Brunswick: Rutgers University Press, 1974), 219–21.

170. It is doubtful that the patriarch and his family can necessarily be considered "rabbinic." Levine, "Bet Še'arim in Its Patriarchal Context."

171. For the dating of Beit She'arim, see Fanny Vitto, "Byzantine Mosaics at Bet She'arim: New Evidence for the History of the Site," *'Atiqot* 28 (1996): 138. For information on the local and diasporic Jews buried there, see Nahman Avigad, *Catacombs 12–23*, vol. 3 of *Beth She'arim: Report on the Excavations During 1953–1958* (New Brunswick: Rutgers University Press, 1976), 259–61.

172. Of note, the *arcosolia* in Beit She'arim often hold more than one body. In several cases these receptacles are large enough to accommodate the burial of three bodies placed perpendicular to the wall and another body placed horizontally at the back of the niche. For more precise information on the dating of these niche types at Beth She'arim, see Avigad, *Catacombs 12–23*, 259. In several sites throughout Palestine, the *kokh* represents the most common type of burial niche. The *kokhim* are often dug at ground level deep into the wall of the cave, and the body is placed perpendicular to the surface of the wall so the feet are facing toward the room.

173. See Amos Kloner and Boaz Zissou, *The Necropolis of Jerusalem in the Second Temple Period* [in Hebrew] (Jerusalem: Yad Izhak Ben-Zvi and Israel Exploration Society, 2003); Fanny Vitto, "Burial Caves from the Second Temple Period in Jerusalem (Mount Scopus, Giv'at Hamivtar, Neveh Ya'aqov)," *'Atiqot* 40 (2000): 65–121; Ann E. Killebrew, "Catalogue of Artifacts," in Hachlili and Killebrew, *Jericho*, 176–91.

174. See Elena Kogan-Zehavi, "Settlement Remains and Tombs at Khirbet Tabaliya" [in Hebrew], *'Atiqot* (2000): 53–79.

175. Of the glass vessels at Hurfeish, Yael Goren-Rosin comments, "It is evident that there was no 'norm' for the number of glass goods per burial, and no particular ratio between the types of vessels left with each burial. The only general tradition that can be discerned is the choice of misshapen and lesser quality vessels. Many of the glass vessels found in the tomb were asymmetrical or slightly misshapen, and thus probably less valuable." Gorin-Rosen, "The Glass Vessels from Burial Cave D at Hurfeish," in *Eretz Zafon: Studies in Galilean Archaeology*, ed. Zvi Gal (Jerusalem: Israel Antiquities Authority, 2002), 166.

176. Virginia Anderson-Stojanović, "The Chronology and Function of Ceramic Unguentaria," *American Journal of Archaeology* 91, no. 1 (1987): 120. Although Anderson-

Stojanović's main concerns are the Hellenistic and early Roman funerary unguentaria from Stobi in Yugoslavian Macedonia, the presence of these bottles is so widespread that Hachlili cites this article in her discussion of Second Temple burials in Israel. Hachlili, *Jewish Funerary Customs*, 383–84; *alabastra* bottles are also found at these sites, but in far fewer quantities (383–85).

177. Hachlili, *Jewish Funerary Customs*, 386; Ann E. Killebrew, "The Pottery," in Hachlili and Killebrew, *Jericho*, 123; Rachel Hachlili and Ann E. Killebrew, "Burial Customs and Conclusions," in Hachlili and Killebrew, *Jericho*, 168.

178. Kloner and Zissou, *Necropolis of Jerusalem*, 60–62.

179. Avni and Greenhut, *Akeldama Tombs*, 123–29.

180. See *b. Sem.* 47a.

181. E.g., at Daburriya, one bottle intact and two others broken (Mordechai Aviam, "Finds from a Burial Cave at Daburriya" [in Hebrew], in Gal, *Eretz Zafon*, 135); at Giv'at Yasaf, one bottle (Hana Abu-Uqsa, "A Burial Cave from the Roman Period East of Giv'at Yasaf" [in Hebrew], *'Atiqot* 33 [1997]: 39–46); at Ḥurfeish, seven bottles found—candlestick, globular, and cylindrical (Gorin-Rosen, "Glass Vessels from Burial Cave D," 160–64); at Kabri, seven bottles (Edna Stern and Yael Gorin-Rosen, "Burial Caves Near Kabri" [in Hebrew], *'Atiqot* 33 [1997]: 1–22); at Kafr Kanna, two candlestick bottles (Hana Abu-Uqsa, "Three Burial Caves at Kafr Kanna" [in Hebrew], in Gal, *Eretz Zafon*); and at Khirbet el-Shubeika, fragments of approximately twenty bottles in two caves; at this site a monastery and burial caves were excavated (Yael Gorin-Rosen, "The Glass Vessels," in Gal, *Eretz Zafon*, 288–322).

182. Dan Barag, "Hanita, Tomb XV: A Tomb of the Third and Early Fourth Century C.E.," *'Atiqot*, English ser., 13 (1978): 10–33.

183. Avigad, *Catacombs 12–23*, 24.

184. Ibid., 68.

185. Dan Barag, "The Glass Vessels," in ibid., 209.

186. Avigad, *Catacombs 12–23*, 62–65, 238–58. See also Levine, "Bet Šeʿarim in Its Patriarchal Context," which argues persuasively that the term "rabbi" at Beit She'arim designates only members of the patriarchate rather than rabbis per se.

187. Israeli, "Glass in the Roman-Byzantine Period"; Dan Barag, "Glass Vessels of the Roman and Byzantine Periods in Palestine" [in Hebrew] (PhD diss., Hebrew University, 1970). Barag also notes the widespread similarity in glass manufacture and use throughout Palestine, indicating that Jews were not much different from others in the region (129).

Chapter 3

1. 2 Sam 12:20; Ps 45:9; Prov 7:17; Ruth 3:3.

2. It is also possible that the practices, implements, and even handling of spices may be different, but this is not readily apparent in the texts or material remains.

3. Egyptian and Mesopotamian evidence dates back to the second or third millennium B.C.E. See J. Kaplan, "Mesopotamian Elements in the Middle Bronze II Culture of Palestine," *Journal of Near Eastern Studies* 30, no. 4 (1971): 293–307.

4. In some cases, Israelite practices, such as the use of the four-horned incense altar, were picked up by other peoples (namely, the Philistines). See Gitin, "Incense Altars."

5. Although the *pi'el* form of *qitter* is often associated with idol worship because of its use in Jeremiah (particularly Jer 44), Diana Edelman points out that the word should not be associated exclusively with aberrant practices. She emphasizes that the act of sacrifice is not the problem; rather, the issue is that people are sacrificing to idols. Edelman, "The Meaning of Qitter," *Vetus Testamentum* 35, no. 4 (1985): 395–404. For more on issues surrounding the late language and the problem of authorship, particularly of such passages as Jer 44, see Yair Hoffman, *Jeremiah: Introduction and Commentary*, 2 vols. [in Hebrew] (Tel Aviv: Am Oved, 2001), 30–32, 44–49, 63–64, 738–40.

6. The term *hiqtir* (הקטיר) is a *hiph'il* form and therefore always transitive. For a more thorough discussion on the two terms, see Edelman, "Meaning of Qitter," 401. For the relationship of the root *q-t-r* to its relative languages, see Max Löhr, *Das Räucheropfer im Alten Testament: Eine archäeologische Untersuchung* (Halle: Max Neimeyer, 1927), 167–71.

7. Menachem Haran and Jacob Milgrom agree that *qetoreth* refers to priestly incense burned in the outer precincts of the Temple—either in censers (Haran) or as frankincense on the sacrificial altar (Milgrom). They also agree that *qetoreth sammim* refers to incense burned on the inner incense altar. Milgrom asserts further that *qetoreth sammim daqqah* is a description of the incense brought into the Holy of Holies on the Day of Atonement. See Menachem Haran, "The Uses of Incense in the Ancient Israelite Ritual," *Vetus Testamentum* 10 (1960): 113–29; Jacob Milgrom, *Leviticus 1–16* (New York: Doubleday, 1991), 1025–26.

8. Hence the messiah is so called because he is God's "anointed one." On *mashaḥ* (משח), see Milgrom, *Leviticus 1–16*, 517–19, 53–55.

9. The *hiph'il* form of this root is also employed as part of an idiom for men's urination: מסיך הוא את־רגליו, "he anointed his feet" (Judg 3:24, see also 1 Sam 24:3).

10. See Kjeld Nielsen, *Incense in Ancient Israel* (Leiden: Brill, 1986), 3–15, 26–27, 18–19. On myrrh, see also *The Assyrian Dictionary of the Oriental Institute of the University of Chicago* (Chicago: Oriental Institute; Glückstadt: J. J. Augustin Verlagsbuchhandlung, 1972), 221–22. For a catalogue by spice, see Miller, *Spice Trade of the Roman Empire*.

11. Pliny, *Naturalis historia*, 12.60.

12. *Assyrian Dictionary of the Oriental Institute*, 222.

13. Nielsen doubts this association and prefers the spice storax for this term. *Incense in Ancient Israel*, 62, 65.

14. This somewhat counterintuitive detail is addressed more fully below.

15. See C. Houtman, "On the Function of the Holy Incense (Exodus XXX 34–8) and the Sacred Anointing Oil (Exodus XXX 22–33)," *Vetus Testamentum* 42, no. 4 (1992): 460.

16. See Chaim Licht, *Ten Legends of the Sages* (Hoboken: KTAV, 1991), 87–117. Steven Fine reviews the evidence for ascendancy of the priesthood in Byzantine Palestine and concludes that liturgical evidence should probably not serve as social evidence. Further, he describes the rabbis' attitude toward the priesthood during the second through fourth centuries as "ambivalent." Steven Fine, "Between Liturgy and Social History: Priestly Power in Late Antique Palestinian Synagogues," *Journal of Jewish Studies* 56, no. 1 (2005): 4. See also Reuven Kimelman, "The Conflict Between the Priestly Oligarchy and the Sages in the Talmudic Period" [in Hebrew], *Zion* 48 (1983): 135–48, who bases his conclusions on rabbinic and priestly social standing by using the literary sources. However, since we seek rabbinic "perception" of the priests, Kimelman's article is useful.

17. Levine, in "Bet Šeʿarim in Its Patriarchal Context," makes the point that anyone of high standing in the community could be referred to as "Rab."
18. See Schwartz, *Imperialism and Jewish Society*.
19. Exod 30:7–9, 34–38, and Lev 16:13.
20. Exod 30:1, 37:25, 35:15, 40:5, and 31:11. Of note, in Ezek 40, no reference to the incense altar appears in the prophet's description of the new Temple.
21. Two terms appear in this list: *besamim* (בשמים), referring to the oil, and *sammim* (סמים), referring to the incense. Both terms may mean "aromatics" or "spices." Nielsen, *Incense in Ancient Israel*, 67, considers *bosem* (בשם) a general term for aromatic spice. Haran, "Uses of Incense," 125, argues that *sammim* might be something added to the mixture of spices rather than a specific spice or spices.
22. Exod 30:22–27, 30–33. Each of the Tabernacle implements and Aaron and his sons are anointed as part of their installation and as evidence of their election and holiness. The term *mashaḥ* (משח) is used. In the proscription against regular Israelites using this oil, the word for "anoint" is *sukh* (סוך) to indicate the type of perfuming used after bathing.
23. The directions in Exodus refer to the structures and architecture of the portable Tabernacle (tent of meeting, ark, etc.) and parallel quite precisely those of the Temple.
24. Exod 30:34–36: "And the Lord said to Moses: 'Take the spices stacte, onycha, and galbanum—these spices and pure frankincense; let there be an equal part of each. Make them into incense, a mixture made of the perfumer, salted, pure, sacred. Beat some of it into powder, and put some before the pact in the tent of meeting, where I will meet with you; it shall be most holy to you.'" On stacte, see Nielsen, who prefers storax (*Incense in Ancient Israel*, 65). On the problems in identifying onycha (*sheḥeleth*, שחלת) as a mollusk containing an aromatic substance or as a substance from the vegetable kingdom, see Feliks, *Trees*, 11n3. See also Nahum Sarna, *Exodus* (Philadelphia: Jewish Publication Society, 1991), 199; Nielsen, *Incense in Ancient Israel*, 66. On galbanum, see Miller, *Spice Trade of the Roman Empire*, 99. On the role of frankincense in other sacrifices and in the incense sacrifice, see Menachem Haran, "'Incense Altars'—Are They?" in *Biblical Archaeology Today, 1990: Proceedings of the Second International Congress on Biblical Archaeology*, ed. Avraham Biran and Joseph Aviram (Jerusalem: Israel Exploration Society and Israel Academy of Sciences and Humanities, 1990), 113–14. On the translation of "salted," see Victor Hurowitz, "Salted Incense—Exodus 30, 35; Maqlû VI 111–113; IX 118–120," *Biblica* 68, no. 2 (1987): 178–94.
25. In the previous verse, 1 Chr 9:29, some of the responsibilities of the Levites are described; they are said to be in charge of "the flour, the wine, the oil, the frankincense, and the spices."
26. Nehemiah returned to Jerusalem in 445 B.C.E. On the possibility of guilds and guild structure in Palestine before the Hellenistic period, see I. Mendelsohn, "Guilds in Ancient Palestine," *Bulletin of the American Schools of Oriental Research* 80 (1940): 17–21. See also Nahum Sarna, "The Psalm Superscriptions and the Guilds," in *Studies in Jewish Religious and Intellectual History: Presented to Alexander Altmann*, ed. Siegfried Stein and Raphael Loewe (Tuscaloosa: University of Alabama Press, 1979), 281–300; Mark Wischnitzer, "Notes to a History of the Jewish Guilds," *Hebrew Union College Annual* 23, part 2 (1950–51): 245–63.
27. In their role as "health care consultants," however, it is possible that female perfumers or apothecaries constituted a loose "guild" of their own. See Meyers, "Guilds and Gatherings."

28. See Houtman, "On the Function of the Holy Incense."

29. Avi Hurvitz, *A Linguistic Study of the Relationship Between the Priestly Source and the Book of Ezekiel: A New Approach to an Old Problem* (Paris: J. Gabalda, 1982), 53–58.

30. *'ishsheh* is probably related to the Ugaritic *'tt*, "gift of devotion." See J. Hoftijzer, "Das sogenannte Feueropfer," *Supplements to Vetus Testamentum* 16 (1967): 114–34. While Propp follows Hoftijzer, Levine employs "burnt offering," "offering by fire." See William C. Propp, *Exodus 19–40* (New York: Doubleday, 2006), 462; Baruch A. Levine, *Numbers 1–20* (New York: Doubleday, 1993), 389.

31. See Menachem Haran, *Temples and Temple-Service in Ancient Israel: An Inquiry into the Character of Cult Phenomena and the Historical Setting of the Priestly School* (Oxford: Clarendon Press, 1978), 17.

32. In Arabic, *laḥm* means "flesh" or "meat," and in Ugaritic, *lḥm* means "bread" or "grain for bread." See Ludwig Koehler and Walter Baumgartner, *The Hebrew and Aramaic Lexicon of the Old Testament*, trans. M. E. J. Richardson (Leiden: Brill, 1996), 526. However, "bread" or "food" is more indicative of the generic nature of the term. See Baruch A. Levine, *Numbers 21–36* (New York: Doubleday, 2000), 370.

33. Other ancient priesthoods are also closely associated with incense. See Michal Artzy, "Pomegranate Scepters and Incense Stand with Pomegranates Found in Priest's Grave," *Biblical Archaeology Review* 16, no. 1 (1990): 48–51.

34. Haran, *Temples and Temple-Service*; Nahum Sarna, *Exploring Exodus: The Heritage of Biblical Israel* (New York: Schocken Books, 1987), 192, 205–6.

35. Sarna, *Exodus*, 156.

36. Jacob Milgrom, "The Compass of Biblical Sancta," *Jewish Quarterly Review* 65, no. 4 (1975): 206.

37. Sarna, *Exodus*, 156.

38. Haran, *Temples and Temple-Service*, 181–84.

39. In commenting on Lev 1:1–9 (sacrifice of the *'olah*), Baruch Levine states, "It is not a rite of expiation that figures in our verse but, rather, protection from God's wrath. Proximity to God was inherently dangerous for both the worshiper and the priests, even if there had been no particular offense to anger Him. The favorable acceptance of the *'olah* signaled God's willingness to be approached and served as a kind of ransom, or redemption, from divine wrath." Baruch A. Levine, *Leviticus* (Philadelphia: Jewish Publication Society, 1989), 7.

40. See Milgrom's three gradations of incense in *Leviticus 1–16*, 1026–28; Haran, "Uses of Incense"; and Haran, *Temples and Temple-Service*, 230–45.

41. On the problems in translating *kapporeth* (כפרת), see Milgrom, *Leviticus 1–16*, 1014.

42. Philo, *On the Special Laws*, in *Philo: In Ten Volumes (and Two Supplementary Volumes)*, trans. F. H. Colson, G. H. Whitaker, and Ralph Marcus (Cambridge: Harvard University Press, 1929), 1.72. The conflicting views of the Pharisees and Sadducees on the burning of incense on the Day of Atonement, its procedure, and its symbolic value are covered in full in Israel Knohl and Shlomo Naeh, "Milluim Ve-Kippurim" [in Hebrew], *Tarbiz* 62, no. 1 (1992): 17–44.

43. On covering the ark, see Milgrom, *Leviticus 1–16*, 1029. On the wrath of God, see Levine, *Leviticus*, 105.

44. Sarna argues that the reason why incense sacrifice is not described during the inauguration of the Tabernacle is that it is not needed. The presence of God, manifested in the cloud, has not yet come to rest upon the Tabernacle. Incense is required only when the cloud appears. Sarna, *Exodus*, 193. As for the purpose of the cloud (serving as a

reminder), this is akin to the incense pans that were hammered and attached to the altar after the Koraḥ episode to serve as a warning to the Israelites regarding encroachment on the priestly duties (Num 17:1–5).

45. Levine, *Leviticus*, 7n38. Levine uses "wrath" somewhat synonymously with uncontrollable "power" or "holiness." The meaning of the term "wrath" (קֶצֶף), as well as its structures, are disputed and therefore deserve separate treatment and study. On the relationship between the terms "wrath" (קֶצֶף) and "anger" (אַף) and the late formulation of "anger" (כַּעַס), see Hurvitz, *Linguistic Study*.

46. Paul Heger, *The Development of Incense Cult in Israel* (Berlin: Walter de Gruyter, 1997), 115–16.

47. As with the gods who "swarm[ed] like flies" around Utnapishtim as he lit incense for them after the flood in the Babylonian flood story. See Benjamin R. Foster, *From Distant Days: Myths, Tales, and Poetry of Ancient Mesopotamia* (Bethesda: CDL Press, 1995), 75. See Victor Hurowitz, "Response: Aspects of Cult and Art in the Land of Israel," in Biran and Aviram, *Biblical Archaeology Today*, 262–64. On the relationship between Utnapishtim and Noah with reference to sacrifice, see Michael Fishbane, *Biblical Myth and Rabbinic Mythmaking* (Oxford: Oxford University Press, 2003), 187n100.

48. With particular reference to *reaḥ niḥoaḥ*, see Fishbane, *Biblical Myth and Rabbinic Mythmaking*, 184–87.

49. On the role of the incense cloud (with a special additive) as a screen to prevent the high priest from seeing God, see Milgrom, *Leviticus 1–16*, 1014–15, 28–30. On the protection from "lethal glory," and the high priest's need for incense in manipulating blood inside the adytum, see Roy Gane, *Cult and Character: Purification Offerings, Day of Atonement, and Theodicy* (Winona Lake, Ind.: Eisenbrauns, 2005), 233–38.

50. On the representation and appeasement of divine anger, see Othmar Keel, *Die Welt der altorientalischen Bildsymbolik und das Alte Testament: Am Beispiel der Psalmen* (Zurich: Benzinger Verlag und Neukirchener Verlag, 1972), 147–48.

51. While it is possible that the deaths of Nadab and Abihu result from their lighting the incense as opposed to a high priest's lighting it, this seems unlikely. The narrative of Lev 10, the resulting proscription from Moses, and Exod 27:21 indicate otherwise.

52. Milgrom, *Leviticus 1–16*, 600–601.

53. Although there is no doubt that the biblical text as it now stands depicts Aaron and Moses as the protagonists, one is reminded of God's declaration: "you will be to me a kingdom of priests, a holy nation" (Exod 19:6).

54. Jacob Milgrom, "Korah's Rebellion: A Study in Redaction," in *De la Tôrah au Messie: Études d'exégèse et d'herméneutique bibliques offertes à Henri Cazelles pour ses 25 années d'enseignement à l'Institut Catholique de Paris, Octobre 1979*, ed. Maurice Carrez, Joseph Doré, and Pierre Grelot (Paris: Desclée, 1981).

55. On the connection of this result to the next rebellion (Num 17), see Jacob Milgrom, "The Rebellion of Korah, Numbers 16–18: A Study in Tradition History," *Society of Biblical Literature Seminar Papers* 27 (1988): 570–73.

56. For a full discussion of קרב in the priestly sources and issues surrounding encroachment (on the priestly functions) in the Koraḥ episode, see Jacob Milgrom, *Studies in Levitical Terminology* (Berkeley and Los Angeles: University of California Press, 1970), 16–22.

57. On the term *karev* as "encroachment" rather than "drawing near," see Milgrom, *Numbers* (Philadelphia: Jewish Publication Society, 1990), 342–43, with reference to Num 3.

58. Literally, the "offerers" (מקריבי), or "those who bring near."

59. See Mayer I. Gruber, *Aspects of Nonverbal Communication in the Ancient Near East* (Rome: Pontifical Biblical Institute, 1980).

60. On the role of intercessor and repentance in the priestly milieu and its similarities with and differences from the prophetic strand, see Jacob Milgrom, "The Priestly Doctrine of Repentance," *Revue Biblique* 82, no. 2 (1975): 201.

61. Cf. Lev 10:6 and Num 17:11. Of the term "wrath" (קֶצֶף), Milgrom notes, "it is a reflex action, an outburst of the Deity resulting from egregious evil. It follows in the wake of idolatry ... rebellion ... war census. ... It is also the inevitable outcome of illicit contact with [the?] sancta. ... However, P effectively restricts the outbreak of divine נגף/קֶצֶף for encroachment upon sancta to the clergy alone." Milgrom, *Studies in Levitical Terminology*, 21n75.

62. See Yochanan Muffs, *Love and Joy: Law, Language, and Religion in Ancient Israel* (New York: Jewish Theological Seminary of America, 1992), 39–40.

63. On "encroachment" and the Temple, see Milgrom, *Studies in Levitical Terminology*, 5ff.

64. Israel Knohl discusses the relationship between the Koraḥ and Uzziah incidents, specifically insofar as both depict the clash between Israel's political leadership and the Temple priesthood. Knohl, *The Sanctuary of Silence: The Priestly Torah and the Holiness School* (Minneapolis: Fortress Press, 1995), 211–12.

65. Literally, "acted treacherously or unfaithfully." Sara Japhet translates this as "done wrong." Japhet, *The Ideology of the Book of Chronicles and Its Place in Biblical Thought* (Frankfurt: Peter Lang, 1989), 427.

66. Milgrom has coined this term with respect to "encroachment on the sancta," but I use it here in both that sense and as encroachment on the rights and authority of the priesthood. Milgrom, *Studies in Levitical Terminology*.

67. See Othmar Keel, *The Song of Songs*, trans. Frederick J. Gaiser (Minneapolis: Fortress Press, 1994), 25–30.

68. By "secular," I mean any image not related to the cult—that is, any nonritualistic terminology. For example, "secular" images include spices, perfume, and incense related to royalty, erotic descriptions, economics, and agriculture. The term is problematic on many levels, not the least of which is an arbitrary separation of "secular" from cultic images. But I would argue that in a primarily religious document, such as the Hebrew Bible, those images that are not inherently connected to the religion or its practice are valuable indicators of other aspects of the culture.

69. See, for example, Jill Munro, *Spikenard and Saffron: The Imagery of the Song of Songs* (Sheffield, U.K.: Sheffield Academic Press, 1995); Ariel Bloch and Chana Bloch, *The Song of Songs: A New Translation* (New York: Random House, 1995); Keel, *Song of Songs*; Shlomo Bahar, "Perfume in the Song of Songs: An Erotic Motive and Sign of Social Class" [in Hebrew], *Shnaton* (2005): 39–52. In her introduction, Edmée Kingsmill reminds us that the Songs cannot reasonably be considered simply a group of love poems or analyzed for its sensuality alone. She argues persuasively that its language, its words, are indelibly connected to the rest of the biblical text; and its inclusion in the Hebrew Bible is inherently purposeful because its metaphors, allusions, and structures refer constantly to the relationship of God and Israel—even the *eros* of God—that draws Israel, the beloved (and therefore each of us), toward the Divine. As I have learned of her volume only recently, after completing this study, I regret that I have not been able to cite her work throughout. See Edmée Kingsmill, *The Song of Songs and Eros of God: A Study in Biblical Intertextuality* (Oxford: Oxford University Press, 2009).

70. The term *reqaḥ* (רקח), "spice mixture" or "spices," appears in Song 8:2, but it refers here to an additive to wine. That said, there is an obvious relationship between the *roqeaḥ* (רוקח), the "one who mixes ointments or spices," and "spiced wine."

71. Rindisbacher, *Smell of Books*, 331.

72. Keel, *Song of Songs*, 26.

73. Translation of the Hebrew is difficult here. If this term is a *hoph'al* imperfect drawn from the root *r-y-q* (ריק), "oil to be poured out," "oil that will be emptied," then it does not agree in gender with its noun ("oil"). It should probably be the *hoph'al* participle *muraq* (מורק), meaning something like "clarified," "purified," or, more commonly, "the best or finest oil." The midrashic understanding is "poured out," which is in line with the Septuagint and Vulgate. See Roland E. Murphy, *The Song of Songs: A Commentary on the Book of Canticles or the Song of Songs* (Minneapolis: Fortress Press, 1990), 125; Koehler and Baumgartner, *Hebrew and Aramaic Lexicon*, 1228. For the problem of translation and the relationship to Ugaritic, see Oswald Loretz, "Die ugaritisch-hebräische Gefäßbezeichnung Trq/Twrq in Canticum 1,3: Liebesdichtung in der westsemitischen Wein- und Olivenkultur," *Ugarit-Forschungen* 36 (2004): 283–89.

74. "*Lereaḥ shemenekhah tovim shemen turaq shemekhah*" (לריח שמניך טובים שמן תורק שמך).

75. Munro, *Spikenard and Saffron*, 48–49; Michael Fox, *The Song of Songs and Ancient Egyptian Love Songs* (Madison: University of Wisconsin Press, 1985), 97.

76. Only in 1:3 does the ambiguous *lereaḥ* (לריח) appear. Murphy, *Song of Songs*, 125.

77. Or "on his couch."

78. Technically "nerd" or "spikenard," *Nardostachys jatamansi*. This spice was traded long before the Persian period in Egypt, Babylonia, and up into Assyria. Miller, *Spice Trade of the Roman Empire*, 88–92.

79. Or "aloe-wood." Ibid., 66.

80. See Marc Z. Brettler, *God Is King: Understanding an Israelite Metaphor* (Sheffield, U.K.: Sheffield Academic Press, 1989), 79. Cheryl Exum argues that Songs 3:6 is about Solomon on his wedding day—with the implication that he is fumigated. J. Cheryl Exum, "Seeing Solomon's Palanquin (Song of Songs 3:6–11)," *Biblical Interpretation* 11, nos. 3–4 (2003): 301–16.

81. One final note on verses 12–13. It is difficult to determine who holds the power in the relationship. On the surface, the king is the most powerful man in the kingdom. In this instance, however, the image of the king as a sachet of myrrh resting between the breasts of the woman depicts his vulnerability. There is a deep undercurrent in these two verses of her strength and sexual prowess. Later in the Songs, the female becomes vulnerable. While she is lost in the city at night and searching for her lover, the watchmen assault her and strip off her clothing (5:7). These shifts in power and vulnerability occur throughout the Songs.

82. The word *ḥantah* (חנטה), "spices," "makes spicy," or "embalms," is difficult to translate. Nearly every translator renders this word as a form of "sweeten" (Bloch and Bloch, *Song of Songs*, 59), "ripen" (Munro, *Spikenard and Saffron*, 24), or "yield" (Murphy, *Song of Songs*, 138–39). Each of these translations is acceptable, for the idea may be of the fig ripening or turning color on the tree. But these choices leave out the obvious translation of the word, which is "to embalm." Because embalming was accomplished with several spices and fragrant oils, the translation of "spices" is more appropriate.

83. In Murphy's view the *hapax legomenon* (פגיה) means the first, unripe fruit. *Song of Songs*, 139.

84. The Hebrew words for "turtledove" and "dove" are not the same (יונה and תור).

85. Note also the vaginal symbolism of "cut figs."

86. J. Cheryl Exum, "A Literary and Structural Analysis of the Song of Songs," *Zeitschrift für die Alttestamentliche Wissenschaft* 85 (1973): 50.

87. Love poetry that conflates the garden and woman (as well as the vineyard) is well known in the literature of the ancient Near East. See Shalom Paul, "A Lover's Garden of Verse: Literal and Metaphorical Imagery in Ancient Near Eastern Love Poetry," in *Tehillah Le-Moshe: Biblical and Judaic Studies in Honor of Moshe Greenberg*, ed. Mordechai Cogan, Barry Eichler, and Jeffrey Tigay (Winona Lake, Ind.: Eisenbrauns, 1977), 99–110.

88. Reading גן with the Septuagint, the Vulgate, and the Peshiṭta.

89. This term is reminiscent of Exod 30:23, in which Moses is told to make the anointing oil out of "choice spices." It is also the same phrase used in the rabbinic legal literature to mean either "chief spices" or "balsam." See chapter 2.

90. Murphy, *Song of Songs*, 156. See also Prov 5:3.

91. Murphy asserts, "This is hardly a reference to the specific odor of cedar, since presumably there was also much vegetation there; Lebanon would be a symbol of all that is fragrant" (*Song of Songs*, 160). This is possible but doubtful. The source of "all things fragrant" is more probably Arabia or Africa, south of Egypt. Caravans heading north passed through Israel from these areas, loaded with spices. The spice trade ran from east to west and from south to north, not the other way around. It is also possible that the woman's garments have a pleasant scent because she has fumigated them with incense. Thus Lebanon is used for its auditory similarity to *lebonah* (לבונה), frankincense—or if not frankincense, then the prized cedars of Lebanon.

92. Munro views the beginning of this verse as the place where the switch in voice from the male to the female occurs (rather than at the end of the verse, as in the translation here). Munro, *Spikenard and Saffron*, 27.

93. Exum, "Literary and Structural Analysis," 64.

94. In 5:1, the woman as garden is taken one step further when the man describes her as *his* own garden: "I have come to my garden, my sister, bride! I gather my myrrh with my spices. I eat my honeycomb with my honey; I drink my wine with my milk." Here the image moves from the sense of smell to that of taste.

95. Exum, however, reads this verse as spoken by the beloved about the male lover. Exum, "Seeing Solomon's Palanquin." While this reading fits well with the verses that follow and while there is precedent for kings being fumigated on their wedding days, Dirksen disagrees. See Peter B. Dirksen, "Song of Songs 3:6–7," *Vetus Testamentum* 39, no. 2 (1989): 219–25.

96. Nielsen, *Incense in Ancient Israel*.

97. Gillis Gereleman, *Ruth, das Hohelied*, ed. Martin Noth and Hans Walter Woff, Biblischer Kommentar, Altes Testament, no. 18 (Neukirchen-Vluyn: Neukirchener, 1965), 159.

98. See Jonathan Culler, *Structuralist Poetics: Structuralism, Linguistics, and the Study of Literature* (Ithaca: Cornell University Press, 1975), 61–74, 113–30.

99. Miller, *Anatomy of Disgust*.

100. For a thorough review of this term and its use and meanings throughout the Bible, see Avrahami, "Sensorium and Its Operation in Biblical Epistemology."

101. See Exod 7:18, 21 (because of fish); Exod 8:10 (because of frogs); Exod 16:20 (because of manna kept overnight); and Isa 50:2 (because of fish).

102. Or "garrison."

103. The term *ba'ash* (באש) is often found with the preposition *beth* (ב), which has a wide semantic range (spatial, temporal, instrumental, etc.). The most typical meanings (including, "in," "at" "with," "against," or "because of") do not really fit with this verb and therefore make the phrase difficult to translate. But the difficulty in translation may provide one clue to the colloquial nature of this term. It is possible that the use of the *beth* (ב) preposition results from the understanding that odor is inhaled. That is, scent is taken into the body via air. In this sense the Israelites stink *inside* the noses of the Philistines. The concept of "stinking in" is repeated in several of the passages cited herein.

104. McCarter translates this as "they had offended David," but he notes the literal meaning as well ("they stank with David"). McCarter also notes that the Septuagint reads, "the people of David were afraid," which the commentator attributes to an understanding of *bosh* (בוש) rather than *ba'ash* (באש). P. Kyle McCarter Jr., *II Samuel* (New York: Doubleday, 1984), 266–67. Note that the *beth* (ב) preposition appears in this verse as well. The Chronicler, however, employs the preposition *'im* (עם) and the *hitpa'el* form of the verb when describing the reek of the Ammonites (1 Chr 19:6).

105. It is possible that a very intuitive understanding of scent is at work in these references—that is, the concept of "smelling fear." In both instances above, it is the assumed victor who smells the stench of the coward or weaker opponent (although Saul does eventually rout the Philistines). It is also possible that the analogy itself is based on reality in that men in hand-to-hand combat would have been able to hear and perhaps even smell the enemy before they could see the enemy. (Job 39:19–25 describes the horse as "smelling" battle from afar and running toward it unafraid.)

106. The use of the *hiph'il* in this instance is causative, and somewhat reflexive, for David, as the subject, has caused himself, as the object, to stink with respect to his own people. In fact, each of these passages demonstrates a reflexivity and "self-description."

107. "To stink," *ba'ash* (באש), appears in this verse in the *niph'al* form as it did in 1 Sam 13:4 and 2 Sam 10:6, where it was the Israelites or the Ammonites who stank. Comparably, the *niph'al* form in this verse indicates that it is Absalom who will stink; he will be odious to his father. However, the preposition ב, which appeared in the other verses to indicate those who will smell the stench, is not used. Instead, the author deftly inserts the direct object marker (את) just before the word "father." This syntax suggests that Absalom (as the subject) will cause his father, David (as the direct object), to stink. The confusing grammar foreshadows the irony that is to come: Absalom will be disgusting (*niph'al* form) to his father and all Israel since he had intercourse with his father's concubines. He will be the outcast (just as his father is the outcast during the episode) and the "other," without power or real protection. The syntax also masks the adviser's words so that his counsel is both true and leads Absalom to ruin.

108. Eduard Kutscher notes that the roots *b-'-sh* (באש) and *b-w-sh* (בוש) are interchanged in the Isaiah scroll. Eduard Y. Kutscher, *The Language and Linguistic Background of the Isaiah Scroll* [in Hebrew] (Jerusalem: Magnes Press, 1959), 169. In reference to each of the examples given here, see also Johanna Stiebert, "Shame and Prophecy: Approaches Past and Present," *Biblical Interpretation* 8, no. 3 (2000): 255–75. Although her discussion centers on Ezek 16, her review of the anthropological data on shame, gender, and public recognition is useful.

109. Genesis 34:30 incorporates many of the same themes. There, Jacob responds to his sons, Simeon and Levi, after they have wiped out Hamor, the Hivite, his son

Shechem, and the entire city, "You have caused trouble for me by causing me to stink among those who dwell in the land, among the Canaanites and among the Perizzites; my men are few in number, and [if] they will be gathered against me, striking me, I and my house will be destroyed." The clustered ideas regarding imminent battle, cowardice, and the "other" are all present in this verse and in the larger context surrounding it. Jacob's intent was to unite with the Shechemites in a good-faith contract. His sons have not only destroyed the contract; they have caused Jacob's house to be treated as outcasts, foreigners. Just as no one trusts the foreigner, so the larger resident population will no longer trust Jacob's word or that of the men of his house. On the issue of the brothers having been "shamed" or having become the "other," a disgrace that would necessitate "revenge," see Claudia Camp, *Wise, Strange, and Holy: The Strange Woman and the Making of the Bible* (Sheffield, U.K.: Sheffield Academic Press, 2000), 279–322.

110. In addition to David and Absalom (1 Sam 26:19), see also the narrative of Jacob and his sons, Simeon and Levi (Gen 34:30).

111. E.g., the cases of David and Saul (1 Sam 26:19) and Israel's striving against Egypt (Exod 5:21).

112. Exod 5:21 may be considered to include men and women, just as the foremen may represent all Israelites. "Community" in the Hebrew Bible, however, is commonly gendered as male.

113. See Camp, *Wise, Strange, and Holy,* 72–89, 323–24; Carol Newsom, "Woman and the Discourse of Patriarchal Wisdom: A Study of Proverbs 1–9," in *Gender and Difference,* ed. Peggy L. Day (Minneapolis: Fortress Press, 1989), 148; Claudia Camp, "What's So Strange About the Strange Woman?" in *The Bible and the Politics of Exegesis: Festschrift for Norman Gottwald,* ed. David Jobling, Peggy L. Day, and Gerald T. Sheppard (Cleveland: Pilgrim Press, 1991), 17–31.

114. This is not necessarily true of the verb "to be ashamed" (*bosh*, בוש), however, which appears in reference to Israel as the adulterous wife or harlot in the books of the Prophets, particularly Jeremiah and Ezekiel.

115. Sexual allusions represented by "eating" appear several times in Proverbs. In this instance, the woman as sword is a devouring and destructive force. Michael Fox translates this passage: "For the strange woman's lips drip honey; her palate is smoother than oil. But her after effect is as bitter as wormwood, sharp as a two-edged sword." Fox, *Proverbs 1–9: A New Translation with Introduction and Commentary,* Anchor Bible, 18A (New York: Doubleday, 2000), 189. But see also p. 192 for his discussion of the literal "sword of mouths."

116. Fox makes clear the use of "strange": "The 'stranger' (*zarah*) is another man's wife.... She is assumed to be a prostitute by all the medieval plain-sense commentators and almost all the modern ones (e.g., Toy, McKane). The LXX apparently read *znh* ('harlot') instead of *zrh* ('stranger') in its Hebrew text of v. 3. This reading could be a scribal change motivated by the same assumption rather than original. In my view the Strange Woman is another man's wife, whose transgression is thus adultery. She is not a prostitute but a wanton amateur of the sort who 'opens her quiver for every arrow,' as Ben Sira puts it." Ibid., 191–92.

117. We are told of the male's assembly (קהל) and congregation (עדה) in Prov 5:14.

118. Cf. the "wicked" woman of 4Q184. Scott C. Jones, "Wisdom's Pedagogy: A Comparison of Proverbs VII and 4Q184," *Vetus Testamentum* 53, no. 1 (2003): 65–80.

119. See Camp, *Wise, Strange, and Holy.*

120. Fox, *Proverbs 1–9*, 192. Of note, in 4Q184 the "wicked woman" is silent. For a complete comparison of the woman from Prov 5 and 7 and 4Q184, see Jones, "Wisdom's Pedagogy." Among other issues, the description of the "wicked woman" is not erotic, she is not a member of the community, and the motif used as a contrast for her is the group "outsider." See also Matthew Goff, "Hellish Females: The Strange Woman of Septuagint Proverbs and 4QWiles of the Wicked Woman (4Q184)," *Journal for the Study of Judaism* 39, no. 1 (2008): 20–45.

121. I would argue further that because all of Songs 4 is so heavily laden with scent imagery, the references to "honey and milk on the tongue" are subtle scent images as well. As a result, the Proverbs passage is already encoded with scent associations. In addition, because the images in both the Songs and Proverbs describe the woman's tongue, a further allusion is made to her breath, which is assuredly a provocative scent producer.

122. With slight emendation, Fox translates this "to guard you from another man's wife." Fox, *Proverbs 1–9*, 227.

123. Cf. 4Q184, in which the "secret" places are compared with the "broad," "light" compared to "darkness," etc. Rick D. Moore, "Personification of the Seduction of Evil: 'The Wiles of the Wicked Woman,'" *Revue de Qumran* 10, no. 4D (1981): 505–19.

124. Of course, in Songs 5:7 the female lover also wanders the streets looking for the male, but she does not find him. See Goff, "Hellish Females," on issues of residence and speech with respect to Prov 7 and its comparators.

125. See also Prov 13:5.

126. *Avot* 1:1.

127. Regardless of their dating, all texts from Isaiah are presented together for ease of reference.

128. In the sense of "vain," "worthless," or "bad." For a complete bibliography on *shaveh*, שוה, see Koehler and Baumgartner, *Hebrew and Aramaic Lexicon*, 1425.

129. Or the lack of it, as expressed in 2 Chr 29:7, in which Hezekiah describes how the previous priests closed the Temple and ceased incense sacrifice.

130. In the priestly literature, cane is only mentioned as an ingredient in the sacred anointing oil (Exod 30:23).

131. Cf. Nielsen, *Incense in Ancient Israel*, 62–63.

132. See Michael Fishbane, *Haftarot* (Philadelphia: Jewish Publication Society, 2002), 148.

133. John L. McKenzie, *Second Isaiah* (Garden City, N.Y.: Doubleday, 1968), 60–61; Fishbane, *Haftarot*, 148–49; John Goldingay, "Isaiah 43, 22–28," *Zeitschrift für die Alttestamentliche Wissenschaft* 110, no. 2 (1998): 173–91.

134. On "clusters" and the units of Isa 66 as a whole and verses 3–4 in particular, see Edwin C. Webster, "A Rhetorical Study of Isaiah 66," *Journal for the Study of the Old Testament* 34 (1986): 93–108.

135. Or "offering up an offering of the blood of a pig."

136. In context of the next verse, "Just as . . . ."

137. Fishbane notes that the legitimate and illegitimate practices appear in pairs. Fishbane, *Haftarot*, 328–29.

138. Benjamin Sommer, *A Prophet Reads Scripture: Allusion in Isaiah 40–66* (Stanford: Stanford University Press, 1998).

139. Isa 56:7, 60:7 and 13, 66:20–23.

140. Fishbane connects the "trembling" people in these verses with "'those who trembled at the teaching/command' of the Lord in Ezra 9:4, [and] 10:3." Fishbane,

Biblical Interpretation in Ancient Israel (Oxford: Oxford University Press, 1985; reprint, 1988), 114n27.

141. Fishbane, *Haftarot*, 328.

142. Literally, "good"; this may also be translated as "pleasing." For more on the function of "good" (טוב) in Jeremiah, see Nielsen, *Incense in Ancient Israel*, 62–63.

143. "Acceptable" in the sense of "producing favor" in order to effect appeasement or forgiveness. "Pleasing" may also be translated as "sweet."

144. Robert P. Carroll, *Jeremiah: A Commentary* (Philadelphia: Westminster Press, 1986), 200–201; William McKane, *Jeremiah* (Edinburgh: T & T Clark, 1996), 148–51.

145. For discussion of the exegetical relationship between Jer 17:19–27 and the Sabbath laws as articulated in Deut 5:12–14 and then in Neh 13:15–21, see Fishbane, *Biblical Interpretation in Ancient Israel*, 129–34.

146. This is a new formulation on Deut 5:12–14, as Fishbane explains: "in Deut. 5:12 the reference is simply to the earlier citation of the command in Exod 20:8; whereas its recurrence in Jer 17:22 follows two prohibitions not found in either Exod 20:8–11 or Deut 5:12–14. In this new context, the statement 'as I commanded your forefathers' does not simply refer to the general prohibition of labour derived from the decalogical command, but is expanded to include a prohibition against bearing burdens into Jerusalem on the Sabbath, and one against removing a burden from one's home on that day." Ibid., 132–33.

147. This would be in line with commentators who suspect an exilic or postexilic (Jerusalem) date for this prophecy. Carroll, *Jeremiah*, 419.

148. On the prophet's critique of the priesthood in Mal 1:6–2:9, using images from the priestly blessing, see Fishbane, *Biblical Interpretation in Ancient Israel*, 332–34.

149. Rather than some form of *qetoreth* (קטורת), the term used in this instance for "incense" is *muqtar* (מקטר)—the *hoph'al* form of the root *q-t-r*; therefore, the sense is "to be turned into rising smoke." Koehler and Baumgartner, *Hebrew and Aramaic Lexicon*, 1095.

150. "And snort at it" (והפחתם אותו); "it" refers to the altar/table. With the verb's root meaning "to blow" or "to breathe" (נפח) in the *hiph'il* form, it would seem that the idiom is onomatopoeic and therefore means that the Israelites, or priests, snorted, sniffed, or blew at the altar/table in derision or disgust. See Andrew Hill, *Malachi* (New York: Doubleday, 1998), 191.

151. God's refusal to smell sacrifices is articulated in Lev 26:31 and Amos 5:21–22.

152. An extraordinarily literal and anthropomorphic image of God consuming sacrifices.

153. The term *bosem* (בשם) could simply mean "spice" here but more probably refers to scented oil or perfume. On Isa 3:16, see also chapter 2.

154. The book of Ezekiel demonstrates priestly concerns in many places, and chapters 40–47 describe in rich detail a new Temple and its environs.

155. This translation is in line with that of Moshe Greenberg, who comments that the last phrase may be an idiom, because the literal translation—"'not coming things [Isa 41:22] and it will not be'—[is] hardly coherent." Further, he notes, "With this and the following verses, compare the cajolery of the adulteress in Prov 7:16, 'I have decked my couch with coverlets, / with striped cloths of the yarn of Egypt. / I have perfumed my bed with myrrh, aloes and cinnamon.' In our verse, shrines (*bamot*) (at which foreign gods were worshiped, II Kings 21:3) replaced the bed—the referent intruding again, recalling Isa 57:7. To be sure, both this and the Isaiah passage are generally thought to

allude to sacred prostitution; O Eissfeldt, who explains all the terms for 'elevations' in our passage as the raised bed or pedestal on which this rite was performed, considers 'harlotry' to have a double meaning (prostitution in the cult of foreign gods; JPOS 16 [1939], 286–92 = Kleine Schriften II, pp. 101–6.)" Greenberg, *Ezekiel 1–20* (New York: Doubleday, 1983), 280.

156. One should note, however, that several scholars view the images of the YHWH cult as added to the phallic and other foreign images. See Walther Zimmerli, *Ezekiel 1* (Philadelphia: Fortress Press, 1979), 344.

157. Mary Shields notes that "the rhetoric used to describe her [Israel's] foreign alliances and her worship of other gods is focused on what she does with her body." Mary E. Shields, "Multiple Exposures: Body Rhetoric and Gender Characterization in Ezekiel 16," *Journal of Feminist Studies in Religion* 14, no. 1 (1998): 5–18.

158. For the grammatical inconsistencies in these verses, see Moshe Greenberg, *Ezekiel 21–37* (New York: Doubleday, 1997), 486; Zimmerli, *Ezekiel 1*, 492.

159. Zimmerli notes that the women may have adorned themselves. *Ezekiel 1*, 492.

160. Although not directly related to our focus, it is important to note the significant work that has been done on the use of metaphor in Ezek 16 by Julie Galambush, *Jerusalem in the Book of Ezekiel: The City as Yahweh's Wife* (Atlanta: Scholars Press, 1992); Linda Day, "Rhetoric and Domestic Violence in Ezekiel 16," *Biblical Interpretation* 8, no. 3 (2000): 205–30; and Peggy L. Day, "Adulterous Jerusalem's Imagined Demise: Death of a Metaphor in Ezekiel XVI," *Vetus Testamentum* 50, no. 3 (2000): 285–309.

161. Whether these qualities are given by God or already belong to the messiah is uncertain.

162. Jesse was the father of David, so this is a clear reference to one of the Davidic line, perhaps Hezekiah.

163. Fishbane explains, "Verse 3a ('he shall sense,' [*va-hariḥo*]) has traditionally been interpreted as an inner perception (Kimḥi; Ibn Ezra), as against the outer senses of sight and of hearing noted in the sequel. Alternatively, the verb may be construed as a denominative, meaning '(God shall) inspire' him (R. Isaiah di Trani; R. Eliezer of Beaugency)." Fishbane, *Haftarot*, 434.

164. These qualities are also considered virtues of the just king (Ps 72:1–2, 4, 7, 12–13; Jer 23:5). See ibid.

165. Cf. הרוח דעת ויראת יהוה and והריחו ביראת יהוה; *Biblia Hebraica Stuttgartensia*, ed. Albrecht Alt, Otto Eisfeldt, Paul Kahle, and Rudolf Kittel (Stuttgart: Deutsche Bibelgesellschaft, 1990), 692. See also George Buchanan Gray, *Isaiah: International Critical Commentary* (New York: Charles Scribner's Sons, 1912), 217. For a thorough review of the interpretations and translations of this verse as well as the anthropological significance of "smelling" as a means of "knowing," see Ian D. Ritchie, "The Nose Knows: Bodily Knowing in Isaiah 11:3," *Journal for the Study of the Old Testament* 87 (2000): 59–73. As something of a corrective to Ritchie and by means of a close syntactical reading of this verse, Avrahami argues for a reading similar to that of the Jewish interpreters, who viewed the messiah as able to judge by "smelling" (Avrahami, "Sensorium and Its Operation in Biblical Epistemology"). Although I take issue with his reformulation of the verse, Jeremiah Unterman gives a concise review of the history of Jewish interpretation of the verse in "The (Non)Sense of Smell in Isaiah 11:3," *Hebrew Studies* 33 (1992): 17–23.

166. Most often this ordering of the senses concerns gods who are not the "real" God. See Deut 4:28 ("There you will serve gods made of the hands of man, of wood and

stone, that cannot see or hear or eat or smell") and Ps 115:5–6 ("They have mouths but do not speak; they have eyes, but do not see; they have ears, but do not hear; they have noses but do not smell").

167. The grammatical structure of the passage presents the senses of sight and hearing as nouns in the "construct form," and only "smelling" occurs in a verbal form. See also the story of Isaac and the blessing of Jacob (Gen 27), in which the blind Isaac must rely on his other senses to determine which son stands before him. His hearing gives him the correct information—this is not his son Esau—but Isaac's sense of touch and smell lead him to bless the disguised Jacob. In fact, scent is what convinces Isaac: "And he smelled the scent of his clothes and he blessed him. He said, 'The scent of my son is like the scent of the field that the Lord has blessed'" (Gen 27:27).

168. Tamar Kadari points out, however, that the overarching metaphor in the Tannaitic material on the Songs is the beloved as Torah. Kadari, "'Within It Was Decked with Love': The Torah as Bride in Tannaitic Exegesis on Song of Songs" [in Hebrew], *Tarbiz* 71 (2002): 391–404.

Chapter 4

1. For more on the provenance and date of *Songs Rabbah*, see chapter 1. No critical edition of *Songs Rabbah* exists. My quotations of the midrashic text are taken from *Song of Songs Rabbah*, Midrash Rabbah, Romm, Wilna edition of 1887, unless otherwise noted. For manuscript evidence of underlying texts, see H. E. Steller, "Preliminary Remarks to a New Edition of Shir Hashirim Rabbah," in *Rashi, 1040–1990: Homage à Ephraim E. Urbach*, ed. Gabrielle Sed-Rajna (Paris: Cerf, 1993), 301–11. See also Kadari, "On the Redaction of Midrash Shir Hashirim Rabbah," which considers the creativity of the editor's enterprise.

2. A "prooftext" is the quotation of a verse from Scripture that is used either to prove or to articulate a rabbi's position.

3. *Songs Rab.* also presents midrashim that appear nowhere else as well as anonymous quotations and attributions. Tamar Kadari has shown decisively that these are probably the creative endeavors of the redactor. See Kadari, "On the Redaction of Midrash Shir Hashirim Rabbah."

4. Similarly, early Christian texts assign the role of the male lover to Jesus and of the beloved to the church. Kadari argues that for the Tannaitic midrashim, the woman is more often compared to the Torah. See Kadari, "'Within It Was Decked with Love.'" Although the metaphors continually shift, I believe that Song of Songs may be the single most interpreted book of the Bible.

5. Gerson Cohen, "The Song of Songs and the Jewish Religious Mentality," in Cohen, *Studies in the Variety of Rabbinic Cultures* (Philadelphia: Jewish Publication Society, 1991), 3–17.

6. Kingsmill would agree with Cohen that the Songs represent a response to the Prophets, but she views this response as grounded in an eschatological presentation of the relationship between God and humans—that is, a representation of future reconciliation and love. Kingsmill, *Song of Songs and Eros of God*.

7. Cf. *Songs Rab.* 8:11.

8. See George W. E. Nickelsburg, *1 Enoch* (Minneapolis: Fortress Press, 2001), 312–28. On the other end, historically, this same association among the righteous and

the garden of the Songs and Eden is also found in *Tg. Cant.* 4:12. See Philip S. Alexander, *The Targum of Canticles, Translated, with a Critical Introduction, Apparatus, and Notes* (Collegeville, Minn.: Liturgical Press, 2003), 140–41.

9. The Shekhinah is the earthly manifestation of God's presence. See *Gen. Rab.* 3:9. See also Ephraim Urbach, *The Sages: Their Concepts and Beliefs*, trans. Israel Abrahams, 2d ed. (Cambridge: Harvard University Press, 1979), 40.

10. Literally, "orchard."

11. *Songs Rab.* 5:1. Such verses as "The king has brought me into his chamber" (Song 1:4) act as a stimulus for the retelling of the famous midrash on the four rabbis who enter *pardes*. See *Songs Rab.* 1:4 and *b. Ḥag.* 14b. On the issue of *pardes* as place or metaphor, see Ephraim Urbach, "Ha-Mesorot 'al Torat ha-Sod be-Tequfat ha-Tannaim" [in Hebrew], in *Studies in Mysticism and Religion Presented to Gershom G. Scholem on His Seventieth Birthday by Pupils, Colleagues, and Friends* (Jerusalem: Magnes Press, 1968), 1–28. See also Gershom Scholem, *Kabbalah* (Jerusalem: Keter, 1974), 18. All of this is reviewed and discussed at length by David Halperin, who also discusses the variety of referents for the garden image, in Halperin, *The Merkabah in Rabbinic Literature* (New Haven, Conn.: American Oriental Society, 1980), 86–92.

12. See Francis Landy, *Paradoxes of Paradise: Identity and Difference in the Song of Songs* (Sheffield, U.K.: Almond, 1983), 183–219.

13. For a more thorough analysis of the comparison of the lovers to fauna in the Songs, see Carol L. Meyers, "Gender Imagery in the Song of Songs," in *A Feminist Companion to the Song of Songs*, ed. Athalya Brenner (Sheffield, U.K.: Sheffield Academic Press, 1993), 197–212.

14. The reference to the lower millstones indicates that even the heaviest of weights could not withstand the water and were destroyed in the flood. The lower millstone is not moved during the milling process and is so heavy that it would be sold with the house. Jastrow, *Dictionary of the Targumim*, 55.

15. The identification of the dove with female Israel creates a subtle allusion to the martyrdom narratives that appear in other parts of *Songs Rab.* Just as the dove happily eats the bitter leaves from God rather than the sweet leaves from Noah, so Israel gladly eats of the bitterness that belief in one God and the commandments entails, rejecting the attempts of non-Jews to seduce her into an easier existence. See chapter 5.

16. There are several parallel sources for this midrash. On the earlier cases, see *Gen. Rab.* 33:6, on Gen 8:10–11 (in which Noah sends the dove out to look for land a second time, and the dove brings back the plucked olive leaf). See also *Lev. Rab.* 31:10, on Lev 24:2 (in reference to the Israelites bringing olive oil for lighting the lamps at the dedication of the Tabernacle). The description of the dove as "killing" the potential of the leaf to grow into a big tree is also found in the other sources—as are the passage from Ezekiel and the argument between the rabbis about what kind of leaf the dove would have brought had she flown to Eden. The identification of Eden as the specific place to which the dove flies, the "bitter" olive branch that comes directly from God's hand, and the counterclaim that the dove would have brought cinnamon or balsam (בלסמון in *Songs Rab.* and פפולוסמון or אופבלסמון in *Gen. Rab.*) had she flown to Eden all indicate the blending of the image of Eden with the garden from the Songs (the only garden mentioned in the Bible as containing fragrant spice trees) and the location of God's habitation.

17. R. Aibu is probably R. Abbahu or R. Abun, third- and fourth-generation Amoraim, respectively. The *Gen. Rab.* version uses the name of R. Abbahu. The other names

in the parallel sources are very similar to each other as well (R. Ṭari and Birai, etc.) and are likely the result of scribal confusion.

18. That the rabbis value particular spices is demonstrated in a *baraita* that reconstructs the ingredients of the Temple incense (see *b. Ker.* 6a) and in chapter 5 of this volume.

19. This glen to the south of Jerusalem is where it is believed that Moloch was worshipped. The place thus becomes the area to which the wicked are sent for punishment in the afterlife, or hell. See *b. 'Erub.* 19a; *b. Sukkah* 32b.

20. The term "evil" (*ra'*, רע) also has the meaning of "bad," in the sense, here, that nothing smells worse.

21. Jastrow says, "than goatskin made hairless by washing" (*Dictionary of the Targumim*, 1555). If Jastrow is correct and this is a reference to the foul odor that arises during the process of hair removal (the step before tanning), then it should be considered a reference to daily life. In rabbinic literature (and throughout the ancient world), the tannery is considered one of the foulest-smelling places and therefore would be situated outside or on the outskirts of the city and downwind. See Weiss, "Location of Jewish Cemeteries in Galilee."

22. The statement attributed to R. Yoḥanan is probably quite ancient. He is a second-generation Amora (ca. 250–90 C.E.), and this statement, attributed to him, also appears in *Gen. Rab.* 65:22.

23. It is unlikely that Esau is equated with Christianity in this passage—particularly given the age of this midrash. That said, Carol Bakhos raises the interesting question of whether Esau necessarily represents Rome. See Bakhos, "Figuring (Out) Esau: The Rabbis and Their Others," *Journal of Jewish Studies* 58, no. 2 (2007): 250–62.

24. Gehenna, or hell, is connected to Esau through a play on words. In the biblical account, when Esau comes back from hunting and brings the dish of game to his father in order to receive the blessing, Isaac asks, "Who then (אפוא) is it who hunted game and brought it to me?" (Gen 27:33). The midrash rereads the enclitic particle as the verb "to bake" (אפה), and so causes Isaac to ask, "Who is baked (נאפה) in this oven?" The midrash then atomizes verse 33 to derive God's response that it is the one "who hunted game."

25. On the *tzaddik* ("righteous one") and odor, see Rudolf Mach, *Der Zaddik in Talmude und Midrasch* (Leiden: Brill, 1957), 103–4. Mach discusses the comparison in *Gen. Rab.* 63 of Esau and Jacob to the rose bush and myrtle. He also considers the issues surrounding the righteous, the world to come, and Paradise.

26. Although this term for "garment" is a standard variation (we expect שמלה), Gen 27:27 employs the word *beged* (בגד).

27. Here one might consider the smells of the kitchen and cooking food that also permeate hair, clothing, furniture, and air. In addition, the hot oven may allude to martyrdom—it may suggest, that is, that Esau, as Rome, is the perpetrator of martyrdoms. See chapter 5.

28. See *Songs Rab.* 2:2, discussed below.

29. See the book of Susanna and the midrashim on the four sages who entered *pardes* (*Songs Rab.* 1:4; *b. Ḥag.* 14b). The place in which Bat Sheva bathes when she is spied by David, who is walking on his rooftop, could also be considered to fit this trope (2 Sam 11:2–3). Of note, in the book of Esther, where so many of the images are inverted, the king retires to the palace garden after Esther's accusation of Haman. Haman then falls prostrate before Esther in the banquet room of her private quarters

(Esth 7:7). Although not all of these places are created in order to appear "natural," each of them raises issues surrounding private versus public space, inside and outside, safe and dangerous, etc.

30. Scholars of rabbinic literature usually define a parable as any expression of comparison (most often to a king) that begins, "To what can X be compared? To a Y . . ." This initial comparison is referred to as the *mashal*. The second part of the parable, which includes an explanation of the *mashal*, is called the *nimshal*. See David Stern, *Parables in Midrash* (Cambridge: Harvard University Press, 1991); Daniel Boyarin, *Intertextuality and the Reading of Midrash* (Bloomington: Indiana University Press, 1990), chapters 2–3.

31. Literally, "field laborer."

32. Or "flower."

33. The parable is quoted in the name of R. Simon, an Amora who was active sometime between 250 and 320 C.E. in Palestine. R. Azariah, a fifth-generation Amora, also in Palestine, recites the midrash in the name of R. Simon's son, R. Judah, a fourth-generation Amora. In consideration of the line of tradents, R. Judah is also known as R. Judah ben Simon ben Pazzi. As such, R. Simon is most probably R. Simon ben Pazzi. The entire cycle of this midrash (six parts in all) appears in *Lev. Rab.* 23:3 with slight emendations. The translation here is from *Songs Rab.* Variations are presented in the notes to the discussion of the text. Because *Lev. Rab.* is thought to have been redacted between 400 and 500 C.E., it would be considered the older source. See Strack and Stemberger, *Introduction to the Talmud and Midrash*, 316–17.

34. As is common in midrashic parables, the king is compared to God in the *nimshal* (the explanation of the parable). See Stern, *Parables in Midrash*, 19–21, 93–101.

35. There is no precise one-to-one correlation between *mashal* and *nimshal*. For more on this issue, see ibid.; Boyarin, *Intertextuality and the Reading of Midrash*, chapter 5.

36. *Lev. Rab.*, "Torah."

37. Or "flower."

38. Literally, "arranged" (סדר).

39. Cf. *Songs Rab.* 8:14.

40. *Lev. Rab.*, "For the merit of the Torah and Israel."

41. Although *Lev. Rab.* is not a Tannaitic text, its reference to "Torah" rather than "Israel" bolsters Kadari's point on the meta-metaphor of the Songs as comparing the woman to "Torah." Kadari, "'Within It Was Decked with Love.'"

42. Having thus brought up the subject of the flood, the midrash continues by portraying the threefold events of rebellion and destruction or punishment: the extinction of the generation of Enosh, the biblical flood story, and the episode of the Tower of Babel. Two of these water references, Enosh and the Tower of Babel, are purely rabbinic formulations; no water appears in those biblical accounts. The explanation for the destruction of the generation of Enosh by means of water is found in *Gen. Rab.* 23:7 (on Gen 4:26), in which R. Simon refers to the "rebellions" of Enosh and Nimrod. In that midrash, R. Levi declares that because these men were so evil, God summoned the sea and destroyed them. The prooftexts R. Levi applies to his argument are Amos 5:8 and 9:6, which twice repeat "He calls for the waters of the sea," thus indicating that there were two floods (that of the generation of Enosh and that of the flood known from the biblical account). The third reference to water, "the generation of the dispersion," refers to the Tower of Babel episode. According to the rabbis, God confuses the language of the builders, so that when they ask for a particular tool or material they are given

something else. The first of these requests is for water: "One would say to his friend, 'Bring me water.' And he would bring him earth. And he would strike him and break his skull. 'Bring me an axe.' And he would bring him a spade" (*Gen. Rab.* 38:10). In this way, the rebellion is put down by means of water. Steven Fraade traces the development of interpretation of Enosh and the generations leading up to the flood. He discusses at length the difference between nonrabbinic portrayals (which are positive) and depictions of Enosh in rabbinic midrashim (which are negative). Fraade, *Enosh and His Generation: Pre-Israelite Hero and History in Postbiblical Interpretation* (Chico, Calif.: Scholars Press, 1984).

43. See also Michael Fishbane's discussion of "soothing odor" in midrashic sources, in which the intended purpose of the ascending odor is to "effect divine mercy." Fishbane, *Biblical Myth and Rabbinic Mythmaking*, 184–87.

44. See *Gen. Rab.* 66:2.

45. See Cohen, "Esau as Symbol."

46. These relationships may not be specified in the midrashim. In addition, because our focus is on textual representation and not on the actual lives or social histories of these women, no distinction is made for social status or other identification (such as religion).

47. May also be translated as "couch," with the sense of reclining in order to eat. See Murphy, *Song of Songs*, 131.

48. Or "bad" (רע).

49. Or "changed."

50. R. Meir is considered a third-generation Tanna. He was a student of R. Ishamel and then of R. Akiba. R. Judah is probably R. Judah bar Ilai, who is of the same generation as R. Meir. See Strack and Stemberger, *Introduction to the Talmud and Midrash*, 84–85.

51. R. Meir may interpret spikenard or "nard" (*nerd*, נרד) as a form of "to descend" (*nered*, נרד), from the root *yarad* (ירד).

52. Cf. *Songs Rab.* 2:2, discussed in the previous section, and *Songs Rab.* 2:3.

53. On negative representations of biblical women, see Judith Baskin, *Midrashic Women: Formations of the Feminine in Rabbinic Literature* (Hanover: University Press of New England, 2002), 54–55; Tirzah Meacham, "Woman More Intelligent Than Man," in *Approaches to Ancient Judaism, New Series*, vol. 5, *Historical, Literary, and Religious Studies*, ed. Herbert W. Basser and Simcha Fishbane (Atlanta: Scholars Press, 1993), 55–65.

54. The narrative structure of the midrash (the language of R. Judah's dissent) may also serve to buttress R. Meir's position. Once in *Gen. Rab.* and several times in *Songs Rab.*, R. Akiba reproves R. Pappus and insists, "Enough!" (see, for example, *Gen. Rab.* 21:5 and *Songs Rab.* 1:9). This midrashic dialogue between R. Akiba and R. Pappus occurs in other sources as well; see Theodor and Albeck, *Midrash Bereshit Rabba*, 200. Each of these admonitions is R. Akiba's response to an occasion on which R. Pappus has expounded on an esoteric matter (the creation of Adam and man's likeness to God or the angels, the manner in which God judges man, the divine chariot, etc.). In each of these encounters, R. Pappus's interpretation could have led to an uncomfortable discussion of abstruse issues and beliefs to which the rabbinic voices only allude in midrash and never discuss openly. See Menachem Kahana, "The Critical Edition of Mekilta De-Rabbi Ishmael in the Light of the Genizah Fragments" [in Hebrew]), *Tarbiz* 55, no. 4 (1986): 504–15. In each instance, R. Akiba attempts to avert or halt such foraging, but he refrains from

attacking R. Pappus directly on each occasion, regardless of how inappropriate the suggestions and implications of Pappus's interpretation may be for public edification. The insinuation is not that R. Akiba disagrees with his colleague but that he strongly desires, and therefore urges, deflection of these topics. R. Judah's employment of comparable language in his dispute with R. Meir is highly reminiscent of the encounters between Rabbis Akiba and Pappus (who are second-generation Tannaim and therefore precede Rabbis Judah and Meir); that is, R. Judah agrees with R. Meir's negative association of Israel with the female whose perfume smells good (and which thereby implies negative attributes). R. Judah's point, that the Songs should be expounded only to praise Israel, reflects that it is somehow different and anomalous. As such, exegesis of the Songs and the ensuing interpretations involving the female should be different in tone and type and of a positive nature.

55. In addition, no appeal to another authority appears after R. Judah's comment.

56. In the manuscript, פילתא. This is *foliatum* (פולייטון, or φουλιᾶτον) a fragrant oil or ointment prepared from leaves (פילון, φύλλον).

57. May also have the sense of "worthy" (כשרות).

58. See the section "Historical Moments and Aroma," below, for more examples of this kind of historicization.

59. R. Yassa could also be R. Yossi or R. Assi, and therefore a third-generation Amora (ca. late third and early fourth centuries C.E.) from Israel.

60. Also known as Abba II, R. bar Yudan is a third-generation Amora. He had contact with R. Abbahu in Caesarea and then with R. Assi in Tiberias. He was originally from Babylonia and studied there with Rav Huna before going to Israel. Strack and Stemberger, *Introduction to the Talmud and Midrash*, 99.

61. Although a literary device, the pun incorporates an understanding that spices did in fact travel by "way of tents," via traveling merchants of the overland spice route.

62. A second-generation Amora from Israel (ca. 250–90 C.E.).

63. Among other passages, see *Songs Rab.* 4:12: "The well [of Miriam]. From where did the Israelites procure wine for drink-offerings all the forty years that they were in the desert? R. Yoḥanan said, 'From the well. From it came most of their enjoyments.' For R. Yoḥanan said, 'The well used to produce for them various kinds of herbs, of vegetables, of trees. The proof of this is that when Miriam died and the well ceased to give its waters to them, they said, *It is no place of seed, or of figs, or of vines* (Num 20:5).'"

64. Strack and Stemberger, *Introduction to the Talmud and Midrash*, 98.

65. As in "all types [of things] entertain you," or "stringed [instruments] entertain you." See discussion on מן (מנן) and מני in Koehler and Baumgartner, *Hebrew and Aramaic Lexicon* 597–602.

66. The term used in the midrash (החקשטות) may mean "to adorn" or "to dress."

67. Judith Baskin, "Woman as Other in Rabbinic Literature," in *In Judaism in Late Antiquity, Part Three: Where We Stand, Issues and Debates in Ancient Judaism*, ed. Jacob Neusner and Alan J. Avery-Peck (Leiden: Brill, 1999), 177–96.

68. It should be noted that this midrash follows directly after another in which woman is described as being more righteous than man.

69. As Judith Baskin notes, "According to this passage, woman is essentially other than man because of the nature of her creation, and the inalterable effects of her shortcomings account for many of her innate shortcomings and social disadvantages. Moreover, the text establishes that it was woman who brought death into the world. By linking the inferior nature of female creation with woman's responsibility for

human mortality, *Gen. Rab.* 17:8 defends Rabbinic sexual politics and the male/female status quo by portraying woman's numerous faults and disadvantages both as divinely ordained and as deserved." Baskin, "Woman as Other in Rabbinic Literature," 179–80. Baskin also discusses this midrash at length in *Midrashic Women*, 65–68.

70. In which the facts are changed for purposes of the lesson; that is, the students and R. Joshua surely know that there is no difference in the posture of male and female babies at birth.

71. Although this type of association is discussed in detail in Lakoff and Johnson's discussion of "systematic" metaphors, it is likely that this metaphor is "unsystematic." That is, because this metaphor does not appear as part of a larger classification of metaphors that describe women (or the "other") as putrefying meat, it is not of a "system" of metaphorical thought within the culture. However, it is also possible that the metaphor about women is derived as a means of describing an oppositional correlative to men. While not a direct subject of this study, men are often described in *Songs Rab.* (and elsewhere) as "of the earth," or in other natural terms: trees, branches, flowers. A more complete study of the descriptions of men, particularly in other midrashic works, would be of value in determining the role of the metaphor about women. George Lakoff, and Mark Johnson, *Metaphors We Live By* (Chicago: University of Chicago Press, 1980), 54–55.

72. See *b. Šab.* 62ab. See chapter 2.

73. See *m. Ber.* 8:6.

74. See *b. Ber.* 53a.

75. Probably R. Ḥiyya bar Abba II, a third-generation Amora from Israel. "Probably the brother of S[himon] b. Abba, immigrated to Palestine from Babylonia in his youth and there became a student chiefly of Yoḥanan." Strack and Stemberger, *Introduction to the Talmud and Midrash*, 99.

76. R. Yoḥanan's comment appears in *y. Ber.* 8:7 (12b) but in the name of R. Abbahu.

77. For a fuller discussion of this passage as well as that of the parallel passage in the *Yerushalmi*, see Deborah Green, "The Scent of a Woman: Rabbinic Attitudes Toward Women's Aromatic Practices" (forthcoming).

78. Meir Bar-Ilan, in reference to this passage, identifies this R. Yossi as a Tanna. See Meir Bar-Ilan, "Witches in the Bible and in the Talmud," in Basser and Fishbane, *Historical, Literary, and Religious Studies*, 12–17.

79. The second-generation Amora from Israel. "Yoḥanan first taught at his birthplace Sepphoris and later at Tiberias . . . by the time of his death in 279 he had been head of an academy (*malakh*) for 80 years." Strack and Stemberger, *Introduction to the Talmud and Midrash*, 94–95. Of note, R. Yoḥanan's comments about women, as depicted in each case studied so far, are either neutral or positive.

80. See also *b. Beṣah* 22b–23a.

81. Baskin, *Midrashic Women*, 117.

82. For more on the status of women in the Talmud, particularly with reference to "witches," see Bar-Ilan, "Witches in the Bible." See also Simcha Fishbane, "Most Women Engage in Sorcery," in Basser and Fishbane, *Historical, Literary, and Religious Studies*, 143–65.

83. See, for example, *t. Kipp.* 2:6; *y. Yoma* 3:9 (41a); *b. Yoma* 38a.

84. Literally, "clear," as in "free from responsibility," since in the biblical scene Moses tells the Reubenites and the Gadites how they must serve in the military before

they settle on the land east of the Jordan. For our purposes, the word is better translated as "clean" or "pure."

85. In the Romm edition, however, the number is 3:5.

86. The House of Garmu also foresees the destruction of the Temple and so refuses to teach the art of making bread.

87. See *t. Kipp.* 2:6. See Lieberman, *Tosefta Ki-Fshuṭah*, 233.

88. "Child" was probably added to the *Songs Rab.* passage so as to align it with the House of Garmu passage. The children of that guild were never seen with fine bread in their hands. "Child" does not appear in any of the Tosefta manuscripts. See Lieberman, *Tosefta Ki-Fshuṭah*, 233.

89. See *Songs Rab.* 1:14 or *y. Šabb.* 6:1 (7c). But see also the discussions of Daniel Boyarin, Tal Ilan, and Judith Baskin with reference to Beruriah, who confounds this depiction of women and whose life ends in suicide. Notably, Boyarin demonstrates that this negative assessment is Babylonian and does not appear in the Yerushalmi. He also emphasizes the connection the rabbinic literature draws between the education of women and their licentiousness. Daniel Boyarin, *Carnal Israel: Reading Sex in Talmudic Culture* (Berkeley and Los Angeles: University of California Press, 1993), 184–92; Tal Ilan, *Mine and Yours Are Hers: Retrieving Women's History from Rabbinic Literature* (Leiden: Brill, 1997), 57–58, 68–73; Baskin, *Midrashic Women*, 81–82.

90. I use this term with caution because none of the women in the rabbinic literature can be considered "historical"; even those who may have lived are in fact only representations of actual people.

91. See *y. Ber.* 8:7 (12b). That said, the Yerushalmi does employ the term דבר אחר, which is read as a negative statement by the Babylonian tradents and may in fact have been negative.

92. Baskin, *Midrashic Women*, 160.

93. Ibid., 117.

94. *Pesiqta de-Rab Kahana* is a homiletic midrash whose chapters follow the liturgical cycle. Although the date of the text is questionable (some scholars date it to the fifth century C.E.), the midrash quoted appears in *Lev. Rab.* as well. The date of *Lev. Rab.* is thought to be between 400 and 500 C.E.; thus the two works are probably contemporaneous. See Strack and Stemberger, *Introduction to the Talmud and Midrash*, 316–22. All passages from *Pesiqta* are from Bernard Mandelbaum, ed. *Pesikta de Rav Kahana According to an Oxford Manuscript, with Variants from All Known Manuscripts and Genizoth Fragments and Parallel Passages*, 2d ed. (New York: Jewish Theological Seminary of America, 1987).

95. A parallel citation is found in *Lev. Rab.* 30:12.

96. Positive rabbinic views of scholars most often include only men. For an interesting discussion of the status of scribes and their relationship to the community in the Tannaitic period, see Martin Goodman, "Texts, Scribes, and Power in Roman Judea," in *Literacy and Power in the Ancient World*, ed. Alan K. Bowman and Greg Woolf (Cambridge: Cambridge University Press, 1994), 99–108.

97. The etrog is a citron, a fruit from Israel used in the rituals associated with Sukkoth. It is slightly larger than a lemon but similar in color and shape. It has a pleasant citrusy-sweet fragrance.

98. In the *Lev. Rab.* passage, this association is reversed and taste appears before scent, thereby rectifying the misalignment in the *Pesiqta* passage.

99. See *Gen. Rab.* 42:1; *Songs Rab.* 1:3.

100. This reading of *turaq* (תורק) is in line with the midrash. See chapter 3 for further discussion of this word.

101. Strack and Stemberger's *Introduction to the Talmud and Midrash* considers Rabbis Eliezer and Joshua second-generation (older group) Tannaim (76–77).

102. On the Babylonian version of R. Eliezer's deathbed scene, which uses the same analogy to an entirely different end, see Shmuel Shepkaru, *Jewish Martyrs in the Pagan and Christian Worlds* (Cambridge: Cambridge University Press, 2006), 89–90.

103. The final line of the midrash—"And it is like filling from a river arm of water and like lighting from candle to candle"—appears to be a late addition as, upon close reading, it does not fit with the rest of the piece.

104. Once we understand the pun, we see that the first part of R. Akiba's comment—"I do not have the strength to say as my teachers do"—expresses his desire to refrain from insulting his teachers (i.e., "I do not have the effrontery to say").

105. *Songs Rab.* 1:3 continues: "Once R. Akiba was delayed in coming to the school. He came and sat outside. A question arose on law. They said, 'The Law is outside.' A question arose again and they said, 'The Torah is outside.' Again, a question arose and they said, 'Akiba is outside. Clear a place for him.' He came and sat before the feet of R. Eliezer. And the school of R. Eliezer was arranged like a race-course and there was one rock there and it was reserved for him to sit on. Once R. Joshua entered and began kissing the rock. He said, 'This rock is like Mount Sinai, and this one who sat on it is like the Ark of the covenant.'"

106. The concept of knowing God and his works intimately through smelling appears as well in Isa 11:2–3, as discussed in chapter 3. Also, compare what may be an addition to the discussion in *b. San.* 93b: "The messiah, as it is written, *The spirit of the Lord will rest on him, a spirit of wisdom and understanding, a spirit of counsel and valor, a spirit of knowledge and awe of the Lord*. And it is written, *And by his smelling in the awe of the Lord*. R. Alexander said, 'It teaches that he loaded him with commandments and sufferings like a great millstone.' Rabba said that he smells certainties, as it is said, *And not by what his eyes see will he judge . . . he will judge the poor with righteousness and he will decide with equity for the impoverished of the land*. Bar Koziba ruled for two and one-half years and said to the rabbis, 'I am the messiah.' They said to him, 'Of the messiah it is written that he smells certainties. Let us see if he smells certainties.' When they saw that he could not smell certainties, they killed him."

107. For example, *b. Ber.* 43b.

108. In personal conversation, Michael Fishbane has pointed out that written *plene* (שמכ"ה) has the numerical equivalent of 365, the number of the negative commandments, by rabbinic reckoning.

109. The entire midrashic cycle for this verse is also found in *Lev. Rab.* 23:1–6. The *lemma* there is: "After the doings of the land of Egypt, in which you dwelt, you shall not do. And after the doings of the land of Canaan, where I will bring you, you shall not do and their laws you shall not follow" (Lev 18:3).

110. In *Lev. Rab.*, "R. Abin."

111. The term is *gav* (גב), which, according to Sokoloff, can mean, "next to," "together with," and "in the case of." Sokoloff, *Dictionary of Jewish Palestinian Aramaic*, 118. In employing Sokoloff's term, however, the word "only" (אלא) must be omitted for the sake of clarity (i.e., "Just as the lily ceases forever only together with its scent"). The Vilna Romm edition of *Lev. Rab.* 23:6 employs the technical term *'al gav* (על גב), "by means of," and so the passage is rendered, "Just as the lily ceases only by means of (על

גב) its scent, so Israel ceases only by means of commandments and good deeds." This may be a late addition, as the opening quotation in Margulies (manuscript based on the British Museum Add. MS 27169) is significantly different: "Another interpretation: *Like a lily among the thorns.* Just as the lily is [created] only for rejoicing (or, happiness), so Israel were created only for commandments and good deeds." Margulies cites the *'al gav* (עַל גַב) construction for the first printings (Constantinople and Venice). Margulies, *Midrash Wayyikra Rabbah,* 533.

112. Also, "favored."

113. In Margulies' critical edition of *Lev. Rab.,* this portion (not quoted in R. Abin's name) appears at the end of our "second" segment. The wording is slightly different there as well. Margulies, *Midrash Wayyikra Rabbah,* 534.

114. R. Berekhiah's statement at the end of this midrash appears as part of the succeeding midrashic unit in *Lev. Rab.* Its amendment in *Songs Rab.* is to connect the *lemma* from Songs with the Leviticus prooftext.

115. The shadow (*tsel,* צל) image is a pun on a word found in the first part of the verse: *ḥavatseleth,* חבצלת, which describes an asphodel, crocus, or narcissus.

116. And with the printed editions of *Lev. Rab.*

117. For more on images like this, see chapter 5.

118. In the Hebrew Bible, this term for "creation" appears only in reference to God's acts of creation.

119. Commingled with the sacrifice of the righteous and the promise of a future redemption, the perfume bottles of Jewish burials may begin to take on some deeper resonances than otherwise understood.

120. And, in some midrashim, the priestly valences of upward, appeasement, exclusivity, and atonement.

121. All references to "history" in this section are to those events the rabbis consider as such (as opposed to our contemporary understanding).

122. *Siyato* (סיעתו), "his escort," in the sense of his traveling force or company.

123. This can also be translated as "God had already anticipated their deliverance." There is no direct object for the verb "to advance," "to anticipate," "to provide against" (הקדים).

124. R. Yudan is a fourth-generation Amora from Israel. Strack and Stemberger, *Introduction to the Talmud and Midrash,* 103.

125. Perhaps a pun on "my spikenard" (נרדי), to be read as "let us go down" (נרד).

126. This midrash is in line with the tradition of the readings of the four nights of Passover; this reading is from the third night. Martin McNamara, Robert Hayward, and Michael Maher, *Targum Neofiti 1, Exodus* (Collegeville, Minn.: Liturgical Press, 1994), Exod 12:42, p. 52; Roger Le Déaut, *La nuit pascale: Essai sur la signification de la Pâque juive à partir du Targum d'Exode XII 42,* Analecta Biblica 22 (Rome: Institut Biblique Pontifical, 1963), 76–87.

127. R. Abbahu is a third-generation Amora from Israel. Strack and Stemberger, *Introduction to the Talmud and Midrash,* 98.

128. Given his role as messenger between Pharaoh and God, Moses could be considered the "fragrance" that wafts forth, except that the prooftext specifically cites God and recounts his action rather than Moses' warning to Pharaoh.

129. This can also mean "refuse"; the verb (סרי) means "to decay" or "to smell offensive."

130. Literally, "they were faint."

131. The Hebrew is סינטומוס, from the Greek συντόμως, "briefly," "concisely." See Lieberman, *Greek in Jewish Palestine*, 79n97.

132. See also *Exod. Rab.* 19:5.

133. However, in *Exod. Rab.* 19:5, God's primary reason for wafting the odor from Eden is to entice the Israelites toward food and thereby toward circumcision. The plague is not the issue; the concern is that no merit for redemption may be found in the Israelites (hence they require circumcision). Of note, the midrash in *Exod. Rab.* is derived from "Awake north wind . . ." (Song 4:16).

134. See further on in *Songs Rab.* 1:12. See also Fishbane, *Biblical Interpretation in Ancient Israel*, 147–51.

135. On this role in Kabbalistic literature, see Peter Schäfer, "Daughter, Sister, Bride, and Mother: Images of the Femininity of God in the Early Kabbala," *Journal of the American Academy of Religion* 68, no. 2 (2000): 221–42.

136. Rindisbacher, *Smell of Books*.

Chapter 5

1. Beds in the sense of "garden terraces." On "graze," cf. Song 2:16 and 4:5, in which "to graze" may be transitive or intransitive; that is, it may mean "to pasture an animal" or "to graze" (i.e., oneself is grazing). As the female is compared to the garden, the male is compared to a gazelle. Murphy, *Song of Songs*, 139.

2. *Songs Rab.* 6:2.

3. Although R. Ḥiyya ben Aviyah's death does not occur with a kiss from God, he may be said to fall into the category of such exemplars: "What is particularly striking about these traditions is that death by divine kiss is a sign of special favor, a mark of grace given to the saintly. Indeed . . . this is particularly the reward granted to the most faithful adherents of the norms and ideals of rabbinic Judaism—the sages themselves. . . . The rapturous death of the righteous by God culminates a lifetime of spiritual labor, of studying the Law and observing the commandments." Michael Fishbane, *The Kiss of God: Spiritual and Mystical Death in Judaism* (Seattle: University of Washington Press, 1994), 18.

4. *Songs Rab.* 6:2.

5. On a literary level, this would be true for the synagogues as well, but in recent years several scholars have pointed to contradictory indications of rabbinic involvement in synagogue life in different periods. The mention of synagogues in the midrash may in fact indicate the midrash's late date. See Lee I. Levine, "The Sages and the Synagogue in Late Antiquity: The Evidence of the Galilee," in Levine, *Galilee in Late Antiquity*, 201–22; Ze'ev Safrai, "The Communal Functions of the Synagogue in the Land of Israel in the Rabbinic Period," in *Ancient Synagogues*, ed. Dan Urman and Paul V. M. Flesher (Leiden: Brill, 1995), 181–204; Fine, *This Holy Place*, 61–67. Michael Swartz has written about the tension in rabbinic depictions in the Mishnah of the high priest and the corresponding "valorization of the priesthood" as found in the Avodah. His reflections are of interest in the ongoing discussion about power, leadership, and influence in the synagogue. Michael D. Swartz, "Sage, Priest, and Poet: Typologies of Religious Leadership in the Ancient Synagogue," in *Jews, Christians, and Polytheists in the Ancient Synagogue*, ed. Steven Fine (London: Routledge, 1999), 101–17.

6. The midrash appears in three places: *b. 'Abod. Zar.* 29b and 35b and *Songs Rab.* 1:2.

7. Although the pronominal suffix on "your oils" (*shemenekhah*, שמניך) could indicate either a masculine or feminine audience, the Masoretic pointing is masculine.

8. It is possible that the passage is appended to the discussion because of its reference to Songs 1:3 and other issues of coherence raised in the midrash (see discussion below).

9. A third-generation Amora from Babylonia. Strack and Stemberger, *Introduction to the Talmud and Midrash*, 101.

10. In Hebrew, פיילטון. See *Songs Rab.* 4:14 and 1:3, below.

11. See also *Songs Rab.* 1:2 for other interpretations.

12. Interpretations and puns on the term "maidens" appear in several places. Among the most familiar are those that involve the phrase "unto death," such as *Mekhilta' de-R. Ishmael*, Shirata, 3; *Siphre Deut.* 443; and *Lev. Rab.* 3:7. All references to *Siphre Deuteronomy* are from Louis Finkelstein, ed., *Sifre on Deuteronomy* (New York: Jewish Theological Seminary of America, 1969).

13. Cf. *b. Ber.* 43b: "Rab Zutra bar Tobiah said, 'Rab said, "Where do we learn to say a blessing over the smelling [of a pleasant scent]?" *As it is said, Let everything that breathes, praise the Lord. Hallelujah* (Psalm 150:6). What is the thing that the soul delights in, but the body does not delight in it? You must say, this is smelling [a fragrant scent].' Rab Zutra bar Tobiah [also] said 'Rab said, "In the future, the young men of Israel (the Munich codex inserts here, "who have not tasted sin") will give forth a good odor like Lebanon, as it is said, *His branches shall spread and his beauty will be like the olive tree, and his fragrance like Lebanon*" (Hos 14:7).'" This comment also appears in *Songs Rab.* 7:14, without attribution to a particular tradent on the verse "The mandrakes give forth fragrance."

14. Surprisingly, in light of other rabbinic legal texts and the biblical literature, one expects the angel of death to be aligned with the beloved, the "man-eating" and destructive female. But the midrash neither draws out nor even implies such a comparison.

15. Issues surrounding rabbinic references to "the next world" are contradictory in terms of what, exactly, the next world is and who may enter it. For a careful consideration of these issues, see Alan F. Segal, *Life After Death: A History of the Afterlife in the Religions of the West* (New York: Doubleday, 2004), 623–28.

16. In *Songs Rab.* 8:8, "R. Berekhiah applied the verse to Abraham our father, '*We have a little sister* (Song 8.8). This is Abraham. . . .' Bar Kappara said, 'It is like a man who sews a tear. While Abraham was still little, he was busy with commandments and good deeds. *She has no breasts.* But the principle [to do] commandments and good deeds had not yet come. *What shall we do for our little sister on the day when she will be spoken for?* On the day that the evil Nimrod sentenced [Abraham] to be lowered into the fiery furnace.'" See also *Gen. Rab.* 38:13 and 39:3. Louis Ginzberg traces this motif throughout the sources. He notes that Abraham the idol destroyer (see *Gen. Rab.* 38:13; see Theodor for parallels) and Abraham the iconoclast (see *b. Pes.* 118a) are two legends combined. Louis Ginzberg, *The Legends of the Jews: I—Bible Times and Characters from the Creation to Jacob*, trans. Henrietta Szold, 2d ed. (Philadelphia: The Jewish Publication Society of America, 1937), 219n50.

17. Or "on his couch."

18. Instances in which a named tradent is in discourse with anonymous rabbis often indicate historical development; that is, the anonymous rabbis are from a later period than R. Eliezer ben Jacob. R. Eliezer is either an older first-generation Tanna or a third-generation Tanna who was a student of R. Akiba. Strack and Stemberger,

Introduction to the Talmud and Midrash, 75, 85. On the role of the redactor as the "anonymous sages," see Kadari, "On the Redaction of Midrash Shir Hashirim Rabbah."

19. Cf. *The Testament of Abraham,* in which God sends the archangel Michael to earth to "bring Abraham up," and the *Apocalypse of Abraham,* in which the angel Iaoel mentions that Michael blesses Abraham.

20. See also *Songs Rab.* 8:9.

21. Employing "my spikenard" (נרדי) as God or as a form of "to go down" (ירד) to refer to God's action of saving Abraham.

22. See *Gen. Rab.* 44:13 on the verse "I am the Lord who took you out of Ur of the Chaldees" (Gen 15:7). Theodor has "R. Leazar ben Jacob" rather than R. Eliezer, but manuscript evidence shows both names. Theodor and Albeck, *Midrash Bereshit Rabba,* 435. See also *Gen. Rab.* 39:8; *Exod. Rab.* 18:5; and *Deut. Rab.* 2:26–27 (just before 30, as the manuscript has no 28–29) in which Amraphel rather than Nimrod is mentioned.

23. For more on the narrative of the three friends and the Prayer of Azariah, see John J. Collins, *Daniel: A Commentary on the Book of Daniel* (Minneapolis: Fortress Press, 1993), 176–207.

24. Or "dedicated," as in sacrificed. On "my name," see below.

25. See Jan Willem van Henten and Friedrich Avemarie, *Martyrdom and Noble Death: Selected Texts from Graeco-Roman, Jewish, and Christian Antiquity* (London: Routledge, 2002), 3; Daniel Boyarin, *Dying for God: Martyrdom and the Making of Christianity and Judaism* (Stanford: Stanford University Press, 1999), 95–96; Arthur J. Droge and James D. Tabor, *A Noble Death: Suicide and Martyrdom Among Christians and Jews in Antiquity* (San Francisco: HarperSanFrancisco, 1992). In each case, the formulaic cadre of the definitions precludes in some way the inclusion of these images. The definition stipulated by Van Henten and Avemarie requires description of the death itself, which is often only alluded to in rabbinic midrashim. In addition, when the death event is described in a midrash, it is not always presented as "torture," as the scholars require. In several instances, the death is described as a sacrifice, and torture is only insinuated or left unexpressed. As seen here, some midrashic martyr scenes are heavily laced with verses from the love poetry of the Songs, so that only the pathos of the deity's response and the piety and love of the righteous martyr are highlighted; the death, therefore, appears peaceful or disappears entirely. These instances would be deleted from the Van Henten–Avemarie catalogue. Boyarin views martyrdom more narrowly and attempts to "perceive the complexities and nuances of its history" in the second through fourth centuries. His requirements include "a ritualized and performative speech act associated with a statement of pure essence. In rabbinic texts, this is the declaration of the oneness of God via the recitation of the 'Hear O Israel' [conception of the martyr] . . . as the fulfilling of a religious mandate per se, and not just the manifestation of a preference 'for violent death' over 'compliance with a decree.' . . . [and] powerful erotic elements . . . to suffer torture and death because [the martyrs] are passionately in love with God, not because they fear his punishment or to demonstrate their Stoic fortitude or apathy. These eroticized elements produce effects that have to do with sex and gender systems as well." Boyarin, *Dying for God,* 95–96. However, this selectivity and specificity leave little room for martyrdom to be viewed as a midrashic literary theme or motif, as the texts of midrash rarely appear in such standard formats. Still, Boyarin's propositions are useful. In the midrashim explicated in this chapter, martyrdom and sacrifice of the body are the direct results of the belief in one God and the act of proselytizing or declaration of such belief. In each case, the death or sacrifice acts

as a theurgic stimulus to the Divine—awakening and arousing the deity to action and immanence. Most often this action incorporates the process of merciful postulation rather than judgment and ultimately effects redemption for the Jews. Therefore, the act of martyrdom or sacrifice may be considered a "religious mandate." And, as already seen in the previous chapter, these acts are born of deep and passionate love on the part of all actors, including God, as expressed in the ardent dialogue of the Songs. On the concept of "motif" (reappropriated here to the subject of martyrdom in rabbinic literature), see Michael Fishbane, "The Well of Living Water," in *Sha'arei Talmon: Studies in the Bible, Qumran, and the Ancient Near East, Presented to Shemaryahu Talmon*, ed. Michael Fishbane and Emanuel Tov (Winona Lake, Ind.: Eisenbrauns, 1992); Shemaryahu Talmon, "The 'Desert Motif' in the Bible and in Qumran Literature," in *Biblical Motifs: Origins and Transformations*, ed. Alexander Altman (Cambridge: Harvard University Press, 1966).

26. See *Songs Rab.* 8:9.

27. See, for example, Justin 2 *Apol.* 12 or *Diogn.* 7:8.

28. See Ign. *Rom.* 2:2; *Mart. Pol.* 15.

29. See below in addition to *Songs Rab.* 3:5 (on Song 3:6) and 4:6. In 4:6, Abraham is described as the mountain of myrrh because he is the foremost of all the righteous. Isaac is described as the hill of frankincense because he was offered up like a handful of frankincense. Jacob is described as the powders of the merchant for his business acumen.

30. This is the verse that follows "While the king . . ." (Song 1:12). Therefore, the midrash on Abraham in the fire and this one appear close together in *Songs Rab.*

31. On the connection among "bitterness," martyrdom, and sacrifice (and references to Abraham), see the discussion on Miriam and her seven sons in Galit Hasan-Rokem, *The Web of Life: Folklore and Midrash in Rabbinic Literature*, trans. Batya Stein, 2d ed. (Stanford: Stanford University Press, 2000), 108–29. Reuven Firestone also comments, "Credit for Abraham's merit of being willing to sacrifice his own son is recalled in Jewish tradition in order to bring atonement even to this day. This is most obvious in the liturgy for the New Year and the Day of Atonement where liturgical poetry often refers to this theme, but it is often included in the liturgy of the daily morning prayers and was earlier associated with Passover (Manns). The merit for the 'aqedah, or the 'binding' of Isaac as it is known in Jewish tradition, is of such magnitude that it is seen in rabbinic literature as the efficient cause of Israel's rescue from affliction throughout history (Levenson:181)." Reuven Firestone, "Merit, Mimesis, and Martyrdom," *Journal of the American Academy of Religion* 66, no. 1 (1998): 97. For a thorough discussion of Abraham's merit, the 'aqedah, and the displacement of Abraham in favor of Isaac in Jewish tradition, see Jon D. Levenson, *The Death and Resurrection of the Beloved Son: The Transformation of Child Sacrifice in Judaism and Christianity* (New Haven: Yale University Press, 1993), 173–99.

32. See *b. Meg.* 13a, which is also quoted in R. Yehudah's name. However, it is unclear whether the rabbi refers to olive oil or myrrh.

33. See also *Songs Rab.* 3:5.

34. The midrash is interesting in its own right because it attempts to wrest control of the Temple precinct from the priests, albeit only after the fact, since the Temple is no longer standing by the time of the midrash. Indeed, this is the only way that the rabbis could gain such a foothold in Temple procedures. In terms of dates, R. Yoḥanan is probably R. Yoḥanan bar Nappaha, a second-generation Amora. R. Huna (also Ḥuna) is

most likely a second-generation Amora from Babylon. See Strack and Stemberger, *Introduction to the Talmud and Midrash*, 94–97.

35. Literally, *foliatum*, φουλιᾶτον, as seen in *b. Avod. Zar.* 35b and *Songs Rab.* 4:14.

36. Cf. *Gen. Rab.* 39:2, on Gen 12:1: "R. Berekhiah expounded *The fragrance of your oils is good; [Oil poured forth, your name. Therefore the maidens love you]* (Song 1:3). R. Berekhiah said, 'To what can Abraham be compared? To a flask of scented oil surrounded by an exact fitting lid, and resting in a corner, and whose scent was not spreading. When it was moved, its scent spread. Thus, said the Holy One, blessed be He, to Abraham, "[Move yourself from place to place and your name will spread in the world.] *Go from [your land and from your birthplace and from the house of your father to the land that I will show you]* (Gen 12:1)."'" The *Songs Rab.* passage is dependent on this version from *Gen. Rab.*, in which R. Berekhiah's remarks are presented as a homiletic interpretation on the verse from Genesis. As for the term "scented oil," Theodor and Albeck transcribe פפלוסימון and it is difficult to know whether this word should be "foliatum" (פולייטון), as in the *Songs Rab.* parable, or אפופלסמון (a miscopying of אפובלסמון). In that case the meaning is "opalbalsam" or "juice of the balsam tree" (ὀποβάλσαμον). Other manuscripts also have *afarsamon* (אפרסמון), which is the transliteration from Greek into Hebrew of opalbalsam. Theodor and Albeck, *Midrash Bereshit Rabba*, 366.

37. Cf. *Gen. Rab.* 30:9 (*b. San.* 108a), in which Noah is compared to a flask of scented oil before his journey because he is the only righteous one of his generation. This midrash also entails a reference to perfume in a graveyard (as discussed with reference to *b. Ber.* 53a).

38. The contextual sense is "persons."

39. The contextual sense is "acquired."

40. This occurs through a hyperliteral reading of the biblical text, reading the term *'asah* (עשה) as "to make" or "to do" rather than the implied meaning of the text, "acquired."

41. The spatial positioning from outside to inside the covenant also echoes the characteristics of scent as seen in reference to the image of the garden in Songs, in which the male lover wants to enter the garden because his beloved's aroma flows out to him.

42. The root "to approach," "to near," is also used to form the word for "sacrifice" or "offering"—that which is brought near—a *qorban* (קרבן). See chapter 3.

43. R. Berekhiah is a fifth-generation Amora from Palestine. Strack and Stemberger, *Introduction to the Talmud and Midrash*, 105.

44. The martyrdom of the righteous is alluded to in the inference of the "two worlds" as this lifetime and the next and in the analogy of the "king's table" as an altar.

45. R. Ḥaninah is difficult to date, as there are several (R. Ḥaninah, a first-generation Amora; R. Ḥaninah ben Pappai/Pappos, a third-generation Amora), including a grandfather and grandson (second- and fourth-generation Amoraim). There is also a fifth-generation Amora, R. Ḥananyah II, who is also referred to as Ḥaninah. While one is tempted to assume that this R. Ḥaninah is the fifth-generation Amora because his comment follows R. Berekhiah's opinion (and R. Berekhiah is a fifth-generation Amora), the work of the redactor is very apparent in this midrash; accordingly, it is difficult to determine a secure date. Strack and Stemberger, *Introduction to the Talmud and Midrash*, 91–106.

46. See Gesenius, sec. 131, item o: "Of a different kind are the cases in which the permutative with its proper suffix follows as a kind of correction of the preceding suffix, e.g., Is 29 *when he* (or rather) *his children see*, &c. (but is clearly a gloss)."

W. Gesenius, *Gesenius' Hebrew Grammar*, 2d English ed., ed. E. Kautzsch, trans. A. E. Cowley (Oxford: Clarendon Press, 1910), 426.

47. In the sense of those who wander toward ruin or error.

48. See also *Songs Rab.* 2:5, 7:8, 7:10, and 8:9. In these midrashim the ancestors are delivered from martyrdom at the last possible moment.

49. "Sanctification of the name" undergoes a development in meaning from "honoring God" to the concept of martyrdom during the period of the Tannaim and continues to develop throughout the centuries. See Shmuel Safrai, "Quiddush Ha-shem be-Toratam Shel Ha-Tannaim" [in Hebrew], *Zion* 44 (1979): 28–42; Urbach, *Sages*, 352–58, 517–21; Yizhak Baer, "The Persecution of 1096" [in Hebrew], in *Sefer Asaf, kovets ma'amarei mehkar mugash lekhvod ha-Rav Prof. Simhah Asaf al-yede yedidav haverav ve-talmidav limlat lo shishim shanah*, ed. Umberto Cassuto (Jerusalem: Mosad ha-Rav Kook, 1953), 126–40. Cf. Shepkaru, *Jewish Martyrs*, 105. See also *Songs Rab.* 2:7.

50. On the verse from Song 1.3 ("Therefore the maidens love you"), Boyarin comments, "It seems to me not too much to suggest, therefore, that R. Akiva's midrashic transformation of maidens into 'until death' alludes to this very verse [Ps 48:15], in which death is transformed into maidens by the midrash. It is not only the two signifiers that can substitute for each other but also their signifieds as well. Death becomes Eros and Eros death." Daniel Boyarin, "'Language Inscribed by History on the Bodies of Living Beings': Midrash and Martyrdom," *Representations* 25 (Winter 1989): 145.

51. "Martyrs do connect the human with the divine through their intercessionary skills, as human sacrifices and witnesses to God. Their stories also reach out to connect people over time and place. A prime function of a martyr's tale is to create an image so compelling that others will want to follow. The martyrology is designed to spread a message about the character, worthiness and truth of both the divine being who inspired such a sacrifice and the one who gave his or her life. Fragrance can be seen as functioning similarly to a martyrology. Like the story, the fragrance emanates out with its presumed proof of divinity and impacts all who perceive it." Suzanne Evans, "The Scent of a Martyr," *Numen: International Review for the History of Religions* 49, no. 2 (2002): 195.

52. "*The Lord smelled the soothing odor* (Gen 8:21). He smelled the scent of Abraham our father going up from the fiery furnace. He smelled the scent of Hananiah, Mishael, and Azariah going up from the fiery furnace (*Gen. Rab.* 34:9)." The midrash asserts that the soothing odor is the scent of the sacrifice of Abraham and the three compatriots. Of note, none of the characters in this episode is saved from fire. Rather, their burning produces the soothing odor. It would seem, then, that the characters are so thoroughly connected with images of sacrifice and martyrdom, and their legends so well known, the reference to soothing odor in Genesis 8 automatically triggers the mention of their names and the "fiery furnace" without further narrative or explication. As such, the "fiery furnace" stands for the altar, and the characters' names come to symbolize righteous martyrdom as a sacrifice. Further, the term "soothing odor" takes on the meaning of soothing divine anger, arousal of the Divine, and immanence as the final result. See also *Gen. Rab.* 25:2 and 33:3 on the name of Noah as connected to the term "soothing odor."

53. Cf. *Gen. Rab.* 47:7: "*And Abraham took Ishmael, his son, and all the sons of his house, and of all [those] purchased with his silver, every male of the men of the house of Abraham, and he circumcised the flesh of their foreskins on this same day when God spoke with him* (Gen 17:23). R. Aibo said, 'In the hour that Abraham circumcised the children of his

house, he erected a hill of foreskins. And the sun shone down, and they became worm-eaten. The smell of them went up before the Holy One, blessed be He, and it was like the ingredients of the incense offering. The Holy One, blessed be He, said, "In the hour that my sons come [to do] transgressions, I will remember for them that smell, and I will be filled with mercy toward them."'"

54. Both of these rabbis are third-generation Amoraim from Palestine who were students of R. Yoḥanan. Strack and Stemberger, *Introduction to the Talmud and Midrash*, 98.

55. Cf. the descriptions of saints and ascetics who employed stench as a means of devotion, instruction, and self-mortification, in Susan Ashbrook Harvey, "On Holy Stench: When the Odor of Sanctity Sickens," *Studia Patristica* 35 (2001): 90–101.

56. A "calming of the soul." Cf. *Songs Rab.* 2:2, the parable of the lily among the brambles.

57. Very few people can actually call a scent to mind as they can with a visual image (i.e., smell the scent without any evidence of its presence). Rather, it is reexperiencing the odor that causes reflective association and recollection.

58. However, tradition fails to transmit the prooftext with R. Levi's comment. The reason for this may be given in the following midrash on Abraham's circumcision: "*In this same day, Abraham was circumcised and [so was] his son Ishmael* (Gen 17:26). R. Abba said, 'He felt [it] and he suffered [pain] so that the Holy One, blessed be He, might double his reward.' R. Levi said, '"Abraham circumcised" is not written; rather, "*he was circumcised*" [is written]. He examined himself and found himself [already] circumcised.' R. Berekhiah said, 'At that time, R. Abba bar Kahana insulted R. Levi. He said to him, "A falsehood and a lie! He felt [it] and he suffered [pain], so that the Holy One, blessed be He, would double his reward!"' (*Gen. Rab.* 47:9)." R. Levi's logic seems indisputable. The biblical verse is written in a passive form and so must indicate that Abraham has no need to circumcise himself. Abraham looks down, sees that he is already circumcised, and so has no need to repeat what has already been done. R. Levi has two justifications for relating the "hill of frankincense" passage from the Songs to Joshua: it contains the prooftext, and God had already circumcised Abraham. However, R. Levi's friend, R. Abba bar Kahana, expresses disdain for the haggadist's suggestion and openly reproves him. The implication of R. Levi's remarks and the response elicited by three rabbis (Abbahu in *Songs Rab.*, Aibo and Abba bar Kahana in *Gen. Rab.*) would suggest that R. Levi's interpretation was considered not only incorrect but improper or offensive. Of interest, the remark by R. Abba bar Kahana is repeated by R. Berekhiah, the fifth-generation Amora from Palestine who consistently introduces strong allusions to and explicit expansions on the theme of suffering (see, in addition to those midrashim cited here, *Gen. Rab.* 94:5).

59. Cf. *Gen. Rab.* 46:2 on circumcision, Abraham, virility, and the cinnamon tree.

60. Fishbane, *Kiss of God*, 87.

61. See *Gen. Rab.* 55:4–56:19. For example, in at least one of these formulations, Isaac dies and is then brought back to life. The literature on Isaac as a sacrifice is extensive. On Isaac as the paradigmatic example of suffering and sacrifice, see Urbach, *Sages*, 502–5. For an excellent treatment of the role of Isaac's sacrifice in the Hebrew Bible and later commentary, particularly with respect to Isaac's "completed" sacrifice, role in atonement, and paradigmatic martyrdom, see Shalom Spiegel, *The Last Trial: On the Legends and Lore of the Command to Abraham to Offer Isaac as a Sacrifice*, trans. Judah Golden (New York: Pantheon Books, 1967), 33–45, 70–120. On the comparison of Isaac's sacrifice to that of Ishmael in Islamic literature, see Firestone, "Merit, Mimesis, and Martyrdom."

62. It is important to remember that the henna referred to in this verse is not the red dye used today; this henna is a spice and appears as part a metonymic list of scent metaphors that the beloved intones to describe her lover.

63. As with Abraham's affiliation with myrrh, Isaac is regularly compared to frankincense. On Songs 3:6, "*Perfumed with myrrh.* This refers to our father Abraham. Just as myrrh is the foremost.... *And frankincense.* This refers to our father Isaac, who was offered like a handful of frankincense on top of the altar. *With all the powders of the merchant.* This refers to our father Jacob" (*Songs Rab.* 3:5). See also *Songs Rab.* 4:6: "Another interpretation. *I will go myself to the mountain of myrrh.* This is Abraham who is the chief of all the righteous. *And to the hill of frankincense.* This is Isaac who was offered like a handful of frankincense on top of the altar."

64. See Shepkaru, *Jewish Martyrs*, 68–69, 104–6.

65. On the issue of righteousness and suffering, and particularly the difference between the Palestinian and Babylonian sources, see Yakov Elman, "The Suffering of the Righteous in Palestinian and Babylonian Sources," *Jewish Quarterly Review* 80, nos. 3–4 (1990): 315–39.

66. James Fernandez, *Persuasions and Performances: The Play of Tropes in Culture* (Bloomington: Indiana University Press, 1986), 5–7, 43, 56.

67. See Schwartz, *Imperialism and Jewish Society*, 103–32; Boyarin, *Dying for God*, 93.

68. See Rindisbacher, *Smell of Books*, on the triangulation of aroma, death, and eros.

Chapter 6

1. These, however, seem to be late midrashim with respect to scent images.
2. Literally, "cause to take an oath."
3. Understanding *tseva'oth* (צבאות) as the "hosts" rather than "gazelles."
4. The patriarchs follow God's "will" (*tsivyoni*, צביוני). The term "matriarchs" refers to the tribes, and Naftali is referred to as a "hind sent forth" in Gen 49:21.
5. The "host" (*tseva'*, צבא) that bears a "sign" ('*ot*, אות).
6. As in 2:17: "Until the day breathes and shadows flee, turn my lover and be like a gazelle or young stag upon the mountains of Bater." See Murphy, *Song of Songs*, 139, 94, 200.
7. *Songs Rab.* 8:14.
8. As in the midrash on Songs 2:17, "gazelle," here *tsivi* (צבי), is read as "host," *tsava'* (צבא).
9. No doubt a reference to the trishagion from Isa 6:3, in which the angels call to one another, "Holy, holy, holy. The Lord of Hosts. His glory fills the earth [קדוש קדוש קדוש יהוה צבאות מלא כל הארץ כבודו]."
10. The *hitpa'el* can also mean "moistened" or "perfumed."
11. These midrashim are probably late formulations, as they are not quoted in any tradent's name. Also, the closest parallels are in *Songs Rab.* or other late midrashic works (i.e., *Pesiqta Rabbati* and *Yalqut Shemoni*). *Pesiqta Rabbati* is from the second half of the ninth century, although much of its material may be much older (some believe the Yelamdenu material is from the year 400, at the latest). *Yalqut Shemoni* is dated to the thirteenth century. See Strack and Stemberger, *Introduction to the Talmud and Midrash*, 326–27 and 84, respectively. For general comparisons, see *Songs Rab.* 4:7, in which the Shekhinah is said to go into exile with Israel, and *Songs Rab.* 4:8, in which God is said

to go into exile with Israel. Cf. also *Songs Rab.* 3:6, in which the merit of the ancestors is discussed in combination with their scent floating up to heaven, and *Songs Rab.* 4:6, in which the scent of Abraham's circumcision floats up to heaven like the fragrance of perfume.

12. This metaphor recalls images both from the Songs and from other rabbinic themes. In the Songs, the female lover says, "Do not stare at me because I am black, for the sun has burned me. The sons of my mother were angry with me. They assigned me as the keeper of the vineyards, [but] my own vineyard I have not kept" (1:6). The verse openly describes the woman as tanned because she has been outside, and it alludes to her lack of chastity (she has been outside where she is not supposed to be and she has not kept her "vineyard"). The commentary in *Songs Rab.* on this verse includes images of Israel as appearing ugly to the other nations (or to herself) but as beautiful to God, or as a woman outcast and tarnished as the result of her sins but a woman who will be cleaned up and restored to her former glory (*Songs Rab.* 1:6). In addition, the interpretations include the biblical images of Israel as sinning through idolatry, as being punished for her sins, but also as being redeemed in the end. Likewise, the midrash hints at Israel's lack of chastity by mentioning that she is soiled by her iniquity, and she asks to be cleaned or purified by God.

13. "To be exiled is to be cut off from the land, from the blessing, from the ancestors, from history, from life, from creation, from reality, from the deity. It is to enter into a new temporal period, palpably different from that which has been before. It is to descend into chaos. . . . To be exiled is to be in a state of chaos, recreation, and death; to return from exile is to be re-created and reborn. For the Temple to have been destroyed is to experience the shattering of the Center, the breaking of the sacred Pole." Jonathan Z. Smith, *Map Is Not Territory: Studies in the History of Religions,* 2d ed. (Chicago: University of Chicago Press, 1993), 120. While the idea that God is with the people during their exile appears sporadically in the Bible, it is fully developed in rabbinic exegesis. Smith discusses this in reference to *Mekhilta' de-Rabbi Ishmael,* Pisha, 14 on Exod 12:41. Ibid., 121.

14. Sokoloff, *Dictionary of Jewish Palestinian Aramaic,* 80.

15. Read this way, this midrash actually retains strong similarities to the biblical imagery, as the priestly source considers the geography of the inner court of the Temple as a place of liminality in which incense sacrifice stimulates two-way communication with the Divine. Sacrifices go up to God, and God's glory comes to rest in the area of the Holy of Holies.

BIBLIOGRAPHY

Abu-Uqsa, Hana. "A Burial Cave from the Roman Period East of Giv'at Yasaf." [In Hebrew.] *'Atiqot* 33 (1997): 39–46.
———. "Three Burial Caves at Kafr Kanna." [In Hebrew.] In *Eretz Zafon: Studies in Galilean Archaeology*, ed. Zvi Gal, 153–61. Jerusalem: Israel Antiquities Authority, 2002.
Ackerman, Diane. *A Natural History of the Senses*. New York: Vintage Books, 1990.
Albeck, Chanokh. *Shishah Sidre Mishnah*. 6 vols. Jerusalem: Bialik Institute and Dvir Co., 1959. Reprint, 1973.
Alexander, Philip S. *The Targum of Canticles, Translated, with a Critical Introduction, Apparatus, and Notes*. Collegeville, Minn.: Liturgical Press, 2003.
Anderson-Stojanović, Virginia. "The Chronology and Function of Ceramic Unguentaria." *American Journal of Archaeology* 91, no. 1 (1987): 105–22.
Arensburg, Baruch, and Patricia Smith. "Appendix: Anthropological Tables." In *Jericho: The Jewish Cemetery in the Second Temple Period*, ed. Rachel Hachlili and Ann E. Killebrew, 192–95. Jerusalem: Israel Antiquities Authority, 1999.
Artzy, Michal. "Pomegranate Scepters and Incense Stand with Pomegranates Found in Priest's Grave." *Biblical Archaeology Review* 16, no. 1 (1990): 48–51.
The Assyrian Dictionary of the Oriental Institute of the University of Chicago. Chicago: Oriental Institute; Glückstadt: J. J. Augustin Verlagsbuchhandlung, 1972.
Aviam, Mordechai. "Finds from a Burial Cave at Daburriya." [In Hebrew.] In *Eretz Zafon: Studies in Galilean Archaeology*, ed. Zvi Gal, 135–39. Jerusalem: Israel Antiquities Authority, 2002.
———. *Jews, Pagans, and Christians in the Galilee: Twenty-Five Years of Archaeological Excavations and Surveys, Hellenistic to Byzantine Periods*. Rochester: University of Rochester Press, 2004.
Avigad, Nahman. *Catacombs 12–23*. Vol. 3 of *Beth She'arim: Report on the Excavations During 1953–1958*. New Brunswick: Rutgers University Press, 1976.
———. "Excavations in the Jewish Quarter, Jerusalem." *Israel Exploration Journal* 22 (1972): 195–200.
Avni, Gideon, and Zvi Greenhut. *The Akeldama Tombs: Three Burial Caves in the Kidron Valley, Jerusalem*. Jerusalem: Israel Antiquities Authority, 1996.
Avrahami, Yael. "The Sensorium and Its Operation in Biblical Epistemology: With Particular Attention to the Senses of Sight and Smell." [In Hebrew.] PhD diss., University of Haifa, 2008.
Baer, Yizhak. "The Persecution of 1096." [In Hebrew.] In *Sefer Asaf, kovets ma'amarei meḥkar mugash lekhvod ha-Rav Prof. Simḥah Asaf al-yede yedidav ḥaverav ve-talmidav limlat lo shishim shanah*, ed. Umberto Cassuto, 126–40. Jerusalem: Mosad ha-Rav Kook, 1953.
Bahar, Shlomo. "Perfume in the Song of Songs: An Erotic Motive and Sign of Social Class." [In Hebrew.] *Shnaton: An Annual for Biblical and Ancient Near Eastern Studies* 15 (2005): 39–52.

Bahat, Dan. "A Synagogue at Beth-Shean." In *Ancient Synagogues Revealed*, ed. Lee I. Levine, 82–85. Jerusalem: Israel Exploration Society, 1981.
Bakhos, Carol. "Figuring (Out) Esau: The Rabbis and Their Others." *Journal of Jewish Studies* 58, no. 2 (2007): 250–62.
Balouka, Marva. "Ceramic Vessels and Objects." In *Sepphoris in Galilee: Crosscurrents of Culture*, ed. Rebecca Martin Nagy, Carol Meyers, Eric Meyers, and Zeev Weiss, 202–6. Winona Lake, Ind.: North Carolina Museum of Art, 1996.
Barag, Dan. "The Glass Vessels." In Nahman Avigad, *Catacombs 12–23*, vol. 3 of *Beth She'arim: Report on Excavations During 1953–1958*, 198–209. New Brunswick: Rutgers University Press, 1976.
———. "Glass Vessels of the Roman and Byzantine Periods in Palestine." [In Hebrew.] PhD diss., Hebrew University, 1970.
———. "Hanita, Tomb XV: A Tomb of the Third and Early Fourth Century C.E." *'Atiqot: English Series* 13 (1978): 10–33.
Bar-Ilan, Meir. "Witches in the Bible and in the Talmud." In *Approaches to Ancient Judaism: New Series*, vol. 5, *Historical, Literary, and Religious Studies*, ed. Herbert W. Basser and Simcha Fishbane, 7–32. South Florida Studies in the History of Judaism 82. Atlanta: Scholars Press, 1993.
Barkay, Gabriel. "The Iron Age II–III." In *The Archaeology of Ancient Israel*, ed. Amnon Ben-Tor, trans. R. Greenberg, 302–73. New Haven: Yale University Press; Tel Aviv: Open University of Israel, 1992.
Baskin, Judith. *Midrashic Women: Formations of the Feminine in Rabbinic Literature*. Hanover: University Press of New England, 2002.
———. "Woman as Other in Rabbinic Literature." In *Judaism in Late Antiquity, Part Three: Where We Stand; Issues and Debates in Ancient Judaism*, ed. Jacob Neusner and Alan J. Avery-Peck, 177–96. Leiden: Brill, 1999.
Biblia Hebraica Stuttgartensia. Edited by Albrecht Alt, Otto Eisfeldt, Paul Kahle, and Rudolf Kittel. Stuttgart: Deutsche Bibelgesellschaft, 1990.
Bloch, Ariel, and Chana Bloch. *The Song of Songs: A New Translation*. New York: Random House, 1995.
Bloch-Smith, Elizabeth. *Judahite Burial Practices and Beliefs About the Dead*. Sheffield, U.K.: Sheffield Academic Press, 1992.
Boyarin, Daniel. *Carnal Israel: Reading Sex in Talmudic Culture*. Berkeley and Los Angeles: University of California Press, 1993.
———. *Dying for God: Martyrdom and the Making of Christianity and Judaism*. Stanford: Stanford University Press, 1999.
———. *Intertextuality and the Reading of Midrash*. Bloomington: Indiana University Press, 1990.
———. "'Language Inscribed by History on the Bodies of Living Beings': Midrash and Martyrdom." *Representations* 25 (Winter 1989): 139–51.
Brakke, David, Michael Satlow, and Steven Weitzman, eds. *Religion and the Self in Antiquity*. Bloomington: Indiana University Press, 2005.
Brand, Yehoshua. *Ceramics in Talmudic Literature*. [In Hebrew.] Jerusalem: Mossad Harav Kook, 1953.
Brenner, Athalya, and Jan Willem van Henten, eds. "Food and Drink in the Biblical Worlds." *Semeia* 86, no. 2 (1999).
Brettler, Marc Z. *God Is King: Understanding an Israelite Metaphor*. Sheffield, U.K.: Sheffield Academic Press, 1989.

Brun, Jean-Pierre. "The Production of Perfumes in Antiquity: The Cases of Delos and Paestum." *American Journal of Archaeology* 104 (2000): 277–308.
Camp, Claudia. "What's So Strange About the Strange Woman?" In *The Bible and the Politics of Exegesis: Festschrift for Norman Gottwald*, ed. David Jobling, Peggy L. Day, and Gerald T. Sheppard, 17–31. Cleveland: Pilgrim Press, 1991.
———. *Wise, Strange, and Holy: The Strange Woman and the Making of the Bible*. Sheffield, U.K.: Sheffield Academic Press, 2000.
Carroll, Robert P. *Jeremiah: A Commentary*. Philadelphia: Westminster Press, 1986.
Caseau, Béatrice. "Euōdia: The Use and Meaning of Fragrances in the Ancient World and Their Christianization (100–900 AD)." PhD diss., Princeton University, 1994.
Classen, Constance, David Howes, and Anthony Synnott. *Aroma: The Cultural History of Smell*. 2d ed. London: Routledge, 1997.
Cohen, Gerson. "Esau as Symbol in Early Medieval Thought." In *Jewish Medieval and Renaissance Studies*, ed. Alexander Altmann, 19–48. Cambridge: Harvard University Press, 1967.
———. "The Song of Songs and the Jewish Religious Mentality." In Cohen, *Studies in the Variety of Rabbinic Cultures*, 3–17. Philadelphia: Jewish Publication Society, 1991.
Cohen, Shaye J. D. "The Place of the Rabbi in Jewish Society of the Second Century." In *The Galilee in Late Antiquity*, ed. Lee I. Levine, 157–73. New York: Jewish Theological Seminary of America, 1992.
Collins, John J. *Daniel: A Commentary on the Book of Daniel*. Minneapolis: Fortress Press, 1993.
Corbin, Alain. *The Foul and the Fragrant: Odor and the French Social Imagination*. Cambridge: Harvard University Press, 1986.
Culler, Jonathan. *Structuralist Poetics: Structuralism, Linguistics, and the Study of Literature*. Ithaca: Cornell University Press, 1975.
Dalby, Andrew. *Empire of Pleasures: Luxury and Indulgence in the Roman World*. London: Routledge, 2002.
Day, Linda. "Rhetoric and Domestic Violence in Ezekiel 16." *Biblical Interpretation* 8, no. 3 (2000): 205–30.
Day, Peggy L. "Adulterous Jerusalem's Imagined Demise: Death of a Metaphor in Ezekiel XVI." *Vetus Testamentum* 50, no. 3 (2000): 285–309.
Dayagi-Mendels, Michal. *Perfumes and Cosmetics in the Ancient World*. Jerusalem: Keter, 1991.
Detienne, Marcel. *The Gardens of Adonis: Spices in Greek Mythology*. 1977. Translated by Janet Lloyd. Princeton: Princeton University Press, 1994.
Dever, William G. "Asherah, Consort of Yahweh? New Evidence from Kuntillet 'Ajrûd." *Bulletin of the American Schools of Oriental Research* 255 (1984): 21–37.
Dirksen, Peter B. "Song of Songs 3:6–7." *Vetus Testamentum* 39, no. 2 (1989): 219–25.
Droge, Arthur J., and James D. Tabor. *A Noble Death: Suicide and Martyrdom Among Christians and Jews in Antiquity*. San Francisco: HarperSanFrancisco, 1992.
Dvorjetski, Estēe. *Leisure, Pleasure, and Healing: Spa Culture and Medicine in the Ancient Eastern Mediterranean*. Leiden: Brill, 2007.
Edelman, Diana. "The Meaning of Qitter." *Vetus Testamentum* 35, no. 4 (1985): 395–404.
Elbogen, Ismar. *Jewish Liturgy: A Comprehensive History*. Translated by Raymond Scheindlin. Based on the original 1913 German edition and the 1972 Hebrew

edition edited by Joseph Heinemann et al. Philadelphia: Jewish Publication Society, 1993.
Eliav, Yaron Z. "The Roman Bath as a Jewish Institution: Another Look at the Encounter Between Judaism and the Greco-Roman Culture." *Journal for the Study of Judaism* 31, no. 4 (2000): 416–54.
———. "Sites, Institutions, and Daily Life in Tiberias During the Talmudic Period." [In Hebrew.] *Mi'tuv T'veria* 10 (1995): 1–106.
Elman, Yakov. "The Suffering of the Righteous in Palestinian and Babylonian Sources." *Jewish Quarterly Review* 80, nos. 3–4 (1990): 315–39.
Engen, Trygg. *The Perception of Odors*. New York: Academic Press, 1982.
Eshel, Hanan. "A Note on 'Miqvaot' at Sepphoris." In *Archaeology and the Galilee: Texts and Contexts in the Graeco-Roman and Byzantine Periods*, ed. Douglas R. Edwards and C. Thomas McCollough, 131–33. Atlanta: Scholars Press, 1997.
Evans, Suzanne. "The Scent of a Martyr." *Numen: International Review for the History of Religions* 49, no. 2 (2002): 193–211.
Exum, J. Cheryl. "A Literary and Structural Analysis of the Song of Songs." *Zeitschrift für die Alttestamentliche Wissenschaft* 85 (1973): 47–79.
———. "Seeing Solomon's Palanquin (Song of Songs 3:6–11)." *Biblical Interpretation* 11, nos. 3–4 (2003): 301–16.
Faure, Paul. *Parfums et aromates de l'antiquité*. Paris: Fayard, 1987.
Feliks, Yehuda. *Trees: Aromatic, Ornamental, and of the Forest*. [In Hebrew.] Jerusalem: Rubin Mass Press, 1997.
Fernandez, James. *Persuasions and Performances: The Play of Tropes in Culture*. Bloomington: Indiana University Press, 1986.
Fine, Steven. "Archaeology and the Interpretation of Rabbinic Literature: Some Thoughts." In *How Should Rabbinic Literature Be Read in the Modern World?* ed. Matthew Kraus, 199–217. Piscataway, N.J.: Gorgias Press, 2006.
———. "Between Liturgy and Social History: Priestly Power in Late Antique Palestinian Synagogues." *Journal of Jewish Studies* 56, no. 1 (2005): 1–9.
———. *This Holy Place: On the Sanctity of the Synagogue During the Greco-Roman Period*. Notre Dame: University of Notre Dame Press, 1997.
Finkelstein, Louis, ed. *Sifre on Deuteronomy*. New York: Jewish Theological Seminary of America, 1969.
Firestone, Reuven. "Merit, Mimesis, and Martyrdom." *Journal of the American Academy of Religion* 66, no. 1 (1998): 93–116.
Fishbane, Michael. *Biblical Interpretation in Ancient Israel*. Oxford: Oxford University Press, 1985. Reprint, 1988.
———. *Biblical Myth and Rabbinic Mythmaking*. Oxford: Oxford University Press, 2003.
———. *Haftarot*. Philadelphia: Jewish Publication Society, 2002.
———. *The Kiss of God: Spiritual and Mystical Death in Judaism*. Seattle: University of Washington Press, 1994.
———. "The Well of Living Water." In *Sha'arei Talmon: Studies in the Bible, Qumran, and the Ancient Near East, Presented to Shemaryahu Talmon*, ed. Michael Fishbane and Emanuel Tov, 3–16. Winona Lake, Ind.: Eisenbrauns, 1992.
Fishbane, Simcha. "Most Women Engage in Sorcery." In *Approaches to Ancient Judaism: New Series*, vol. 5, *Historical, Literary, and Religious Studies*, ed. Herbert W. Basser and Simcha Fishbane, 143–65. South Florida Studies in the History of Judaism 82. Atlanta: Scholars Press, 1993.

Fonrobert, Charlotte Elisheva, and Martin S. Jaffee. *The Cambridge Companion to the Talmud and Rabbinic Literature*. Cambridge: Cambridge University Press, 2007.
Foster, Benjamin R. *From Distant Days: Myths, Tales, and Poetry of Ancient Mesopotamia*. Bethesda: CDL Press, 1995.
Fox, Michael. *Proverbs 1–9: A New Translation with Introduction and Commentary*. Anchor Bible 18A. New York: Doubleday, 2000.
———. *The Song of Songs and Ancient Egyptian Love Songs*. Madison: University of Wisconsin Press, 1985.
Fraade, Steven. *Enosh and His Generation: Pre-Israelite Hero and History in Postbiblical Interpretation*. Chico, Calif.: Scholars Press, 1984.
Freud, Sigmund. *Civilization and Its Discontents*. Translated by James Strachey. New York: W. W. Norton, 1962.
Galambush, Julie. *Jerusalem in the Book of Ezekiel: The City as Yahweh's Wife*. Society of Biblical Literature Dissertation Series 130. Atlanta: Scholars Press, 1992.
Galor, Katharina. "The Stepped Water Installations of the Sepphoris Acropolis." In *The Archaeology of Difference: Gender, Ethnicity, Class, and the "Other" in Antiquity; Studies in Honor of Eric M. Meyers*, ed. Douglas R. Edwards and C. Thomas McCollough, 201–13. Boston: American Schools of Oriental Research, 2007.
Gane, Roy. *Cult and Character: Purification Offerings, Day of Atonement, and Theodicy*. Winona Lake, Ind.: Eisenbrauns, 2005.
Gereleman, Gillis. *Ruth, das Hohelied*. Edited by Martin Noth and Hans Walter Woff. Biblischer Kommentar, Altes Testament, no. 18. Neukirchen-Vluyn: Neukirchener, 1965.
Gesenius, W. *Gesenius' Hebrew Grammar*. 2d English ed. Edited by E. Kautzsch. Translated by A. E. Cowley. Oxford: Clarendon Press, 1910.
Ginzberg, Louis. *The Legends of the Jews: I—Bible Times and Characters from the Creation to Jacob*. Translated by Henrietta Szold. 2d ed. Philadelphia: Jewish Publication Society of America, 1937.
Gitin, Seymour. "Incense Altars from Ekron, Israel, and Judah: Context and Typology." *Eretz-Israel* 20 (1989): 52–67.
Glare, P. G. W., ed. *Oxford Latin Dictionary*. Combined ed. Oxford: Clarendon Press, 1982.
Goff, Matthew. "Hellish Females: The Strange Woman of Septuagint Proverbs and 4QWiles of the Wicked Woman (4Q184)." *Journal for the Study of Judaism* 39, no. 1 (2008): 20–45.
Goldingay, John. "Isaiah 43, 22–28." *Zeitschrift für die Alttestamentliche Wissenschaft* 110, no. 2 (1998): 173–91.
Goodenough, Erwin R. *Jewish Symbols in the Greco-Roman Period*. Vols. 1–13. New York: Pantheon Books, 1953–68.
Goodman, Martin. "The Roman State and the Jewish Patriarch in the Third Century." In *The Galilee in Late Antiquity*, ed. Lee I. Levine, 127–39. New York: Jewish Theological Seminary, 1992.
———. "Texts, Scribes, and Power in Roman Judea." In *Literacy and Power in the Ancient World*, ed. Alan K. Bowman and Greg Woolf, 99–108. Cambridge: Cambridge University Press, 1994.
Gorin-Rosen, Yael. "The Glass Vessels." In *Eretz Zafon: Studies in Galilean Archaeology*, ed. Zvi Gal, 288–322. Jerusalem: Israel Anitquities Authority, 2002.
———. "The Glass Vessels from Burial Cave D at Hurfeish." In *Eretz Zafon: Studies in Galilean Archaeology*, ed. Zvi Gal, 140–66. Jerusalem: Israel Antiquities Authority, 2002.

Gray, George Buchanan. *Isaiah: International Critical Commentary.* New York: Charles Scribner's Sons, 1912.
Green, Deborah. "Sweet Spices in the Tomb: An Initial Study on the Use of Perfume in Jewish Burials." In *Commemorating the Dead: Texts and Artifacts in Context; Studies of Roman, Jewish, and Christian Burials*, ed. Laurie Brink and Deborah Green, 145–73. Berlin: Walter de Gruyter, 2008.
Greenberg, Moshe. *Ezekiel 1–20.* Anchor Bible 22. New York: Doubleday, 1983.
———. *Ezekiel 21–37.* Anchor Bible 22A. New York: Doubleday, 1997.
Gruber, Mayer I. *Aspects of Nonverbal Communication in the Ancient Near East.* Studia Pohl 12/1. Rome: Biblical Institute Press, 1980.
Guggenheimer, Heinrich. *The Jerusalem Talmud: First Order; Zeraim (Tractate Berakhot).* Berlin: Walter de Gruyter, 2000.
Hachlili, Rachel. *Ancient Jewish Art and Archaeology in the Land of Israel.* Leiden: Brill, 1988.
———. *Jewish Funerary Customs, Practices, and Rites in the Second Temple Period.* Leiden: Brill, 2005.
Hachlili, Rachel, and Ann E. Killebrew, eds. *Jericho: The Jewish Cemetery in the Second Temple Period.* Jerusalem: Israel Antiquities Authority, 1999.
Halperin, David. *The Merkabah in Rabbinic Literature.* New Haven, Conn.: American Oriental Society, 1980.
Haran, Menachem. "'Incense Altars'—Are They?" In *Biblical Archaeology Today, 1990: Proceedings of the Second International Congress on Biblical Archaeology*, ed. Avraham Biran and Joseph Aviram, 237–47. Jerusalem: Israel Exploration Society and Israel Academy of Sciences and Humanities, 1990.
———. *Temples and Temple-Service in Ancient Israel: An Inquiry into the Character of Cult Phenomena and the Historical Setting of the Priestly School.* Oxford: Clarendon Press, 1978.
———. "The Uses of Incense in the Ancient Israelite Ritual." *Vetus Testamentum* 10 (1960): 113–29.
Harvey, Susan Ashbrook. "On Holy Stench: When the Odor of Sanctity Sickens." *Studia Patristica* 35 (2001): 90–101.
———. *Scenting Salvation: Ancient Christianity and the Olfactory Imagination.* Berkeley and Los Angeles: University of California Press, 2006.
Hasan-Rokem, Galit. *The Web of Life: Folklore and Midrash in Rabbinic Literature.* Translated by Batya Stein. 2d ed. Stanford: Stanford University Press, 2000.
Hegel, G. W. F. *Ästhetik.* Edited by Friedrich Bassenge. 2 vols. Berlin: Das Europäische Buch, 1985.
Heger, Paul. *The Development of Incense Cult in Israel.* Berlin: Walter de Gruyter, 1997.
Hertz, Robert. *Death and the Right Hand.* 1907. Translated by Rodney Needham and Claudia Needham. Reprint, Glencoe, Ill.: Free Press, 1960.
Hezser, Catherine. *The Social Structure of the Rabbinic Movement in Roman Palestine.* Tübingen: Mohr Siebeck, 1997.
Hill, Andrew. *Malachi.* Anchor Bible 25D. New York: Doubleday, 1998.
Hirsch, Alan R. "Nostalgia, the Odors of Childhood, and Society." *Psychiatric Times* 9, no. 8 (1992): 29–30.
Hirschfeld, Yizhar. "Early Roman Manor Houses in Judea and the Site of Khirbet Qumran." *Journal of Near Eastern Studies* 57, no. 3 (1998): 161–89.
———. *Hammat Gader Excavations: 1979–1982.* Jerusalem: Israel Exploration Society, 1997.

Hoffman, Yair. *Jeremiah: Introduction and Commentary.* 2 vols. [In Hebrew.] Tel Aviv: Am Oved, 2001.
Hoftijzer, J. "Das sogenannte Feueropfer." *Supplements to Vetus Testamentum* 16 (1967): 114–34.
Holum, Kenneth G. "Identity and the Late Antique City." In *Religious and Ethnic Communities in Later Roman Palestine,* ed. H. Lapin, 155–77. Potomac: University Press of Maryland, 1998.
Holum, Kenneth G., Robert L. Hohlfelder, Robert J. Bull, and Avner Raban. *King Herod's Dream: Caesarea on the Sea.* New York: W. W. Norton, 1988.
Houtman, C. "On the Function of the Holy Incense (Exodus XXX 34–8) and the Sacred Anointing Oil (Exodus XXX 22–33)." *Vetus Testamentum* 42, no. 4 (1992): 458–65.
Howes, David. "Olfaction and Transition." In *The Varieties of Sensory Experience: A Sourcebook in the Anthropology of the Senses,* ed. David Howes, 128–47. Toronto: University of Toronto Press, 1991.
Hurowitz, Victor. "Response: Aspects of Cult and Art in the Land of Israel." In *Biblical Archaeology Today, 1990: Proceedings of the Second International Congress on Biblical Archaeology,* ed. Avraham Biran and Joseph Aviram. Jerusalem: Israel Exploration Society and Israel Academy of Sciences and Humanities, 1990.
———. "Salted Incense—Exodus 30,35; Maqlû VI 111–113; IX 118–120." *Biblica* 68, no. 2 (1987): 178–94.
Hurvitz, Avi. *A Linguistic Study of the Relationship Between the Priestly Source and the Book of Ezekiel: A New Approach to an Old Problem.* Cahiers de la Revue Biblique. Paris: J. Gabalda, 1982.
Ilan, Tal. *Mine and Yours Are Hers: Retrieving Women's History from Rabbinic Literature.* Leiden: Brill, 1997.
Israeli, Yael. "Glass in the Roman-Byzantine Period." [In Hebrew.] In *Ancient Glass in the Israel Museum: The Eliyahu Dobkin Collection and Other Gifts,* ed. Yael Israeli, 93–342. Jerusalem: Israel Museum, 2003.
Japhet, Sara. *The Ideology of the Book of Chronicles and Its Place in Biblical Thought.* Frankfurt: Peter Lang, 1989.
Jastrow, Marcus. *Dictionary of the Targumim, Talmud Babli, Yerushalmi, and Midrashic Literatures.* New York: Judaica Press, 1903.
Jones, Scott C. "Wisdom's Pedagogy: A Comparison of Proverbs VII and 4Q184." *Vetus Testamentum* 53, no. 1 (2003): 65–80.
Josephus. *Jewish Antiquities.* Translated by H. St. J. Thackeray et al. 10 vols. Cambridge: Harvard University Press, 1926–65.
———. *The Jewish War.* Translated by H. St. J. Thackeray. 3 vols. Cambridge: Harvard University Press, 1927–97.
Kadari, Tamar. "On the Redaction of Midrash Shir Hashirim Rabbah." [In Hebrew.] PhD diss., Hebrew University, 2004.
———. "'Within It Was Decked with Love': The Torah as Bride in Tannaitic Exegesis on Song of Songs." [In Hebrew.] *Tarbiz* 71 (2002): 391–404.
Kahana, Menachem. "The Critical Edition of Mekilta De-Rabbi Ishmael in the Light of the Genizah Fragments." [In Hebrew.] *Tarbiz* 55, no. 4 (1986): 489–524.
Kaplan, J. "Mesopotamian Elements in the Middle Bronze II Culture of Palestine." *Journal of Near Eastern Studies* 30, no. 4 (1971): 293–307.
Keel, Othmar. *The Song of Songs.* Translated by Frederick J. Gaiser. Continental Commentary. Minneapolis: Fortress Press, 1994.

———. *Die Welt der altorientalischen Bildsymbolik und das Alte Testament: Am Beispiel der Psalmen*. Zurich: Benziger Verlag und Neukirchener Verlag, 1972.

Killebrew, Ann E. "Catalogue of Artifacts." In *Jericho: The Jewish Cemetery in the Second Temple Period*, ed. Rachel Hachlili and Ann E. Killebrew, 176–91. Jerusalem: Israel Antiquities Authority, 1999.

———. "The Pottery." In *Jericho: The Jewish Cemetery in the Second Temple Period*, ed. Rachel Hachlili and Ann E. Killebrew, 115–33. Jerusalem: Israel Antiquities Authority, 1999.

Kimelman, Reuven. "The Conflict Between the Priestly Oligarchy and the Sages in the Talmudic Period." [In Hebrew.] *Zion* 48 (1983): 135–48.

Kingsmill, Edmée. *The Song of Songs and Eros of God: A Study in Biblical Intertextuality*. Oxford: Oxford University Press, 2009.

Kister, Menahem. *Avoth De-Rabbi Nathan: Solomon Schechter Edition, with References to Parallels in the Two Versions and to the Addenda in the Schechter Edition*. New York: Jewish Theological Seminary of America, 1997.

Kloner, Amos, and Boaz Zissou. *The Necropolis of Jerusalem in the Second Temple Period*. [In Hebrew.] Jerusalem: Yad Izhak Ben-Zvi and Israel Exploration Society, 2003.

Knohl, Israel. *The Sanctuary of Silence: The Priestly Torah and the Holiness School*. Minneapolis: Fortress Press, 1995.

Knohl, Israel, and Shlomo Naeh. "Milluim Ve-Kippurim." [In Hebrew.] *Tarbiz* 62, no. 1 (1992): 17–44.

Koehler, Ludwig, and Walter Baumgartner. *The Hebrew and Aramaic Lexicon of the Old Testament*. Translated by M. E. J. Richardson. Leiden: Brill, 1996.

Kogan-Zehavi, Elena. "Settlement Remains and Tombs at Khirbet Tabaliya." [In Hebrew.] *'Atiqot* (2000): 53–79.

Kraemer, David. *The Meanings of Death in Rabbinic Judaism*. London: Routledge, 2000.

Krauss, Samuel. *Talmudische Archäologie*. Vols. 1–3. Leipzig: Buchhandlung Gustav Fock, 1910. Reprint, New York: Arno Press, 1979.

Kutscher, Eduard Y. *The Language and Linguistic Background of the Isaiah Scroll*. [In Hebrew.] Jerusalem: Magnes Press, 1959.

Lakoff, George, and Mark Johnson. *Metaphors We Live By*. Chicago: University of Chicago Press, 1980.

Landy, Francis. *Paradoxes of Paradise: Identity and Difference in the Song of Songs*. Sheffield, U.K.: Almond, 1983.

Lapin, Hayim. *Economy, Geography, and Provincial History in Later Roman Palestine*. Tübingen: Mohr Siebeck, 2001.

———. "Rabbis and Cities in Later Roman Palestine." *Journal of Jewish Studies* 50, no. 2 (1999): 187–207.

Lauterbach, Jacob. "The Origin and Development of Two Sabbath Ceremonies." *Hebrew Union College Annual* 15 (1940): 367–424.

Le Déaut, Roger. *La nuit pascale: Essai sur la signification de la Pâque juive à partir du Targum d'Exode XII 42*. Analecta Biblica 22. Rome: Institut Biblique Pontifical, 1963.

Levenson, Jon D. *The Death and Resurrection of the Beloved Son: The Transformation of Child Sacrifice in Judaism and Christianity*. New Haven: Yale University Press, 1993.

Levine, Baruch A. *Leviticus*. JPS Torah Commentary. Philadelphia: Jewish Publication Society, 1989.

———. *Numbers 1–20*. Anchor Bible 4. New York: Doubleday, 1993.

———. *Numbers 21–36*. Anchor Bible 4A. New York: Doubleday, 2000.
Levine, Lee I. "The Archaeological Finds and Their Relationship to the History of the City." In *Excavations at Caesarea Maritima: 1975, 1976, 1979—Final Report*, ed. Lee I. Levine and Ehud Netzer, 178–86. Jerusalem: Institute of Archaeology, Hebrew University of Jerusalem, 1986.
———. "Bet Šeʿarim in Its Patriarchal Context." In *"The Words of a Wise Man's Mouth Are Gracious" (Qoh 10, 12): Festschrift for Günter Stemberger on the Occasion of His Sixty-Fifth Birthday*, ed. Mauro Perani, 197–225. Berlin: Walter de Gruyter, 2005.
———. *Caesarea Under Roman Rule*. Leiden: Brill, 1975.
———. *The Rabbinic Class of Roman Palestine*. Jerusalem: Yad Izhak Ben-Zvi, 1989.
———. "The Sages and the Synagogue in Late Antiquity: The Evidence of the Galilee." In *The Galilee in Late Antiquity*, ed. Lee I. Levine, 201–22. New York: Jewish Theological Seminary, 1992.
Licht, Chaim. *Ten Legends of the Sages*. Hoboken: KTAV, 1991.
Lieber, Andrea. "God Incorporated: Feasting on the Divine Presence in Ancient Judaism." PhD diss., Columbia University, 1998.
Lieberman, Saul. *Greek in Jewish Palestine*. New York: Jewish Theological Seminary of America, 1942. Reprint, 1994.
———. *Hayerushalmi Kiphshuto: A Commentary, Based on MS. of the Yerushalmi, and Works of the Rishonim and Midrashim in MSS in Rare Ed. 1,1, Sabbath Erubin Pesahim*. Jerusalem: Hotsaʾat Darom, 1934.
———. "Some Aspects of After Life in Early Rabbinic Literature." In *Harry Austryn Wolfson Jubilee Volume*, 495–532. Jerusalem: American Academy for Jewish Research, 1965.
———. *The Tosefta: According to Codex Vienna, with Variants from Codex Erfurt, Ms. Schocken and Editio Princeps (Venice 1521)*. 4 vols. New York: Jewish Theological Seminar of America, 1988–95.
———. *Tosefta Ki-Fshuṭah: A Comprehensive Commentary on the Tosefta*. New York: Jewish Theological Seminary of America, 1992.
Löhr, Max. *Das Räucheropfer im Alten Testament: Eine archäeologische Untersuchung*. Halle: Max Neimeyer, 1927.
Loretz, Oswald. "Die ugaritisch-hebräische Gefäßbezeichnung Trq/Twrq in Canticum 1,3: Liebesdichtung in der westsemitischen Wein- und Olivenkultur." *Ugarit-Forschungen* 36 (2004): 283–89.
Mach, Rudolf. *Der Zaddik in Talmude und Midrasch*. Leiden: Brill, 1957.
Magness, Jodi. *The Archaeology of Qumran and the Dead Sea Scrolls*. Grand Rapids, Mich.: William B. Eerdmans, 2002.
———. "The Burials of Jesus and James." *Journal of Biblical Literature* 124, no. 1 (2005): 121–54.
———. "Qumran Pottery." In *Methods of Investigation of the Dead Sea Scrolls and the Khirbet Qumran Site: Present Realities and Future Prospects*, ed. Michael O. Wise, Norman Golb, John J. Collins, and Dennis Pardee, 39–50. Annals of the New York Academy of Sciences 22. New York: New York Academy of Sciences, 1994.
Mandelbaum, Bernard, ed. *Pesikta de Rav Kahana According to an Oxford Manuscript, with Variants from All Known Manuscripts and Genizoth Fragments and Parallel Passages*. 2d ed. New York: Jewish Theological Seminary of America, 1987.
Mann, Jacob. "Rabbinic Studies in the Synoptic Gospels." *Hebrew Union College Annual* 1 (1924): 323–55.

Margulies, Mordecai, ed. *Midrash Wayyikra Rabbah: A Critical Edition Based on Manuscripts and Genizah Fragments with Variants and Notes*. Jerusalem: Jewish Theological Seminary of America, 1958.
Marks, Lawrence. *The Unity of the Senses: Interrelations Among the Modalities*. New York: Academic Press, 1978.
Mazar, Amihai. *Archaeology of the Land of the Bible: 10,000–586 B.C.E.* Anchor Bible Reference Library. New York: Doubleday, 1990. New ed., 1992.
McCarter, P. Kyle, Jr. *II Samuel*. Anchor Bible 9. New York: Doubleday, 1984.
McKane, William. *Jeremiah*. Edinburgh: T & T Clark, 1996.
McKenzie, John L. *Second Isaiah*. Anchor Bible 20. Garden City, N.Y.: Doubleday, 1968.
McNamara, Martin, Robert Hayward, and Michael Maher. *Targum Neofiti 1, Exodus*. Collegeville, Minn.: Liturgical Press, 1994.
Meacham, Tirzah. "Woman More Intelligent Than Man." In *Approaches to Ancient Judaism: New Series*, vol. 5, *Historical, Literary, and Religious Studies*, ed. Herbert W. Basser and Simcha Fishbane, 55–65. South Florida Studies in the History of Judaism 82. Atlanta: Scholars Press, 1993.
Mendelsohn, I. "Guilds in Ancient Palestine." *Bulletin of the American Schools of Oriental Research* 80 (1940): 17–21.
Meyers, Carol L. "Fumes, Flames, or Fluids? Reframing the Cup-and-Bowl Question." In *Boundaries of the Ancient Near Eastern World: A Tribute to Cyrus H. Gordon*, ed. Meir Lubetski, Clare Gottlieb, and Sharon Keller, 30–39. Sheffield, U.K. Sheffield Academic Press, 1998.
———. "Gender Imagery in the Song of Songs." In *A Feminist Companion to the Song of Songs*, ed. Athalya Brenner, 197–212. Sheffield, U.K.: Sheffield Academic Press, 1993.
———. "Guilds and Gatherings: Women's Groups in Ancient Israel." In *Realia Dei: Essays in Archaeology and Biblical Interpretation in Honor of Edward F. Campbell, Jr. at His Retirement*, ed. Prescott H. Williams and Theodore Hiebert, 154–84. Atlanta: Scholars Press, 1999.
Meyers, Eric M. "The Ceramic Incense Shovels from Sepphoris: Another View." In *"I Will Speak the Riddles of Ancient Times": Archaeological and Historical Studies in Honor of Amihai Mazar on the Occasion of His Sixtieth Birthday*, ed. Aren M. Maeir and Pierre de Miroschedji, 865–78. Winona Lake, Ind.: Eisenbrauns, 2006.
———. "Roman Sepphoris in Light of New Archaeological Evidence." In *The Galilee in Late Antiquity*, ed. Lee I. Levine, 321–38. New York: Jewish Theological Seminary, 1992.
———. "The Use of Archaeology in Understanding Rabbinic Materials." In *Texts and Responses: Studies Presented to Nahum N. Glatzer on the Occasion of His Seventieth Birthday by His Students*, ed. Michael Fishbane and Paul Flohr, 28–42. Leiden: Brill, 1975.
Meyers, Eric M., A. Thomas Kraabel, and James Strange. *Ancient Synagogue Excavations at Khirbet Shema', Upper Galilee, Israel, 1970–1972*. Durham: Duke University Press, 1976.
Meyers, Eric M., Carol Meyers, and James Strange. *Excavations at the Ancient Synagogue of Gush Halav*. Winona Lake, Ind.: Eisenbrauns, 1990.
Meyers, Eric M., James Strange, and Carol Meyers. *Excavations at Ancient Meiron*. Cambridge, Mass.: American Schools of Oriental Research, 1981.

Milgrom, Jacob. "The Compass of Biblical Sancta." *Jewish Quarterly Review* 65, no. 4 (1975): 205–16.

———. "Korah's Rebellion: A Study in Redaction." In *De la Tôrah au Messie: Études d'exégèse et d'herméneutique bibliques offertes à Henri Cazelles pour ses 25 années d'enseignement à l'Institut Catholique de Paris, Octobre 1979*, ed. Maurice Carrez, Joseph Doré, and Pierre Grelot, 135–46. Paris: Desclée, 1981.

———. *Leviticus 1–16*. Anchor Bible 3. New York: Doubleday, 1991.

———. *Numbers*. JPS Torah Commentary. Philadelphia: Jewish Publication Society, 1990.

———. "The Priestly Doctrine of Repentance." *Revue Biblique* 82, no. 2 (1975): 186–205.

———. "The Rebellion of Korah, Numbers 16–18: A Study in Tradition History." *Society of Biblical Literature Seminar Papers* 27 (1988): 570–73.

———. *Studies in Levitical Terminology*. Berkeley and Los Angeles: University of California Press, 1970.

Miller, J. Innes. *The Spice Trade of the Roman Empire: 29 BC to AD 641*. Oxford: Clarendon Press, 1969.

Miller, Stuart S. "Stepped Pools and the Non-Existent Monolithic 'Miqveh.'" In *The Archaeology of Difference: Gender, Ethnicity, Class, and the "Other" in Antiquity; Studies in Honor of Eric M. Meyers*, ed. Douglas R. Edwards and C. Thomas McCollough, 215–34. Boston: American Schools of Oriental Research, 2007.

———. *Studies in the History and Traditions of Sepphoris*. Leiden: Brill, 1984.

Miller, William Ian. *The Anatomy of Disgust*. Cambridge: Harvard University Press, 1997.

Moore, Rick D. "Personification of the Seduction of Evil: 'The Wiles of the Wicked Woman.'" *Revue de Qumran* 10, no. 4D (1981): 505–19.

Muffs, Yochanan. *Love and Joy: Law, Language, and Religion in Ancient Israel*. New York: Jewish Theological Seminary of America, 1992.

Munro, Jill. *Spikenard and Saffron: The Imagery of the Song of Songs*. Sheffield, U.K. Sheffield Academic Press, 1995.

Murphy, Roland E. *The Song of Songs: A Commentary on the Book of Canticles or the Song of Songs*. Minneapolis: Fortress Press, 1990.

Narkiss, Mordechai. "Origins of the Spice Box." *Journal of Jewish Art* 8 (1981): 28–41.

Naveh, Joseph. *On Stone and Mosaic: The Aramaic and Hebrew Inscriptions from Ancient Synagogues*. [In Hebrew.] Jerusalem: Ha-Ḥeverah le-Hakirat Erets Yisrael ve-'Atikoteiha, 1978.

Neusner, Jacob. *Judaism in Society: The Evidence of the Yerushalmi; Toward a Natural History of a Religion*. Chicago: University of Chicago Press, 1983.

Newman, Cathy. "Perfume: The Essence of Illusion." *National Geographic*, October 1998, 94–119.

Newsom, Carol. "Woman and the Discourse of Patriarchal Wisdom: A Study of Proverbs 1–9." In *Gender and Difference*, ed. Peggy L. Day, 142–60. Minneapolis: Fortress Press, 1989.

Nickelsburg, George W. E. *1 Enoch*. Minneapolis: Fortress Press, 2001.

Nielsen, Kjeld. *Incense in Ancient Israel*. Leiden: Brill, 1986.

Patrich, Joseph. "Agricultural Development in Antiquity: Improvements in Cultivation and Production of Balsam." In *Qumran: The Site of the Dead Sea Scrolls; Archaeological Interpretations and Debates*, ed. Katharina Galor, Jean-Baptiste Humbert, and Jürgen Zangenberg, 241–48. Leiden: Brill, 2006.

Patrich, Joseph, and Benny Arubas. "A Juglet Containing Balsam Oil (?) from a Cave Near Qumran." *Israel Exploration Journal* 39 (1989): 43–59.
Paul, Shalom. "A Lover's Garden of Verse: Literal and Metaphorical Imagery in Ancient Near Eastern Love Poetry." In *Tehillah Le-Moshe: Biblical and Judaic Studies in Honor of Moshe Greenberg*, ed. Mordechai Cogan, Barry Eichler, and Jeffrey Tigay, 99–110. Winona Lake, Ind.: Eisenbrauns, 1977.
Philo. *On the Special Laws*. In *Philo: In Ten Volumes (and Two Supplementary Volumes)*, trans. F. H. Colson, G. H. Whitaker, and Ralph Marcus. Cambridge: Harvard University Press, 1929.
Pliny. *Naturalis historia*. Translated by H. Rackham. 4 vols. Cambridge: Harvard University Press, 1945–2000.
Pollak, Rachel. "Glass from the Sediments of the Inner Harbour." In *Caesarea Papers 2: Herod's Temple, the Provincial Governor's Praetorium and Granaries, the Later Harbor, a Gold Coin Hoard, and Other Studies*, ed. K. G. Holum, A. Raban, and J. Patrich, 323–32. Portsmouth, R.I.: Journal of Roman Archaeology, 1999.
Propp, William C. *Exodus 19–40*. Anchor Bible 2A. New York: Doubleday, 2006.
Rahmani, L. Y. *A Catalogue of Jewish Ossuaries in the Collections of the State of Israel*. Jerusalem: Israel Antiquities Authority, Israel Academy of Sciences and Humanities, 1994.
Rindisbacher, Hans J. *The Smell of Books: A Cultural-Historical Study of Olfactory Perception in Literature*. Ann Arbor: University of Michigan Press, 1992.
Ritchie, Ian D. "The Nose Knows: Bodily Knowing in Isaiah 11:3." *Journal for the Study of the Old Testament* 87 (2000): 59–73.
Rubin, Nissan. *The End of Life: Rites of Burial and Mourning in the Talmud and Midrash*. [In Hebrew.] Jerusalem: Hakkibutz Hameuchad, 1997.
Rutgers, Leonard Victor. "Incense Shovels at Sepphoris?" In *Galilee Through the Centuries: Confluence of Cultures*, ed. Eric M. Meyers, 177–98. Winona Lake, Ind.: Eisenbrauns, 1999.
Safrai, Shmuel. "Quiddush Ha-shem be-Toratam Shel Ha-Tannaim." [In Hebrew.] *Zion* 44 (1979): 28–42.
Safrai, Ze'ev. "The Communal Functions of the Synagogue in the Land of Israel in the Rabbinic Period." In *Ancient Synagogues*, ed. Dan Urman and Paul V. M. Flesher, 181–204. Leiden: Brill, 1995.
———. *The Economy of Roman Palestine*. London: Routledge, 1994.
Sarna, Nahum. *Exodus*. JPS Torah Commentary. Philadelphia: Jewish Publication Society, 1991.
———. *Exploring Exodus: The Heritage of Biblical Israel*. New York: Schocken Books, 1987.
———. "The Psalm Superscriptions and the Guilds." In *Studies in Jewish Religious and Intellectual History: Presented to Alexander Altmann*, ed. Siegfried Stein and Raphael Loewe, 281–300. Tuscaloosa: University of Alabama Press, 1979.
Satlow, Michael. *Tasting the Dish: Rabbinic Rhetorics of Sexuality*. Atlanta: Scholars Press, 1995.
Schäfer, Peter. "Daughter, Sister, Bride, and Mother: Images of the Femininity of God in the Early Kabbala." *Journal of the American Academy of Religion* 68, no. 2 (2000): 221–42.
Schäfer, Peter, and Hans-Jürgen Becker, eds. *Synopse zum Talmud Yerushalmi*. Vol. 1. Tübingen: J. C. B. Mohr (Paul Siebeck), 1991.
Scholem, Gershom. *Kabbalah*. Jerusalem: Keter, 1974.

Schwabe, Moshe, and Baruch Lifshitz. *The Greek Inscriptions.* Vol. 2 of *Beth She'arim: Report on the Excavations During 1953–1958.* New Brunswick: Rutgers University Press, 1974.
Schwartz, Seth. *Imperialism and Jewish Society, 200 B.C.E. to 640 C.E.* Princeton: Princeton University Press, 2001.
Segal, Alan F. *Life After Death: A History of the Afterlife in the Religions of the West.* New York: Doubleday, 2004.
Shepkaru, Shmuel. *Jewish Martyrs in the Pagan and Christian Worlds.* Cambridge: Cambridge University Press, 2006.
Shields, Mary E. "Multiple Exposures: Body Rhetoric and Gender Characterization in Ezekiel 16." *Journal of Feminist Studies in Religion* 14, no. 1 (1998): 5–18.
Sivertsev, Alexei. *Private Households and Public Politics in Third–Fifth-Century Jewish Palestine.* Tübingen: Mohr Siebeck, 2002.
Smith, Jonathan Z. *Map Is Not Territory: Studies in the History of Religions.* 2d ed. Chicago: University of Chicago Press, 1993.
Sokoloff, Michael, ed. *A Dictionary of Jewish Palestinian Aramaic of the Byzantine Period.* Ramat-Gan, Israel: Bar-Ilan University Press, 1992.
Sommer, Benjamin. *A Prophet Reads Scripture: Allusion in Isaiah 40–66.* Stanford: Stanford University Press, 1998.
Sperber, Dan. *Rethinking Symbolism.* Translated by Alice Morton. Cambridge: Cambridge University Press, 1975.
Sperber, Daniel. *Roman Palestine, 200–400: Money and Prices.* Ramat-Gan, Israel: Bar-Ilan University Press, 1974.
Spiegel, Shalom. *The Last Trial: On the Legends and Lore of the Command to Abraham to Offer Isaac as a Sacrifice.* Translated by Judah Golden. New York: Pantheon Books, 1967.
Steller, H. E. "Preliminary Remarks to a New Edition of Shir Hashirim Rabbah." In *Rashi, 1040–1990: Homage à Ephraim E. Urbach,* ed. Gabrielle Sed-Rajna, 301–11. Paris: Cerf, 1993.
Stern, David. *Parables in Midrash.* Cambridge: Harvard University Press, 1991.
Stern, Edna, and Yael Gorin-Rosen. "Burial Caves Near Kabri." [In Hebrew.] *'Atiqot* 33 (1997): 1–22.
Stern, E. Marianne, and Birgit Schlick-Nolte. *Early Glass of the Ancient World: 1600 B.C.–A.D. 50.* Osfildern: Verlag Gerd Hatje, 1994.
Stiebert, Johanna. "Shame and Prophecy: Approaches Past and Present." *Biblical Interpretation* 8, no. 3 (2000): 255–75.
Stoddart, D. Michael. *The Scented Ape: The Biology and Culture of Human Odour.* Cambridge: Cambridge University Press, 1990.
Strack, H. L., and G. Stemberger. *Introduction to the Talmud and Midrash.* Translated by Markus Bockmuehl. London: T & T Clark, 1991.
Strange, James F., Thomas R. W. Longstaff, and Dennis E. Groh. *Excavations at Sepphoris,* vol. 1, *University of South Florida Probes in the Citadel and Villa.* Leiden: Brill, 2006.
Swartz, Michael D. "Sage, Priest, and Poet: Typologies of Religious Leadership in the Ancient Synagogue." In *Jews, Christians, and Polytheists in the Ancient Synagogue,* ed. Steven Fine, 101–17. London: Routledge, 1999.
Talmon, Shemaryahu. "The 'Desert Motif' in the Bible and in Qumran Literature." In *Biblical Motifs: Origins and Transformations,* ed. Alexander Altman, 31–63. Cambridge: Harvard University Press, 1966.

Theodor, J., and Ch. Albeck, eds. *Midrash Bereshit Rabba.* Jerusalem: Shalem Books, 1996.
Theophrastus. *Historia plantarum.* Translated by A. F. Hort. Cambridge: Harvard University Press, 1926.
Unterman, Jeremiah. "The (Non)Sense of Smell in Isaiah 11:3." *Hebrew Studies* 33 (1992): 17–23.
Urbach, Ephraim. "Ha-Mesorot 'al Torat ha-Sod be-Tequfat ha-Tannaim." [In Hebrew.] In *Studies in Mysticism and Religion Presented to Gershom G. Scholem on His Seventieth Birthday by Pupils, Colleagues, and Friends,* 1–28. Jerusalem: Magnes Press, 1967.
———. *The Sages: Their Concepts and Beliefs.* Translated by Israel Abrahams. 2d ed. Cambridge: Harvard University Press, 1979.
Van Gennup, Arnold. *The Rites of Passage.* 1909. Translated by Monika B. Vizedom and Gabrielle L. Caffe. Chicago: University of Chicago Press, 1960.
Van Henten, Jan Willem, and Friedrich Avemarie. *Martyrdom and Noble Death: Selected Texts from Graeco-Roman, Jewish, and Christian Antiquity.* London: Routledge, 2002.
Vitto, Fanny. "Burial Caves from the Second Temple Period in Jerusalem (Mount Scopus, Giv'at Hamivtar, Neveh Ya'aqov)." *'Atiqot* 40 (2000): 65–121.
———. "Byzantine Mosaics at Bet She'arim: New Evidence for the History of the Site." *'Atiqot* 28 (1996): 137–41.
Webster, Edwin C. "A Rhetorical Study of Isaiah 66." *Journal for the Study of the Old Testament* 34 (1986): 93–108.
Weiss, Zeev. "Hellenistic Influences on Jewish Burial Customs in the Galilee During the Mishnaic and Talmudic Period." [In Hebrew.] *Eretz Israel* 25 (1996): 356–64.
———. "The Location of Jewish Cemeteries in Galilee in the Mishnaic and Talmudic Periods." [In Hebrew.] In *Graves and Burial Practices in Israel in the Ancient Period,* ed. I. Singer, 230–40. Jerusalem: Yad Izhak Ben-Zvi, 1994.
Weiss, Zeev, and Ehud Netzer. "Zippori—1994–1995." *Excavations and Surveys in Israel* 18 (1998): 22–27, 31–38.
Wilson, Donald A., and Richard J. Stevenson. *Learning to Smell: Olfactory Perception from Neurobiology to Behavior.* Baltimore: Johns Hopkins University Press, 2006.
Wischnitzer, Mark. "Notes to a History of the Jewish Guilds." *Hebrew Union College Annual* 23, part 2 (1950–51): 245–63.
Wolff, Esther. "Notes on the Act of Perfuming Clothes and on the Cypriot Origin of Minoan and Greek Perfumery." In *From Aphrodite to Melusine: Reflections on the Archaeology and History of Cyprus,* ed. Matteo Campagnolo and Marielle Martiniani-Reber, 41–47. Geneva: La Pomme d'Or, 2007.
Yadin, Yigal. *Bar-Kokhba: The Rediscovery of the Legendary Hero of the Last Jewish Revolt Against Imperial Rome.* New York: Random House, 1971.
Yegül, Fikret. *Baths and Bathing in Classical Antiquity.* New York: Architectural History Foundation, 1992.
Zimmerli, Walther. *Ezekiel 1.* Philadelphia: Fortress Press, 1979.
Zuckermandel, M. S. *Tosephta: Based on Erfurt and Vienna Codices.* Jerusalem: Wahrmann Books, 1970.
Zwickel, Wolfgang. *Räucherkult und Räuchergeräte: Exegetische und archäologische Studien zum Räucheropfer im Alten Testament.* Freiburg, Switzerland: Universitätsverlag, 1990.

SOURCE INDEX

HEBREW BIBLE

Genesis
3:23–24, 121
4:26, 241 n. 42
8, 253 n. 52
8:10–11, 239 n. 16
8:21, 253 n. 52
12:1, 182–83, 252 n. 36
12:2, 183
12:5, 183, 184
15:7, 176, 177, 250 n. 22
17:23, 253 n. 53
17:23–27, 189
17:26, 254 n. 58
18:1–5, 179, 184
18:2, 179
27, 122, 238 n. 167
27:27, 122, 238 n. 167, 240 n. 26
27:33, 122, 240 n. 24
34:30, 233 n. 109, 234 n. 110
49:21, 255 n. 4

Exodus
5:21, 96, 234 nn. 111, 112
7:18, 232 n. 101
7:21, 232 n. 101
8:10, 232 n. 101
11:4–8, 165
12:21–28, 165
12:29, 164
12:41, 256 n. 13
12:43, 164
12:44, 165
12:48, 165
16:20, 232 n. 101
19:6, 229 n. 53
20:1, 161
20:8, 236 n. 146
20:8–11, 236 n. 146
24:7, 130
24:16, 161, 162
25:2, 70
25:6, 70
25–31, 70
27:21, 229 n. 51
29:18, 72
30, 69
30:7–9, 75, 227 n. 19
30:23, 121, 232 n. 89, 235 n. 130
30:22–33, 70, 227 n. 22
30:34, 68, 181
30:34–36, 71, 227 n. 24
30:34–37, 104
30:34–38, 227 n. 19
30:37–38, 71
31:11, 227 n. 20
32, 131–32
32:4, 130
32:6, 131
32:18, 131
35:15, 227 n. 20
37:25, 227 n. 20
40:5, 227 n. 20
40:34–38, 74

Leviticus
1:1–9, 228 n. 39
1:4, 74
10, 77–78, 228 n. 51
10:2, 77, 80
10:3, 78
10:6, 78, 230 n. 61
10:9, 77
16:12–13, 74
16:13, 227 n. 19
17:13–14, 202
18:3, 157, 246 n. 109, 247 n. 114
23:40, 148
24:2, 229 n. 16
26:31, 236 n. 151

Numbers
16, 77
16:5, 79
16:9, 79
16:20–21, 80
16:32, 79, 80
16:35, 79, 80
17, 77, 82–83
17:1–5, 80, 228 n. 44
17:6, 80
17:7, 80
17:10, 80
17:11, 80, 230 n. 61
20:5, 243 n. 63
28:2, 72
32:22, 144

Deuteronomy
4, 10
4:11, 161
4:12, 161
4:28, 237 n. 166
5:12, 236 n. 146
5:12–14, 236 nn. 145, 146
33:5, 161

Joshua
5:2–3, 165
5:3, 189, 191, 192

Judges, 3:24, 222 n. 9, 226 n. 9

1 Samuel
8:13, 72
9, 101
10:10, 101
13:4, 233 n. 107
13:14, 95
24:3, 222 n. 9, 226 n. 9
26:19, 234 nn. 110, 111, 112
27:12, 95

2 Samuel
10:6, 95, 233 n. 107
11:2–3, 240 n. 29
12, 101
12:20, 225 n. 1
16:21, 95–96

1 Kings
10:2, 87
10:10, 87, 215 n. 50
10:25, 87
21, 101

2 Kings
2:3, 101
19:1–4, 163
19:35, 163
20:13, 87
21:3, 236 n. 155

Isaiah
1:13, 103, 105
2:4, 104

Isaiah (continued)
3:16, 110, 236 n. 153
3:24, 110
6:3, 255 n. 9
9:24, 87
11:2, 112, 113
11:2–3, 246 n. 106
11:3, 113, 237 nn. 163, 165
29:23, 186
29:24, 186
39:2, 87
41:22, 236 n. 155
43:7, 143
43:22, 103
43:22–24, 103–4
43:23, 103
43:23–24, 106
43:24, 103, 104, 105
50:2, 232 n. 101
56:7, 235 n. 139
57:7, 236 n. 155
60:7, 235 n. 139
60:13, 235 n. 139
61:9, 156–57
66, 105, 235 n. 134
66:1, 105
66:2, 105
66:3, 104
66:3–4, 235 n. 134
66:4, 104, 105
66:5, 105
66:6, 105–6
66:20–23, 235 n. 139
Jeremiah
6:1–19, 106
6:20, 104, 106
17:19–27, 236 n. 145
17:22, 236 n. 146
17:24–27, 106–7
23:5, 237 n. 164
44, 226 n. 5
Ezekiel
16, 131, 233 n. 108, 237 n. 160
16:9–13, 110
16:16, 110
16:18–19, 110, 111
16:20, 111
16:20–21, 111
22:24, 120
23, 131
23:40–41, 111
23:42, 111
27:22, 108

37:19, 104
40, 227 n. 20
40–47, 236 n. 154
Hosea
2:4–7, 110
14:6, 156
14:7, 249 n. 13
Amos
5:8, 241 n. 42
5:21–22, 236 n. 151
9:6, 241 n. 42
Malachi
1:6, 108, 109
1:6–2:9, 236 n. 148
1:8, 108
1:11, 108–9
1:12, 109
1:12–13, 109
1:14, 109
2:2, 109
Psalms
29:10, 125, 126
44:23, 203
45, 135
45:9, 87, 134, 135, 225 n. 1
48:15, 253 n. 50
72:1–2, 237 n. 164
72:4, 237 n. 164
72:7, 237 n. 164
72:12–13, 237 n. 164
115:5–6, 237 n. 166
141:2, 205
150:6, 249 n. 13
Proverbs
1–7, 98
3:4, 144
5, 98, 235 n. 120
5:3, 98, 232 n. 90
5:3–4, 98
5:5–9, 98
5:14, 234 n. 117
6:24–25, 99
6:25, 98
7, 110, 131, 199, 235 nn. 120, 124
7:10–11, 99
7:12, 99
7:13, 98
7:14–15, 100
7:16, 236 n. 155
7:17, 121, 225 n. 1
7:17–18, 99
7:19–20, 100

10:7, 143, 144
11:2, 122, 123
13:5, 235 n. 125
31, 145
Job, 39:19–25, 233 n. 105
Song of Songs
1:2, 173
1:2–3, 90
1:3, 85–87, 90, 150, 154–56, 173, 182–84, 231 n. 76, 249 n. 8, 252 n. 36, 253 n. 50
1:4, 239 n. 11
1:6, 89, 256 n. 12
1:12, 85, 86, 130, 160, 162, 176, 178, 252 n. 30
1:13, 86, 179, 180–81, 192
1:13–14, 193
1:14, 86, 192
1:15, 120
2:2, 124, 125, 156, 185
2:4, 132
2:7a, 202
2:12, 88
2:12–13, 231 n. 81
2:13, 85, 87–88
2:14, 88
2:16, 248 n. 1
2:17, 255 nn. 6, 8
3:6, 92, 93, 143, 231 n. 80, 255 n. 63
4, 89–90, 91, 92, 99, 123, 234 n. 118, 235 n. 121
4:5, 248 n. 1
4:6, 92, 118, 189, 190, 191, 251 n. 29
4:10, 85, 90
4:10–16, 92
4:11, 85, 90, 91, 92, 98, 122
4:12, 90, 134
4:12–16, 91–92, 118
4:13, 90
4:14, 90, 121, 133
4:15, 90, 99, 134, 135
4:16, 90, 93, 160, 248 n. 133
5, 91
5:1, 92–93, 99, 232 n. 94
5:2, 88
5:5, 88, 91, 93
5:6, 88
5:7, 231 n. 81, 235 n. 124
5:13, 91, 93
5:14, 93
6:2, 170–71

SOURCE INDEX 273

6:2–3, 88
7:9, 85
7:13, 88
7:13–14, 89
7:14, 85, 88
8:2, 231 n. 70
8:8, 249 n. 16
8:14, 204
Ruth, 3:3, 225 n. 1
Ecclesiastes, 10:1, 71–72
Esther, 2:12, 87
Daniel, 3, 177
Ezra
  9:4, 235 n. 140
  10:3, 235 n. 140
Nehemiah
  3:8, 71
  13:15–21, 236 n. 145
1 Chronicles
  9:29, 227 n. 25
  9:30, 71
  19:6, 233 n. 104
2 Chronicles
  9:1, 87
  9:9, 87
  9:24, 87
  16:14, 87
  26, 77
  26:3–4, 81
  26:16, 81
  26:18, 82
  26:19–21, 81
  29:7, 235 n. 129
  32:27, 87

MISHNAH
Berakot
  3:1, 222 n. 139, 223 n. 153
  6:6, 46, 219 n. 97
  8:5, 48, 220 n. 113
  8:6, 56, 58, 215 n. 44, 217 n. 68, 244 n. 73
Kil'ayim, 9:4, 222 n. 137
Ma'aśer Šeni, 5:12, 222 n. 137
Šabbat
  6:3, 221 n. 133
  6:10, 223 n. 164
  8:1, 221 n. 131
  9:6, 221 n. 133
  22:6, 219 n. 92
  23:4, 222 n. 137
  23:5, 56, 222 nn. 137, 138, 223 n. 150

Yoma, 3:11, 142–43
Beṣah, 2:7, 219 n. 105
Ta'anit, 1:6, 222 n. 148
Megillah
  3:3, 222 n. 140, 223 n. 153
  4:3, 222 nn. 139, 140, 223 n. 153
Mo'ed Qaṭan
  1:5, 222 n. 143
  1:6. 222 n. 142
  3:8, 222 n. 140, 223 n. 153
Ketubbot, 4:4, 222 n. 140
Baba Meṣi'a, 6:1, 222 n. 140
Baba Batra
  6:3, 216 n. 57
  6:7, 222 n. 139, 223 n. 153
  6:8, 222 n. 142, 223 n. 153
Sanhedrin
  2:1 (2:3), 222 n. 139
  2:3, 223 n. 153
  6:6, 222 n. 143
'Eduyyot, 3:11, 219 n. 105
'Abodah Zarah, 2:5, 173
Avot, 1:1, 235 n. 126
Menaḥot, 10:9, 222 n. 140, 223 n. 153
Ḥullin, 4.7, 223 n. 164

TOSEFTA
Berakot
  2:20, 42
  5:29, 217 n. 73
  5:30, 220 nn. 113, 115
  5:32, 217 n. 70, 218 n. 89
Demai
  1:22, 218 n. 91
  1:23, 218 n. 91
Terumot, 10:10, 218 n. 91
Šebi'it
  5:12, 216 n. 63
  6:9, 218 n. 91
Šabbat
  5:9, 222 n. 135
  9:11, 221 n. 133
  16:9, 218 n. 91
  16:14, 218 n. 91
  16:16, 218 nn. 90, 91
  17, 222 n. 140
  17:18, 222 n. 138, 223 n. 151
  62a–b, 221 n. 134
Šeqalim, 1:12, 57, 223 nn. 156, 159
Kippurim, 2:6, 244 n. 83, 245 n. 87

Beṣah (Yom Tov), 2:14, 47, 220 n. 108
Niddah, 9:16, 57

TALMUD YERUSHALMI
Berakot
  2:8 (5c), 218 n. 83
  6:6 (10d), 46, 216 n. 54, 219 n. 102
  8:1 (12a), 220 n. 113
  8:5 (12b), 49, 216 n. 55, 217 n. 73, 220 n. 116
  8:6 (12b), 217 n. 69, 220 n. 111, 223 n. 160
  8:7 (12b), 217 n. 69, 220 n. 111, 244 n. 76, 245 n. 91
  9:5 (14d), 218 n. 86
Kil'ayim, 9:3 (32b), 41, 218 n. 87
Šabbat
  1:2 (3a), 218 n. 84
  6:1 (7c), 245 n. 89
  8:1 (11b), 221 n. 131
  8:6 (11c), 221 n. 132
'Erubin, 9:4 (25d), 215 n. 47
Yoma
  3:9 (41a), 244 n. 83
  4:5 (41d), 216 nn. 59, 64
Šeqalim, 2:7 (47a), 223 n. 156
Ketubbot, 12:3 (35a), 41, 218 n. 87
Baba Batra, 6:1 (15b), 216 n. 57

TALMUD BAVLI
Berakot
  43, 219 n. 98
  43a, 217 n. 72, 219 n. 103
  43b, 38, 46, 216 n. 56, 217 n. 74, 75, 219 n. 101, 246 n. 107, 249 n. 13
  51b, 220 n. 113
  52b, 220 n. 117
  53a, 139, 215 n. 44, 217 n. 70, 219 n. 101, 220 n. 111, 223 nn. 161, 162, 244 n. 74, 252 n. 37
Šabbat
  18a, 220 n. 112
  26a, 215 n. 53
  62ab, 221 n. 134, 244 n. 72
  62b, 212 n. 1
'Erubin, 19a, 240 n. 19
Pesaḥim, 118b, 249 n. 16

Yoma, 38a, 244 n. 83
Sukkah, 32b, 240 n. 19
Beṣah
    22b, 220 n. 109
    22b–23a, 244 n. 80
Megillah, 13a, 30, 251 n. 32
Ḥagigah, 14b, 239 n. 11, 240 n. 29
Baba Batra, 53b, 43, 219 n. 93
Sanhedrin
    108a, 252 n. 37
    93b, 246 n. 106
'*Avodah Zarah*
    29b, 248 n. 6
    35b, 173–74, 248 n. 6, 252 n. 35
Keritot, 6a, 240 n. 18

MIDRASH

Mekhilta de-R. Ishmael
    Pisha 14, 256 n. 13
    Shirata 3, 249 n. 12
Siphre Deuteronomy, 443, 249 n. 12
Genesis Rabbah
    3:9, 119, 239 n. 9
    17:8, 137, 243 n. 69
    21:5, 242 n. 54
    23:7, 241 n. 42
    25:2, 253 n. 52
    30:9, 252 n. 37
    33:3, 253 n. 52
    33:6, 239 n. 16
    34:9, 189, 253 n. 52
    38:10, 241 n. 42
    38:13, 249 n. 16
    39:2, 252 n. 36
    39:3, 249 n. 16
    39:8, 177, 250 n. 22
    42:1, 209 n. 1, 245 n. 99
    44:13, 250 n. 22
    46:2, 254 n. 59
    47:7, 189, 253 n. 53
    47:9, 254 n. 58
    55:4–56:19, 254 n. 61
    62:2, 173, 242 n. 44
    63, 240 n. 25
    65:22, 240 n. 22
    71:8, 135
    86:3, 30
    94:5, 254 n. 58
Exodus Rabbah
    18:5, 250 n. 22
    19:5, 248 n. 132

Leviticus Rabbah
    3:7, 249 n. 12
    16:1, 213 n. 3
    18:3, 246 n. 109
    23:1–6, 246 n. 109
    23:3, 241 n. 233
    23:6, 246 n. 111
    30:12, 245 n. 94
    31:10, 239 n. 16
Deuteronomy Rabbah, 2:26–27, 250 n. 22
Pesikta de-Rab Kahana, 27:9, 148–49, 245 n. 94
Song of Songs Rabbah
    1:2, 248 n. 6, 249 n. 11
    1:3, 150, 154, 182, 193, 202, 245 n. 99, 246 n. 105, 249 n. 10
    1:4, 239 n. 11, 240 n. 29
    1:6, 256 n. 12
    1:9, 242 n. 54
    1:12, 161, 162–63, 164, 165, 176, 248 n. 134
    1:13, 179, 192, 193
    1:14, 181, 192, 193, 201, 245 n. 89
    1:15, 120
    2:2, 124, 125, 153, 156, 157, 240 n. 28, 242 n. 52, 247 n. 114, 254 n. 56
    2:3, 242 n. 52
    2:4, 132
    2:5, 253 n. 48
    2:7, 202, 253 n. 49
    2:13, 153
    3:5, 251 nn. 29, 33, 255 n. 63
    3:6, 143–44, 255 n. 11
    4:6, 189, 255 nn. 11, 63
    4:7, 255 n. 11
    4:8, 255 n. 11
    4:10, 153
    4:11, 122
    4:12, 243 n. 63
    4:14, 134, 160, 249 n. 10, 252 n. 35
    5:1, 119, 239 n. 11
    6:2, 248 nn. 2, 4
    7:8, 253 n. 48
    7:10, 253 n. 48
    7:14, 249 n. 13
    8:8, 249 n. 16
    8:9, 119, 249 n. 16, 250 n. 20, 251 n. 26, 253 n. 48

    8:11, 238 n. 7
    8:14, 205, 206, 241 n. 39, 255 n. 7
    160, 232 n. 91

OTHER RABBINIC SOURCES

Avot d'Rabbi Natan (A)
    6, 209 n. 1
    18.5, 34–36, 216 n. 55, 217 n. 66
Avot d'Rabbi Natan (B), 13, 209 n. 1
Semaḥot (Ebel Rabbati)
    2:9, 216 n. 57
    8:2, 224 n. 166
    8:4, 224 n. 166
    12:9, 223 n. 156
    47a, 225 n. 180
Targum of Canticles, 4:12, 238 n. 8

OTHER ANCIENT SOURCES

3 Maccabees
    5:2, 216 n. 57
    45, 216 n. 57
Dead Sea Scrolls, 4Q184, 234 n. 118, 235 nn. 120, 123
Theophrastus, *Historia plantarum*, 9.6.2, 32, 215 n. 48
Pliny, *Naturalis historia*
    12.60, 68
    12.111–12, 32–33, 215 n. 49
    12.111–23, 215 n. 49
Josephus, *Jewish Antiquities*
    8:174, 215 nn. 5, 51
    9:7, 215 n. 51
Josephus, *Jewish War*
    1:136–41, 215 n. 51
    1:358–62, 215 n. 51
    4:402–5, 215 n. 52
    4:467–72, 215 n. 51
Ignatius
    Letter to the Romans, 2:2, 251 n. 28
    Martyrdom of Polycarp, 15, 251 n. 28
Justin the Martyr
    Diognetus, 7:8, 251 n. 27
    Second Apology, 12, 251 n. 27

GENERAL INDEX

Aaron, 96, 227 n. 22, 229 n. 53
Aaronide priesthood, 78–82, 166, 227 n. 22
Abba, R., 38
Abba bar Kahana, R., 254 n. 58
Abba bar Yudan, R., 134, 243 n. 60
Abbahu, R., 135, 136, 164, 165, 166, 173, 189, 191, 239 n. 17, 243 n. 60, 244 n. 76, 247 n. 127
Abihu, death of, 77–78, 79, 80, 229 n. 51
Abiram, 79
Abraham, 168, 191, 209 n. 5, 250 n. 19, 252 n. 36, 253 n. 53, 254 n. 58, 255 n. 63. *See also* Isaac, Abraham's sacrifice of; martyrdom, Abraham's near
   suffering of, 175–88, 189, 193, 195–96, 200
Absalom, 95–96, 97, 98, 233 n. 107, 234 n. 110
Abtinas, House of, 142–47, 152, 167, 181
Abun, R., 156, 157
Achish, 95–96, 97
Ackerman, Diane, 6–8
Adam, 121, 124, 137, 242 n. 54
adornments, 53, 55, 221 n. 133, 237 n. 159
adulteress, 98–100, 234 n. 116, 236 n. 155
   Israel as, 110–12, 114, 131, 234 n. 114, 237 n. 157
adytum. *See* Holy of Holies
Ahab (king), 101
Aibu, R., 120, 121
Akeldama tombs, 60–61
Akiba, R., 34, 150, 151, 152, 154–55, 161, 162, 174, 201, 216 n. 63, 223 n. 156, 242 nn. 50, 54, 246 nn. 104, 105, 249 n. 18, 253 n. 50
Albeck, Chanokh, 221 n. 133, 252 n. 36
Alexander, R., 246 n. 106
aloes, 87, 99, 133, 134, 135, 236 n. 155
altars, 44, 109, 158, 252 n. 44. *See also* kings, tables of
   incense, 20, 70, 73, 75, 76, 78, 213 n. 6, 225 n. 4, 227 n. 20, 228 n. 44
   sacrificial, 188, 200, 226 n. 7
Ammi, R., 19
Ammonites, 95, 233 nn. 104, 107
Amoraic period, 17, 193
Amraphel, 250 n. 22
Anderson-Stojanovic, Virginia, 224 n. 176
angels, 255 n. 9. *See* death, angel of; Michael
animals, 160, 162, 219 n. 104

anointed one, 4, 226 n. 8. *See also* messiah
   in prophetic literature, 112–13, 114,
anointing. *See also* bodies, anointing; hair, anointing
   of kings, 4, 67, 87, 97, 99
   of priests, 69, 110, 227 n. 22
   rabbis' experience with, 34, 39, 42, 43, 62–63, 119
   terms for, 34, 66–68, 67
aphrodisiac, incense as, 21, 28
apothecaries, 34, 71–72, 216 n. 61, 227 n. 27
Arabia, spice culture in, 22, 67
Aristotle, 9
Ark of the Covenant, 73, 74, 76, 246 n. 105
aroma/aromatics, 13–14, 178. *See also* fragrance; incense; perfume; spices
   in biblical literature, 2–3, 4, 63, 64–118; erotic images, 83–100, 114; pastoral images, 84, 87–88, 93, 115, 118–19; priestly literature, 64, 68–83, 94, 102–3, 111, 128, 167, 172; prophetic literature, 100–113; in Song of Songs, 84–89, 117–18, 200
   for burials, 55–62
   culture of, 20–28, 138
   in homes, 45–53, 55
   love's relationship to, 196, 197
   in Palestine, 28–62
   prescription and, 69–73
   in rabbinic literature, 1–4, 64–65, 68, 69, 83–84, 116–68, 173, 182, 197–98, 200; geographic references, 118–28, 167, 171–72, 205, 206; historical moments and, 159–66, 167, 168, 249 n. 18; the other in, 128–47, 167; rabbinic values in, 147–59, 164, 167
   rabbis' experiences with, 14, 19–63, 127
   terms for, 32–34, 66–73, 227 n. 21
   uses of, 45–53, 55, 135–36
   valences of, 114, 147, 209 n. 4
arousal, 100, 121, 165, 166, 207
   from perfume, 86–87, 89, 91, 93, 146, 175, 185, 199, 200
Arubas, Benny, 28
Asa (king), 87
Assi, R., 47, 48, 243 nn. 59, 60. *See also* Yassa, R.

Assyrians, 162–63
atonement. *See also* Day of Atonement; repentance; sacrifices
  in biblical literature, 108, 114, 159
  incense and, 73–77, 82–83, 175, 199
  in rabbinic literature, 69, 170
  for sins, 149, 169, 188–95, 196
attraction, 163, 167, 173, 207
  of perfume, 121, 178, 184
  in Song of Songs, 94, 195
Augustine, of Hippo , 9
authority, 97, 113
  priestly, 69, 71, 77–83, 112, 230 n. 66
  rabbinic, 69, 131, 153, 155, 156
Avemarie, Friedrich, 250 n. 25
Avigad, Nahman, 61
Avrahami, Yael, 237 n. 165
Axel, Richard, 210 n. 19
Azariah (friend of Daniel), 176–78, 182, 186–89, 253 n. 52
Azariah, R., 81, 82, 124, 179, 241 n. 33

Ba, R., 49
Babylonia, 14, 32, 212 n. 42
Bakhos, Carol, 240 n. 23
Balouka, Marva, 51–52
balsam, 19, 47, 55, 214 n. 30, 216 n. 59
  in biblical literature, 84, 120, 121, 232 n. 89
  production of, 28, 32–33, 215 n. 53
  in rabbinic literature, 121, 173, 179, 239 n. 16, 252 n. 36
  terms for, 32, 67, 216 n. 63
Barag, Dan, 61–62, 225 n. 187
baraitot, 16, 138, 212 n. 39
Bar Kappara (Qappara), R., 34, 249 n. 16
Bar Kokhba
  revolt, 30, 31, 201, 202–3, 215 n. 38
  Bar Koziba, 246 n. 106
Baskin, Judith, 142, 146–47, 148, 243 n. 69
bathhouses/bathing, 24, 218 nn. 81, 91, 240 n. 29
  aromatics in, 198, 207
  Greek, 21–22
  rabbis' use of, 31, 39–43, 63, 87, 218 n. 82, 219 n. 95
  Roman, 23, 27
  Stepped (*miqvah*), 52–53, 217 n. 79
  terms for, 34, 67
Bat Sheva, bathing incident, 240 n. 29
bed, woman as, 99–100
Beit Midrash, 137, 150, 151
Beit She'arim, 59–62, 224 nn. 171, 186
beloved, the, 116, 175, 232 n. 95, 238 n. 4
  as garden, 64, 121–22, 238 n. 168, 252 n. 41
  Israel as, 114–15, 118, 131, 205, 207, 230 n. 69

  in Song of Songs, 123, 124, 133, 143, 156
Ben Kamzar, R., 143
Berekhiah, R., 157, 161, 162, 185, 186, 193, 194, 195, 201, 202, 247 n. 114, 249 n. 16, 252 nn. 36, 43, 45, 254 n. 58
Bible. *See* Hebrew Bible
blessings, 219 n. 101, 223 n. 161
  over spices, 36–37, 46–49, 220 n. 117
  for pleasant scents, 138–42, 217 n. 70, 218 n. 89, 219 n. 96, 249 n. 13
blossoms
  in rabbinic literature, 117, 118, 124–28, 169, 199
  in Song of Songs, 88, 89, 92, 170–75
bodies, anointing, 21–22, 42, 55, 56, 83–84, 123, 150, 223 n. 156
  oils for, 31, 37–39, 53, 64–65, 70, 71, 198, 227 n. 22, 232 n. 89, 235 n. 130
  scraping, 21, 24, 38, 43
bottles, perfume, 29, 50, 221 n. 133, 247 n. 119. *See also* containers, perfume; unguentaria
Boyarin, Daniel, 245 n. 89, 250 n. 25, 253 n. 50
breathing, terms for, 66, 68, 113, 236 n. 150. *See also* inhaling, act of
Brun, Jean-Pierre, 216 n. 62
Buck, Linda, 210 n. 19
burials, 55–62. *See also* grave goods; tombs
  incense used for, 28, 57–58, 59, 198
  oils used for, 31, 223 n. 156, 224 n. 166
  perfume used for, 57, 59, 61, 62, 170, 198, 247 n. 119
  spices used for, 36–37, 57–58, 223 n. 162, 231 n. 82
burners, incense, 20, 50, 219 n. 106
Byzantine period, 4, 6, 69, 226 n. 16
  aromatics in, 2, 14, 28–62, 193, 198, 214 n. 26

Caesarea (Palestine), 28, 29–30
calf, golden, episode of, 130, 131–32, 165
Canaanites, 21, 66, 157, 233 n. 109, 246 n. 109
cane (spice), 70, 133, 235 n. 130
  in prophetic books, 102, 104, 105, 106
Caseau, Béatrice, 14
cassia, 70, 87, 134, 135
caves, burial, 59–60, 224 n. 171
censers, 221 n. 130, 226 n. 7
charity, terms for, 148
children, 111, 144, 145, 186, 245 n. 88
Christianity, 9–10, 240 n. 23
  scent in, 14, 16–17, 32
  treatment of the Jews, 196, 201–3
cinnamon, 24, 129
  in biblical literature, 70, 84, 99, 120, 121, 236 n. 155
  in rabbinic literature, 121, 133, 239 n. 16

circumcision, 165, 166, 190
  redemption through, 200, 202, 248 n. 133
  as sacrifice, 188–92, 196
  scent of, 117, 207, 253 n. 53, 254 n. 58
Classen, Constance, 13–14, 210 n. 22, 211 n. 27
clothing
  fragrance of, 122, 123
  fumigation of, 31, 38–39, 48, 52, 64–65, 87, 129, 134–35, 139–41, 160, 168, 198, 217 n. 76, 232 n. 91
cloud
  incense, 73, 74, 76, 228 n. 44
  on Mt. Sinai, 161–62
Cohen, Gerson, 118, 238 n. 6
commandments, 99, 101, 148, 174, 246 n. 108
  acceptance of, 117, 126, 131, 133, 136, 167, 239 n. 15
  observance of, 107, 156, 171, 190, 196, 246 n. 111, 248 n. 3, 249 n. 16
  reception on Sinai, 125, 127, 153, 154–55, 158, 160–62
comparison, language of, 7–8, 83, 84–89, 90, 241 n. 30. See also metaphors; metonyms; similes
consuming, 80, 81–82, 94, 236 n. 152. See also eating, imagery of
containers, perfume, 5, 20–22, 24, 28, 45, 53. See also bottles, perfume; unguentaria
conversion. See gentiles, conversion of
Corbin, Alain, 13
corruption, moral, 39, 41, 133, 137–38. See also evil
cosmetics, 53, 54, 60, 214 n. 32
covenant, 101–2, 185, 200. See also Ark of the Covenant
  observance of, 107, 114, 188
  oil of, 55, 188
  scent of, 127, 252 n. 41
creation, 125, 126, 143, 158, 247 n. 118
  of woman, 136–37, 243 n. 69
cultic practices, 30–31, 64, 71, 72, 107, 111, 235 n. 137. See also incense, cultic; rituals
  images of, 230 n. 68, 237 n. 156
  terms from, 103, 104–6, 108–9
culture
  fragrance's relationship to, 8–14, 15, 214 n. 30
  spice, 20–28
Cypriots, 213 n. 4

Daniel (prophet), friends of. See Azariah; Hananiah; Mishael
Darwin, Charles, 211 n. 27
date palms, 148, 149
Dathan, 79

David (king), 95–96, 101, 234 nn. 110, 111, 240 n. 29
  bad odors and, 97, 233 nn. 104, 106, 107
  messiah descended from, 112, 237 n. 162
Dayagi-Mendels, Michal, 21–22
Day of Atonement, 65, 188, 199, 226 n. 7, 251 n. 31
  incense used on, 70, 74, 76, 82
Dead Sea, 215 n. 38, 216 n. 59
death, 169–96, 207, 248 n. 3. See also burials; martyrdom; sacrifices
  angel of, 163, 173–75, 195, 249 n. 14
  fragrance of, 59, 158, 182, 197
  love and, 190, 191, 253 n. 50
  odors of, 62, 164, 168, 201, 204
  in rabbinic literature, 169–75, 195, 250 n. 25
desire, 24, 173, 175, 184, 195, 206
  sexual, 99, 137, 152, 168
Detienne, Marcel, 15
dove (flood story), 120–21, 128, 232 n. 84, 239 nn. 15, 16. See also flood, story of
downtrodden, the, concern for, 105, 107, 108, 114

eating, imagery of, 91, 93–94, 149, 166, 234 n. 115. See also consuming
Edelman, Diana, 226 n. 5
Eden, Garden of, 119–24, 128, 165–66, 204–6, 238 n. 8, 239 n. 16, 248 n. 133
Edomite, Esau as, 31, 122, 123, 128
Egypt, 22, 67, 164, 246 n. 109
  Israel's redemption from, 97, 153, 156–57, 164, 165–66, 246 n. 109
Ein Gedi (Palestine), 33, 192, 215 n. 53
Eleazar (son of Aaron), 78
Eleazar, R., 35–36, 47
elect, God's, 97, 105, 108, 167, 172, 186, 190. See also anointed one; kings; priests; rabbis
Eliezer, R., 1–2, 53, 137, 150, 152, 161, 167, 176–77, 190, 202, 203, 246 nn. 101, 105, 249 n. 18, 250 n. 22
Elijah (prophet), 101
embalming, 67, 231 n. 82. See also burials
emotions, 103, 210 n. 22
  scents' effects on, 5, 6–7, 12, 13, 84, 85, 156, 168, 191
Enosh, generation of, 125, 241 n. 42
eros, 13, 65–66, 156, 194–95, 230 n. 69, 253 n. 50
eroticism, 11–12, 168
  in biblical literature, 83–100, 126–27
  in rabbinic literature, 145, 158, 169, 172, 175, 180, 185
  in Song of Songs, 127, 159, 166, 171–72
Esau, 156, 238 n. 167, 240 nn. 24, 25
  as Edomite, 31, 122, 123, 128
  Jacob and, 31, 121–23, 128, 166

Esau (*continued*)
  as Roman, 122, 128, 129, 156, 157, 240 nn. 23, 27
Eshel, Hanan, 217 n. 79
Essenes, 28, 214 n. 30
Esther, 30, 87, 240 n. 29
etrogs, 149, 151, 245 n. 97
Evans, Suzanne, 253 n. 51
Eve, 121, 124, 137
everything man, 194, 196, 201
evil, 230 n. 61. *See also* corruption, moral; odors, bad; other, female
  odor, 122, 130, 240 n. 20, 242 n. 48
exclusivity, 65, 158, 175, 190, 195, 199
  priestly, 69, 72, 73, 77, 78–80, 81, 167, 169
Exum, J. Cheryl, 91–92, 231 n. 80, 232 n. 95
Ezekiel (prophet), 108, 110–11, 120, 234 n. 114, 239 n. 16

Feliks, Yehuda, 215 n. 53, 216 n. 59
Fernandez, James, 195
festivals, 47–48, 129, 158, 159
figs/fig trees, 84, 87–89, 231 n. 82, 232 n. 85, 243 n. 63
Fine, Steven, 226 n. 16
Firestone, Reuven, 251 n. 31
Fishbane, Michael, 235 nn. 137, 140, 236 n. 146, 237 n. 163, 242 n. 43, 246 n. 108
flasks, 35, 54. *See also* containers, perfume
flood, story of, 125, 126, 189, 229 n. 47, 241 n. 42. *See also* dove
flowers. *See* blossoms
flowing, in Song of Songs, 89–94, 98–99
fountains, 90–92, 94, 99–100, 121, 134–36
Fox, Michael, 98, 234 nn. 115, 116
Fraade, Steven, 241 n. 42
fragrance, 24, 27, 220 n. 118. *See also* oils, fragrance of; perfume
  in biblical literature, 1–3, 63, 69, 82–83, 114, 115, 121
  death and, 169–96, 197
  ephemerality and, 197–207
  giving forth, 86–89, 161–62
  in homes, 45–55
  in rabbinic literature, 2–3, 15, 63, 116–68, 182–84, 206
  rabbis' experiences with, 31–32, 116–17, 197–98
  secular images of, 84, 102
  in Song of Songs, 85–87, 89, 91–94, 100, 205
  terms for, 32–34, 36, 68, 163
  wafting, 88–93, 112, 114, 121, 142, 155, 176, 187, 195, 199
frankincense, 24, 34, 67–68, 216 n. 57. *See also* incense, Temple
  in biblical literature, 196, 199
  hill of, 189, 190, 191–92, 251 n. 29, 254 n. 58
  in prophetic literature, 102, 103, 104, 105, 106, 107
  in Song of Songs, 92, 133, 160, 232 n. 91, 255 n. 63
Freud, Sigmund, 11, 12, 211 n. 27
fumigation, 119, 221 n. 130. *See also* clothing, fumigation of; homes, fumigation of
  incense used for, 21, 129, 135
  in Song of Songs, 84, 92, 100
  on wedding day, 231 n. 80, 232 n. 95
funerals. *See* burials

galbanum, 24, 71
Galen, 214 n. 26, 215 n. 53
Galilee, the, 28, 30, 31, 40, 53, 61–62, 198, 202
Gallus (emperor), 212 n. 42
Galor, Katharina, 217 n. 79
garden
  in rabbinic literature, 116, 117, 118–28, 168, 170–72
  in Song of Songs, 64, 88–94, 97, 114, 133–36, 199, 204–5, 207, 232 nn. 87, 94, 238 n. 8, 239 n. 16, 248 n. 1, 252 n. 41
Garmu, House of, 142–43, 245 n. 86
Gehenna. *See* hell
gentiles, 140, 141, 218 n. 91
  conversion of, 178, 179, 181–88, 189, 190, 193, 196, 200
  spices of, 36–37, 217 n. 71, 220 n. 113
geographic references, 118–28, 171–72
Gereleman, Gillis, 93
Ginzberg, Louis, 249 n. 16
glass/glassmaking, 22, 213 n. 17, 220 n. 121, 224 n. 175, 225 n. 187. *See also* bottles, perfume; unguentaria
God, 94, 237 n. 163, 250 n. 25, 253 n. 51
  abode of, 119–21
  acceptance of sacrifices, 72–73, 106, 109, 114, 187, 236 n. 152
  appeasing anger of, 75–76, 80–82, 108, 114, 127, 159, 163, 187, 188, 191, 195, 228 n. 39, 229 n. 45, 230 n. 61, 236 n. 143, 253 n. 52
  communication with, 4, 69, 74–76, 82, 105, 146, 256 n. 15
  covenant of, 101–2, 107, 114, 127, 155
  honoring, 109, 253 n. 49
  humanity's relationship with, 72–73, 76, 152, 169, 238 n. 6
  immanence of, 114, 166, 170, 171, 178, 187, 195, 197–207, 250 n. 25, 253 n. 52
  Israel's relationship with, 101–2, 104, 110, 127, 156, 162, 194–95, 201–7, 230 n. 69, 239 n. 15

GENERAL INDEX 279

knowledge of, 156, 246 n. 106
as male lover, 118, 130–31, 171, 178, 190, 193–94, 203
name of, 155, 156, 174, 183
nearness of, 79–80, 81, 82, 175, 228 n. 39
presence of, 10, 75–76, 82, 105, 161–63, 190, 228 n. 44, 239 nn. 9, 16, 256 n. 13
good deeds, 148, 149, 157–58, 246 n. 111, 249 n. 16
grain, sacrifice of, 74, 104, 105, 106, 107, 108, 109
grave goods, 20–21, 22, 58–62, 223 n. 165, 224 n. 175. *See also* burials; tombs
Great Revolt, 32, 33
Greece, 21–22, 24, 214 n. 22
Greenberg, Moshe, 236 n. 155
Guggenheimer, Heinrich, 46, 217 n. 69, 219 n. 98, 223 n. 161

Hachlili, Rachel, 60
Hadrian (emperor), 31
hair, anointing, 24, 27, 38, 39, 123, 168, 198
Haman (Book of Esther), 240 n. 29
Hammat Gader hot springs, 218 n. 81
Hamor, the Hivite, 233 n. 109
Ḥanan, R., 153
Ḥananiah (friend of Daniel), 176–78, 182, 186–89, 253 n. 52
Ḥananiah (perfumer), 71
Ḥaninah, R., 58
Ḥaninah (Ḥananyah II), R., 186, 187, 202, 252 n. 45
Ḥaninah bar Pappa, R., 202, 203
Haran, Menachem, 226 n. 7, 227 n. 21
harlots, 99, 110, 236 n. 155
Harvey, Susan Ashbrook, 14, 16, 32
havdalah ceremony, 48–49
hearing, sense of, 8, 10, 12, 57, 113, 237 n. 163, 238 n. 167
heaven, 105, 119–21, 204–5, 206, 249 n. 15
Hebrew Bible
aromatic images in, 2–3, 4, 63, 64–118; erotic, 83–100, 114; priestly literature, 64, 68–83, 102, 128; prophetic literature, 100–113; "secular," 230 n. 68; scent terms in, 66–73
Genesis, 16
rabbinic interpretations of, 2–3, 102, 209 n. 3
Song of Songs, 209 n. 5, 230 n. 69, 238 nn. 4, 6, 242 n. 54
Torah, 99, 102, 128, 238 n. 4, 241 n. 41, 246 n. 105; study of, 1–2, 125, 126, 127, 149, 150–52, 167
Hegel, Georg Wilhelm Friedrich, 10
Heger, Paul, 75
hell, 121–23, 240 n. 24
henna, 86, 192–93, 194, 196, 255 n. 62

Herod (king), 29
Herod Antipas (king), 30
Hezekiah (king), 87, 162–64, 235 n. 129, 237 n. 162
high priests, 73, 74, 76, 82, 188, 229 n. 51, 248 n. 5
Hillel, House of, 36, 42, 48–49, 219 n. 101, 220 n. 117
Hirschfeld, Yizhar, 28, 214 n. 30
Hisda, R., 173
historical moments, 6, 159–66, 167, 168, 249 n. 18
Ḥiyya bar Abba II, R., 38, 63, 139, 203, 244 n. 75
Ḥiyya ben Aviyah, R., 170, 171, 174, 248 n. 3
Ḥiyya the Elder, R., 41–42
Ḥizkiyah, R., 58
holiness, 69, 73, 76, 227 n. 22, 253 n. 49
Holy of Holies, 73–75, 82, 110, 226 n. 7, 256 n. 15
homes
aromatics in, 45–53, 55, 198, 207, 240 n. 27
fumigation of, 45–46, 47, 52, 123
incense used in, 24, 28, 53, 219 n. 96
Hosea (prophet), 110
Howes, David, 13–14, 210 n. 22, 211 n. 27
humanity, God's relationship with, 72–73, 76, 152, 169, 238 n. 6. *See also* God, Israel's relationship with
Huna, Rav, 181, 243 n. 60, 251 n. 34
Hunya, R., 183
hypocaust water heating systems, 24, 31, 40, 41. *See also* bathhouses/bathing

idolatry, 31, 129, 226 n. 5, 237 n. 166. *See also* calf, golden, episode of
incense used for, 36–37, 39, 65, 140
Israel's, 101, 104, 111, 237 n. 157, 240 n. 19, 256 n. 12
scents related to, 63, 142
spices used for, 36–37, 139–40, 144, 217 n. 71, 220 n. 118
Ignatius, sacrifice of, 178
impulsivity, 66, 199, 207. *See also* irrationality
incense, 55, 69, 75, 82, 123, 219 n. 96, 229 n. 51. *See also* altars, incense; burners, incense; censers; frankincense; shovels, incense
atonement and, 73–77, 82–83, 175, 199
in biblical literature, 64–118, 158–59, 181, 199, 207
blessing, 46, 48–49
for burials, 28, 57–58, 59, 198
burning, 20, 28, 196, 221 n. 129
cultic, 65, 67, 76–77, 92
fumigation with, 21, 129, 135
in homes, 46, 198
idolatrous, 36–37, 39, 65, 140

incense (*continued*)
  instructions for use, 70, 71, 78
  lighting, 23, 47, 48–49, 69, 75, 82, 123, 219 n. 96, 229 n. 51
  in priestly literature, 167, 169, 175, 187, 200
  in prophetic literature, 102, 103, 104, 107, 108, 109, 111, 112
  in rabbinic literature, 15, 16, 77, 117, 178–81, 187, 189, 198
  rabbis' experience with, 14, 62–63, 167–68
  ritual, 30–31, 39, 75, 78, 79, 80
  secular images of, 111, 213 n. 6, 230 n. 68
  in Song of Songs, 92, 97
  spices in, 136, 143, 178, 180, 195
  Temple, 34, 65–66, 71, 110, 142, 143–44, 146, 180–81, 226 n. 7, 227 n. 24, 240 n. 18
  terms for, 32–34, 66–68, 227 n. 21, 236 n. 149
  wafting, 81, 112, 170, 198
  in witchcraft, 139, 140, 220 n. 118
incense, sacrificial, 28, 66, 106, 160, 162, 175, 227 n. 24, 228 n. 44, 235 n. 129, 253 n. 53
  atonement with, 185, 187, 190–92, 199, 256 n. 15
  soothing odors of, 72–77, 82–83, 114, 167, 194–96
inhaling, act of, 89, 125, 127, 141, 233 n. 103. *See also* breathing, terms for
intimacy, sexual, 13, 93, 94
irrationality, 173, 175, 185. *See also* impulsivity
Isaac (son of Abraham), 240 n. 24, 255 n. 63
  Abraham's sacrifice of, 176, 179, 192–93, 196, 200, 201, 206, 251 nn. 29, 31, 254 n. 61
  blessing of Jacob by, 122, 123, 238 n. 167, 240 n. 24
Isaac, R., 19
Ishmael (son of Abraham), 253 n. 53, 254 n. 58
Ishmael, R., 41–42, 173, 174, 242 n. 50
Israeli, Yael, 62
Israel/Israelites. *See also* God, Israel's relationship with; Jews
  as adulteress, 110–12, 114, 118, 131, 234 n. 114, 237 n. 157
  aromatics in, 28–62, 64–66, 71
  as beloved, 114–15, 118, 129–30, 131, 230 n. 69
  exiles of, 133–36, 204–7, 256 n. 13
  as flowers, 125, 156
  idolatry of, 101, 104, 217 n. 71, 237 n. 157, 240 n. 19, 256 n. 12
  Jacob as, 122, 123
  odors of, 95–98, 126, 233 nn. 103, 107
  redemption of, 153, 156–59, 175, 200, 247 nn. 119, 123, 248 n. 133, 256 n. 12
  righteousness of, 64, 169

  sacrifices of, 79–81, 104, 187, 193–94
  spices in, 20–21, 66, 93
  as woman, 130–38, 166, 242 n. 54
Ithamar (son of Aaron), 78

Jacob, 167, 192, 233 n. 109, 234 n. 110, 251 n. 29, 255 n. 63
  descendants of, 186, 196
  Esau and, 31, 121–23, 128, 166
  Isaac's blessing of, 122, 123, 238 n. 167, 240 n. 24
Jacob, R., 37, 217 n. 69
Jacob bar Aḥa, R., 58
jars. *See* containers, perfume
Jastrow, Marcus, 217 n. 65, 219 nn. 106, 107, 240 n. 21
Jeremiah (prophet), 106, 234 n. 114
Jeremiah, R., 37, 46
Jesse, 112, 237 n. 162
Jesus Christ, 193, 194, 238 n. 4
Jews, 201–7. *See also* Israel/Israelites; Judaism
  aromatics' use by, 140, 141, 142, 144, 147
  redemption of, 186, 190–91, 192, 196, 250 n. 25
Johnson, Mark, 244 n. 71
Josephus, 33, 214 n. 30
Joshua (prophet), 165, 189, 191, 196, 200, 254 n. 58
Joshua, R., 41, 136–37, 146, 150, 173, 174, 244 n. 70, 246 nn. 101, 105
Judah, R., 34–36, 49, 124, 130, 131, 132, 133, 134, 136, 165, 241 n. 33, 242 nn. 50, 54, 243 n. 55
Judah ha-Nasi (patriarch), 30
Judaism, 9–10, 14, 15, 102, 112, 248 n. 3. *See also* Jews; rabbinic literature; rabbis
Judea, balsam production in, 32–33
juglets/jugs. *See* containers, perfume
Julian (emperor), 212 n. 42
justice, 102, 189, 190, 193, 194, 196, 201, 207

Kadari, Tamar, 238 nn. 3, 4, 168, 241 n. 41
Kant, Immanuel, 10
Keel, Othmar, 85
Kimelman, Reuven, 226 n. 16
kings, 102, 159, 160, 162, 231 n. 81, 232 n. 95, 237 n. 164
  anointing, 4, 67, 87, 97, 199
  tables of, 158, 159, 252 n. 44
Kingsmill, Edmée, 230 n. 69, 238 n. 6
Kloner, Amos, 60, 223 n. 156
knowledge
  acquisition of, 1, 3, 9, 113
  of God, 156, 246 n. 106
  perfume of, 32, 55, 152–53, 175, 195

rabbinic, 36, 39, 151
kokh/kokhim. See tombs; burials
Koraḥ rebellion, 79–81, 228 n. 44
Kraemer, David, 59
Kutscher, Eduard, 233 n. 108

Lakoff, George, 244 n. 71
lamps, 36–37, 49, 56, 58, 220 n. 117
Lapp, Eric, 51, 52
laws, 163, 164, 248 n. 3. *See also* commandments; Sabbath, laws of
Leazar ben Jacob, R., 250 n. 22
Lebanon, fragrance of, 91–92, 122, 123, 232 n. 91, 249 n. 13
Levi (son of Jacob), 233 n. 109, 234 n. 110
Levi, R., 120, 189, 191, 241 n. 42, 254 n. 58
Levi, Hygros b., 143
Levine, Baruch A., 74, 227 n. 17, 228 n. 39
Levites, 79–81, 227 n. 25
Lieberman, Saul, 59, 216 n. 63, 217 n. 72, 219 n. 107, 221 n. 133
lilies
  in rabbinic literature, 172, 175, 185, 246 n. 111, 254 n. 56
  in Song of Songs, 84, 88, 91, 124, 153, 156–58, 167, 170–71
limbic system, 6–7, 12, 84
love
  death and, 173, 190, 191, 253 n. 50
  of God, 156, 159, 166, 194, 238 n. 6
  in rabbinic literature, 116, 180
  scent and, 86–87, 197, 204
  in Song of Songs, 180, 182, 195, 250 n. 25
lover, female. *See also* women
  Israel as, 129–30, 190
  in Song of Songs, 89, 92, 97, 118–19, 170–71, 178, 206, 235 n. 124, 248 n. 1
lover, male, 136, 175, 238 n. 4. *See also* men
  God as, 118, 130–31, 171, 178, 190–91, 193–94, 203
  in Song of Songs, 87, 93, 118–19, 121–24, 133, 143, 156, 161, 170–71, 184, 199, 248 n. 1, 252 n. 41
loving kindness, acts of, 148, 153

Mach, Rudolf, 240 n. 25
maḥtah. See shovels, incense
maidens, 249 n. 12
  conversion of, 181–88
  in Song of Songs, 85, 150, 154, 252 n. 36, 253 n. 50
manna, spices from, 64, 134–36, 160
Margulies, Mordecai, 246 n. 111

marketplaces, 2, 17, 19–20, 30–31, 34–39, 198, 207
martyrdom, 192–95, 202–3, 240 n. 27, 252 n. 44
  Abraham's near, 176–85, 189, 196, 200, 201, 206, 249 n. 16, 250 n. 21, 251 n. 30, 253 n. 52
  of Daniel's friends, 176–78, 182, 186–89, 253 n. 52
  in rabbinic literature, 169, 170, 194, 195, 202, 203, 239 n. 15, 250 n. 25, 253 n. 48
  as sacrifice, 158, 159, 207, 253 n. 51
matriarchs, 129, 135, 138, 153, 202, 255 n. 4
McCarter, P. Kyle, Jr., 233 n. 104
medicines, 14, 28, 55, 214 n. 26, 218 n. 91
Meir, R., 53, 57, 130, 131, 132, 133, 137, 165, 242 nn. 50, 51, 54
memory, scents' evocation of, 5, 6–7, 12, 84–89, 93, 100, 191, 195, 197, 209 n. 6, 254 n. 57
men, 27, 148–49, 152, 234 n. 112, 244 n. 71, 245 n. 96. *See also* everything man; lover, male; other, the, male
mercy, 189, 190, 200, 201, 207, 242 n. 43
messiah, 4, 112–114, 128, 158, 226 n. 8, 237 n. 165, 246 n. 106. *See also* anointed one
metaphors, 5, 7, 244 n. 71
  in biblical literature, 66, 92, 93, 168
  layering of, 64, 102, 112, 114–15, 118, 147, 150, 153, 155, 157, 159, 167, 195, 199–200, 204
  in rabbinic literature, 168, 182, 184, 192
metonyms, 5, 83, 85, 89, 90, 105, 167, 255 n. 62
Meyers, Carol L., 221 n. 129, 223 n. 163
Meyers, Eric M., 52
Michael (archangel), 176, 177, 250 n. 19
Midrash, 209 n. 3, 255 n. 11
  Genesis Rabbah, 16, 118, 192, 209 n. 5
  Leviticus Rabbah, 241 nn. 33, 41, 245 n. 94
  Pesiqta de-Rab Kahana, 245 n. 94, 255 n. 11
  Song of Songs Rabbah, 16, 117–18, 209 n. 5, 238 n. 3, 255 n. 11
  Yalqut Shemoni, 255 n. 11
Milgrom, Jacob, 226 n. 7, 230 nn. 61, 66
Miller, William Ian, 7–8, 13, 216 n. 59
millstones, 239 n. 14, 246 n. 106
miqvah/miqva'ot. See bathhouses/bathing, stepped pools
miracles, 160, 186, 187
Miriam, 243 n. 63
Mishael (friend of Daniel), 176–78, 182, 186–89, 253 n. 52
Mishnah, 16, 31–32, 212 n. 39
Moses, 232 n. 89, 244 n. 84
  deliverance of Israel, 96, 149, 164–65, 247 n. 128
  priesthood and, 78, 79, 80, 229 n. 53
Murphy, Roland E., 90–91, 232 n. 91

myrrh
  Abraham and, 182–83, 185, 186–87, 192–93, 195–96, 255 n. 63
  in biblical literature, 70, 87, 99, 199, 236 n. 155
  mountains of, 92, 118–19, 189, 251 n. 29
  in rabbinic literature, 34, 143, 178–81, 190, 195, 251 n. 32
  in Song of Songs, 86, 91, 92, 93, 100, 133, 160, 231 n. 81
  terms for, 194
  uses of, 19, 24, 67–68, 129, 191
  in the wilderness, 134, 135
myrtle, 149, 219 n. 101, 220 n. 114, 240 n 25

Nabataea, spice trade of, 22
Nadab, death of, 77–78, 79, 80, 229 n. 51
Naftali (son of Jacob), 255 n. 4
Naḥman, R., 57, 173, 174
nard/nerd. *See* spikenard
Nathan (prophet), 101
Nathan, R., 57
natural world, 83–84, 87–89, 99–100, 124, 172
Near East, spices in, 22, 67, 93
Nebuchadnezzar (king), 176, 186
Nehemiah (prophet), 227 n. 26
niches, burial. *See* tombs
Nielsen, Kjeld, 216 n. 59, 226 n. 13
Nimrod (king), 176–78, 185, 241 n. 42, 249 n. 16, 250 n. 22
Noah, 239 nn. 15, 16, 252 n. 37, 253 n. 52. *See also* flood, story of

odors, 4–14, 132, 210 n. 19, 233 n. 103
  recognition of, 209 nn. 6, 9, 211 n. 30
  terms for, 68, 85–86
odors, bad, 11, 94–95, 100, 240 nn. 20, 21. *See also* evil; stinking
  covering up, 57, 219 nn. 99, 101, 223 n. 161
  of the other, 94–95, 100, 123
  of scholars, 1–2, 152, 167, 190
  women's, 137–38
odors, pleasant, 76, 97, 158, 166, 190, 236 n. 142
  Abraham's, 182–84, 186–87
  blessings for, 138–42, 217 n. 70, 218 n. 89, 219 n. 96, 249 n. 13
  of rabbinic teachings, 4, 36, 219 n. 102
  in Song of Songs, 124, 125
odors, soothing, 169–96, 201. *See also* incense, sacrificial, soothing odor of; sacrifices, soothing odor of
  for God, 170, 201, 242 n. 43
  of incense, 73–77, 110–11, 114
  in priestly literature, 127, 128

oils, 46, 111, 146, 170, 188, 232 n. 89. *See also* bodies, anointing
  in bathhouses, 41–42, 218 n. 87
  for burials, 62, 198, 223 n. 156, 224 n. 166, 231 n. 82
  extraction of, 213 n. 4, 216 n. 62
  fragrance of, 85–86, 90, 150–53, 154, 156, 173–75, 182–86, 243 n. 56, 252 nn. 36, 37
  perfumed, 71, 185
  pouring out, 117, 150–52, 155, 231 n. 73
  in rabbinic literature, 153, 200
  rabbis' experience with, 43, 62–63, 168
  in Song of Songs, 85–86, 90, 91, 92, 93–94, 97, 249 n. 7
  terms for, 33, 67, 227 n. 21, 236 n. 153
  uses of, 21–22, 24, 27–28, 214 n. 26, 217 n. 72, 218 n. 91, 219 n. 99, 101
ointments, 36, 62, 70, 146, 221 n. 133
olfaction, 5–14, 191, 207, 210 n. 19, 211 n. 29. *See also* smell, sense of
  in humans, 167, 211 n. 30
  limbic system and, 6–7, 12, 84
  in rabbinic literature, 3, 4, 49, 63, 116–18
olive oil, 70, 239 n. 16, 251 n. 32
opalbalsam, 32, 252 n. 36. *See also* balsam
orchards, in rabbinic literature, 124–28. *See also* trees
Oshaiyah, R., 203
ossuraies. *See* tombs
other, the, 89, 233 n. 107
  Abraham as, 181–88
  aroma of, 94–100, 123
  in biblical literature, 123, 128–29
  female, 98-100, 114, 136–37, 139, 147, 199, 243 n. 69, 244 n. 71, 256 n. 12
  inside *vs.* outside, 97, 109, 128–30, 141, 142, 145
  male, 114, 129
  in rabbinic literature, 117, 123, 128–47

Palestine, aromatics in, 14, 28–62, 215 n. 53
Papa, R., 38
Pappus, R., 242 n. 54
parables, 241 nn. 30, 34
Passover, 47, 163, 164, 165, 166, 200, 251 n. 31
patriarchs, 193, 202, 224 n. 170, 225 n. 186, 255 n. 4
Patrich, Joseph, 28
perfume, 11, 93, 96, 174–75, 214 n. 30, 230 n. 68. *See also* fragrance; women, perfume use by
  in biblical literature, 2, 64–118, 187, 207
  for burials, 57, 59, 61, 62, 170, 247 n. 119

containers for, 20–21, 22
death and, 170–75
erotic images of, 65–66, 126–27
myrrh used in, 178, 180, 236 n. 153
the other and, 128–47
production of, 213 n. 4, 216 n. 62
in rabbinic literature, 116, 117, 132–33, 167, 173, 175, 178–81, 187, 189, 198
rabbis' experiences with, 36, 41–42, 127, 152–53, 167–68, 173, 207
in Song of Songs, 4, 86–87, 89, 91, 133, 178
spices in, 134–36, 195
terms for, 32–34, 66–68, 221 n. 133, 223 n. 154
uses of, 14, 24–25, 30, 32
valences of, 15, 132–33, 156, 165–66, 190, 199–200
wafting, 4, 167, 170
perfumers, 34, 71, 72. *See also* apothecaries
Pharisees, 74
pheromones, 8, 12, 13
Philistines, 95, 213 n. 6, 225 n. 4, 233 nn. 103, 105
piety, 107, 166, 250 n. 25
plagues, 80, 81, 82–83, 164
Plato, 9
pleasure, 9, 63, 159, 169, 175
Polycarp, sacrifice of, 178
pomegranate trees, 88, 89
Potiphar (priest), 30
potpourri, 52, 221 n. 129
practices, religious, 9–10, 204. *See also* cultic practices; rituals
prayer, 205, 206, 251 n. 31
priests, 168, 199, 226 n. 16, 248 n. 5, 251 n. 34. *See also* Aaron, Aaronide priesthood; Abtinas, House of
    anointing, 67, 69, 70, 71, 110, 199, 227 n. 22
    authority of, 69, 71, 77–83, 112, 230 n. 66
    literature of, 64, 68–83, 94, 103, 111, 167, 172
    prophetic critiques of, 102, 109
    rabbis' relationship to, 69, 226 n. 16
    relationship to God, 108, 146, 194
    role in sacrifices, 73–77, 78
    in Sepphoris, 52, 53
prophetic literature, 100–113, 175, 234 n. 114, 238 n. 6
Proust, Marcel, 5
purity, 74, 77, 122, 148
pyxis, 27. *See also* containers, perfume

Qumran site, 28, 214 n. 30, 215 n. 38

Rabban Gamaliel, 47, 48, 216 n. 59, 218 n. 82, 219 n. 106

rabbinic literature, 100, 112–15
    aromatic images in, 1–4, 14–17, 64–65, 68–69, 83–84, 116–68, 173, 182, 197–98, 200; geographic references, 118–28, 167, 171–72, 205, 206; historical moments and, 159–66, 167, 168, 249 n. 18; the other in, 128–47, 167; rabbinic values in, 147–59, 164, 167
    death in, 170–75
    on spices, 33, 34, 36–37, 172, 198, 206, 220 n. 118
rabbis, 69, 102, 251 n. 34. *See also* teacher-student relationship
    aromatics' experiences of, 14, 19–63, 207
    authority of, 69, 131, 153, 155, 156
    bathhouse use, 31, 39–43, 63, 218 n. 82, 219 n. 95
    centers of, 28–29, 30
    perfume experiences, 36, 41–42, 127, 152–53, 167–68, 173, 207
    righteousness of, 194, 201
    use of term, 16, 212 n. 41, 225 n. 186, 227 n. 17
    values of, 117, 147–59, 164, 172, 173, 175, 196
    worldview of, 14, 15, 188
Rachel (matriarch), 135
Rashi (Rabbi Shlomo Yitzhaki), 219 n. 101
Rebekah (matriarch), 129, 153
redemption, 74, 189, 228 n. 39
    divine immanence and, 195, 204–7
    Israel's, 153, 156–59, 162–66, 175, 200, 247 nn. 119, 123, 248 n. 133, 256 n. 12
    of Jewish community, 192, 196, 203, 250 n. 25
    martyrdom as, 185, 186, 187, 202–3
    in prophetic literature, 101, 103, 106, 112–13
    in rabbinic literature, 170, 193–94
religion, 9–10, 14, 30–31, 204. *See also* Christianity; Judaism
repentance, 106, 153, 188, 189, 192. *See also* atonement
resins, 33–34, 46, 146, 216 n. 59
restriction, incense related to, 77, 78, 81
righteous, the, 148, 153–59, 167–69, 199, 238 n. 8, 240 n. 25, 246 n. 106, 247 n. 119, 248 n. 3
    Abraham's embodiment of, 176, 179–80, 183, 188, 196, 251 n. 29, 31, 255 n. 63
    martyrdom of, 194, 201, 252 n. 44
    reward for, 173, 175
    scent of, 64, 170–72, 186-87, 195, 252 n. 37
    suffering of, 185, 192, 200
Rindisbacher, Hans J., 9, 10, 13, 168
Ritchie, Ian D., 237 n. 165
rituals, 9, 114, 166, 170, 192. *See also* cultic practices; incense, ritual

Romans
  aromatics' use by, 19, 28–62, 64–65, 198
  Esau as, 122, 128, 129, 156, 157, 240 n. 23, 27
  rabbis' opinions of, 30–31, 128
roses, 124, 125, 240 n. 25
royalty, 87, 94, 108, 111, 114. *See also* kings
Rutgers, Leonard Victor, 52

Sabbath
  laws of, 34, 43, 53, 55, 56, 107, 221 n. 133, 236 n. 146
  lighting incense on, 42, 47, 48–49, 158
sacrifices, 2, 70, 169–96, 250 n. 25, 252 n. 42. *See also* altars, sacrificial; grain, sacrifice of; incense, sacrificial; Isaac, Abraham's sacrifice of; martyrdom; redemption
  in biblical literature, 65, 159, 169, 206–7
  God's acceptance of, 72–73, 106, 109, 114, 187, 236 n. 152
  human, 200, 253 n. 51
  in priestly literature, 178, 187, 188, 194–95
  prophetic critique of, 103–9, 111
  in rabbinic literature, 83, 170, 178, 205–7
  role of priests in, 73–77, 78
  soothing odor of, 4, 68–69, 72, 82, 117, 158, 167, 188–96, 205–6, 253 n. 52
  Temple, 160, 161
Sadducees, 74
Safrai, Ze'ev, 33, 215 n. 53
Samuel (prophet), 95
Sanhedrin, 119
Sarna, Nahum, 73, 74–75, 228 n. 44
Saul (king), 95, 101, 233 n. 105, 234 n. 111
scent, 11–14, 12, 28, 63, 155, 206, 252 n. 41. *See also* emotions, scents' effects on; memory, scents' evocation of
  antinomies of, 116, 122–23, 129
  applied to the other, 128–29
  in biblical literature, 199, 235 n. 121
  descriptions of, 5, 7–8
  in priestly literature, 172, 199
  in prophetic literature, 103, 108, 110
  in rabbinic literature, 3, 117, 123, 160–66, 195, 198, 201
  of scholarship, 167, 170, 174–75
  secular images of, 103, 108
  in Song of Songs, 84–89, 93–94, 119, 202
  terms for, 65, 97, 209 n. 4
  upward movement of, 163, 190
  wafting, 131, 141–42, 207
  women's, 11, 93, 97, 129–30
scholars/scholarship, 1–2, 36, 117, 151–52, 172, 176, 194
  scent of, 148–53, 167, 170, 174–75, 190, 195
scraping bodies, 21, 24, 38, 43
Scripture. *See* Hebrew Bible
seduction, 2, 166
  in biblical literature, 111–12, 167
  of perfume, 129, 187, 199, 200
  by women, 98–100, 114, 143
Semaḥot, 58
Sennacharib, 162–63
senses, 6, 8–10, 12, 210 n. 13, 237 n. 166. *See also* hearing, sense of; sight, sense of; smell, sense of; taste, sense of
Sepphoris (Palestine), 28, 30, 40, 50–53, 217 n. 79, 221 n. 130
Shammai, House of, 36, 42, 48–49, 219 n. 101
Sheba, 106
  queen of, 33, 87, 108
Shekhinah, 239 n. 9
Sheshet, R., 38
Shields, Mary E., 237 n. 157
Shimon, R., 154, 170, 171–72
shovels, incense, 50–53, 215 n. 38, 221 n. 130
sight, sense of, 9–10, 12, 57, 113, 210 n. 22, 211 n. 27, 237 n. 163, 238 n. 167
Simeon (son of Jacob), 233 n. 109, 234 n. 110
Simeon ben Nanos, R., 223 n. 156
similes, 5, 7, 83, 84, 85, 92, 169, 179
Simon, R., 124, 241 nn. 33, 42
sins
  atonement for, 149, 169, 188–95, 196
  original, 124, 138
  prophets' condemnation of, 103, 104–5, 106, 107
slaves, 43, 96–97, 108–9, 129, 165, 219 n. 95
smell, sense of, 5–13, 46, 124, 211 n. 27, 28, 232 n. 94, 237 n. 165, 238 n. 167. *See also* olfaction
  scholarship and, 148–53, 246 n. 106
smelling, act of, 8, 37, 46, 49, 68, 113, 149, 156
Smith, Jonathan Z., 256 n. 13
smoke
  column of, 92, 143, 145, 161, 162
  of incense, 46, 47, 76, 92
  sacrificial, 66, 68–69, 75, 103
  upward movement of, 105, 114, 131, 236 n. 149
Sokoloff, Michael, 206, 246 n. 111
Solomon (king), 33, 87, 94, 108, 154, 231 n. 80
Sperber, Dan, 8
spices. *See also individual spices*
  in biblical literature, 64, 65–66, 70, 94, 102, 107, 108, 230 n. 68
  blessings for, 36–37, 46–47, 49, 220 n. 117, 223 n. 162

for burials, 56, 57–58, 231 n. 82
culture of, 20–28
in Garden of Eden, 120–21
handling, 221 n. 133, 225 n. 2
for idolatry, 36–37, 139–40, 144, 217 n. 71, 220 n. 118
incense made from, 136, 143, 178, 180, 195
lighting, 49, 136, 141, 178, 180, 195
mountain of, 204–5, 206, 207
in rabbinic literature, 33, 34, 36–37, 116–68, 172, 198, 206, 220 n. 118
rabbis' experience with, 14, 41–42, 62, 195, 240 n. 18
in Song of Songs, 4, 84, 86–87, 89–94, 97, 99–100, 118–20, 167, 170–71, 195, 204–5
terms for, 32–34, 66–68, 71, 216 n. 63, 223 n. 154, 226 n. 13, 227 n. 21, 231 nn. 70, 82, 236 n. 153
uses of, 42, 48, 52, 55, 223 n. 161
in the wilderness, 134–36
spice trade, 34–39, 72, 108, 217 n. 65, 232 n. 91, 243 n. 61
Near East, 14, 22, 66
in rabbinic literature, 216 n. 63, 217 n. 70
in Song of Songs, 93, 94, 143
spikenard, 24
fragrance of, 160, 161–62, 165, 176, 177
in rabbinic literature, 130, 131, 132
in Song of Songs, 86, 89, 100, 164, 167, 178
terms for, 163, 231 n. 78, 242 n. 51, 247 n. 125, 250 n. 21
spirit, use of term, 113. *See also* breathing, terms for
Stemberger, G., 223 n. 163
stinking, 95–98, 114, 129, 233 nn. 103, 106, 107, 109. *See also* odors, bad
Strack, H. L., 223 n. 163
Strange, James F., 52
strigil. *See* bodies, scraping
students, 37–38, 117, 173, 174–75. *See also* teacher-student relationship
suffering, 18, 169–96, 207
of Abraham, 175–88, 189, 193, 195–96, 200
in rabbinic literature, 148, 169, 170, 189
Sukkoth (holiday), 148, 245 n. 97
Swartz, Michael, 248 n. 5
synagogues, 52–53, 215 n. 53, 220 n. 121, 221 n. 130, 248 n. 5
synesthesia, 210 n. 13
Synnott, Anthony, 13–14, 210 n. 22, 211 n. 27

Tabernacle, 74, 132. *See also* Temple
dedication of, 227 n. 22, 228 n. 44, 239 n. 16

implements used in, 70, 227 n. 22
priestly service in, 79, 80
sacrifices in, 74, 105, 160
Talmuds
Bavli, 4, 19, 31–32
Yerushalmi, 4, 16, 30, 31–32
Tannaitic period, 17, 212 n. 39, 217 n. 69, 238 n. 4, 241 n. 41, 253 n. 49
Tarfon, R., 34
Taryi, R., 120
taste, sense of, 7, 10, 11, 211 n. 28, 232 n. 94, 245 n. 98
teacher-student relationship, 1–2, 36, 117, 151–52
Temple, 102, 206, 236 n. 154, 251 n. 34. *See also* Holy of Holies; incense, Temple; Tabernacle
closing of, 235 n. 129
destruction of, 30, 102, 112, 144, 204, 205, 245 n. 86, 256 n. 13
levels of holiness in, 69, 73–75, 76
sacrifices in, 160, 161
second, 30, 53, 60, 227 n. 20
synagogue depictions of, 52–53, 221 n. 130
Ten Commandments. *See* commandments
thanatos, 13, 194, 195
Theodor, J., 250 n. 22, 252 n. 36
theology, geographic, 118–28
Theophrastus, 215 n. 53
thorns, 124–26, 153, 156, 159, 247 n. 111
Tiberias (Palestine), 28, 30, 40–41
Titus (emperor), 32
tombs, 56, 59–60, 224 n. 171. *See also* burials; grave goods
Torah. *See* Hebrew Bible
Tosefta, 16, 31–32, 118
touch, sense of, 8, 10
Tower of Babel, 241 n. 42
tradents, 16, 31, 118, 203, 212 n. 41, 241 n. 33, 249 n. 18, 255 n. 11. *See also* rabbis
tranquility, 65, 68, 254 n. 56
Tree of Knowledge, 120, 121, 124
trees, 148–49. *See also* balsam; figs/fig trees
in Song of Songs, 88, 89, 119, 124–28, 239 n. 16

unctorium, 41–42, 218 n. 87
unguentaria, 21, 23, 24, 25, 26, 44, 49–50, 224 n. 176
as grave goods, 59, 60–61, 62, 215 n. 38
Utnapishtim, 229 n. 47
Uzziah (king), 77, 81–82, 230 n. 64

Van Henten, Jan Willem, 250 n. 25
Vespasian (emperor), 32

vials, perfume. *See* containers, perfume
vines/vineyards, in Song of Songs, 89, 192, 256 n. 12

wafting. *See* fragrance, wafting; incense, wafting; perfume, wafting
war, 162–66, 233 n. 105
well-being, feelings of, 146, 207
West, the, attitudes toward scent, 10–11, 13
wilderness, Israel's wandering in, 133–36
willow trees, 148, 149
wine, 46
    burial uses of, 223 n. 156, 224 n. 166
    in rabbinic literature, 46, 132–33
    spiced, 33, 216 n. 57, 231 n. 70
witchcraft, 139, 140, 142, 146, 220 n. 118
women, 217 n. 76. *See also* lover, female; other, the, female
    as apothecaries, 34, 71–72, 72, 216 n. 61, 227 n. 27
    in biblical literature, 83–84, 115, 167, 234 n. 112
    carrying spices, 53, 55
    creation of, 136–37, 243 n. 69
    idealized, 129, 130–38, 142, 145, 147, 199–200
    perfume use by, 19–20, 24, 38, 53, 55, 114, 132, 134–38, 142–47, 152, 217 n. 77, 242 n. 54
    in Proverbs, 98, 100, 131, 235 n. 120
    in rabbinic literature, 130–47, 245 nn. 89, 90
    real, 129, 138–47, 199
    in Song of Songs, 64, 88–94, 100–101, 110, 114, 121–22, 132–34, 231 n. 81, 232 nn. 87, 94, 241 n. 41

Yannai, R., 154, 155, 156, 174
Yassa (Assi), R., 40–41, 134, 243 n. 59. *See also* Assi, R.
Yegül, Fikret, 214 n. 21
Yehuda bar Simon, R., 202, 203
Yehuda ben Isaiah, R., 34, 179–80, 251 n. 32
Yoḥanan, R., 38, 120, 122, 123, 134, 135, 136, 139, 140, 181, 182, 220 n. 117, 240 n. 22, 243 n. 63, 244 nn. 75, 76, 79, 251 n. 34, 254 n. 54
Yoḥanan ben Zakkai, R., 1–2
Yossi, R., 58, 139, 140, 142, 243 n. 59
Yudan, R., 162, 163, 164

Ze'ira, R., 46
Ze'ira, Rav, 219 n. 98
Zimmerli, Walther, 237 n. 159
Zutra bar Tobiah, R., 249 n. 13

www.ingramcontent.com/pod-product-compliance
Lightning Source LLC
Chambersburg PA
CBHW021356290426
44108CB00010B/266